Differential Diagnosis of Gastric Diseases

KEIICHI KAWAI, M.D.
HIROMICHI TANAKA, M.D.

IGAKU SHOIN LTD. TOKYO
SPRINGER-VERLAG BERLIN · HEIDELBERG · NEW YORK
1974

Keiichi Kawai, M. D.
Professor, Department of Preventive Medicine, Kyoto Prefectural University of Medicine.

Hiromichi Tanaka, M. D.
Associate Professor, Department of Internal Medicine (Director: Professor Dr. K. Ishihara), Tottori University School of Medicine; Director, Division of Endoscopy.

PUBLISHERS
© First edition, 1974 by IGAKU SHOIN LTD., 5-24-3 Hongo Bunkyo-ku, Tokyo.
Softcover reprint of the hardcover 1st edition 1974
Sole distribution rights for Europe (including the United Kingdom) granted to SPRINGER-VERLAG Berlin · Heidelberg · New York.

ISBN-13: 978-3-642-65767-2 e-ISBN-13: 978-3-642-65765-8
DOI: 10.1007/978-3-642-65765-8

Preface

This book is intended to systematically explain our clinical experience with gastric diseases. We have concentrated on how to avoid overlooking changes on the gastric walls and how to improve diagnostic differentiation of these changes on the basis of the findings.

It is difficult to differentiate malignancy from benignancy when the change is a minor or a very small one. Because of this, we have thoroughly classified protruding lesions and excavated lesions for diagnosis. The criterion adopted for classification is the commonly observed unevenness of each gastric area. If the change protrudes higher than normal from the mucous membrane, it is classified as a protruding lesion, and if it is deeper seated, as an excavated lesion. Differentiation follows diagnosis of the presence of disease. The whole process has been described concretely.

There often are small size changes which have not been detected by cautious x-ray examinations and are discovered by endoscopic observations. This book describes the techniques of endoscopic and radiologic examinations and the principles of macroscopic diagnosis based on our experiences.

If the detected change is a protruding lesion, the following findings are necessary for differentiation: 1) size and shape, 2) height, 3) nodular appearance over the protuberant surface, 4) color tone, and 5) morphology of the protuberance. In an excavated lesion: 1) size and shape, 2) depth, 3) nodular appearance at the bottom of the excavation, 4) color tone, 5) border region of the excavation, and 6) nature of the mucous folds.

Repeated examinations are indispensable in order to accurately judge the findings obtained. For this purpose roentgenological examinations and endoscopic observations are both required. In the section on case presentations, interpretation and explanation of the diagnostic processes have been given following the order of the above mentioned checkpoints.

Roentgenology and endoscopy are macroscopic. Thus, they have certain limitations when dealing with minute changes which present few macroscopic findings specific for the disease. Cytology and biopsy are required for definitive diagnosis. The book contains demonstrative descriptions of gastric biopsies under direct vision and discrimination of varied cases, including presentation of cases in which diagnoses are impossible except by gastric biopsies.

January, 1974

Authors

Acknowledgments

Progress in the diagnoses of gastric diseases in the past ten years has been remarkable. X-ray diagnosis in gastroenteropathy has advanced technically through clinical application of the double contrast radiography which was developed by Prof. H. SHIRAKABE. This has been the main reason for success in raising roentgenological diagnosis to the limit of its effectiveness on a macroscopic level. Mechanical improvement of gastroenterological radiography through application of the rotating anode has also been important.

In addition, the remarkable development of endoscopic diagnosis must be mentioned. Such a significant advancement would not have been possible without the often unappreciated continuing efforts of the Olympus Optical Co., Ltd. and the Machida Endoscopic Co., Ltd. At the same time we are extremely grateful to our predecessors, S. TASAKA, D. KONDO and others, for their ceaseless efforts.

Such unprecedented progress attracted international attention to Japan from all of the scholars of the digestive organs. The success of endoscopic diagnosis was especially significant because it appeared simultaneously with the current problem of *Differential Diagnosis of Gastric Diseases.*

Historically, histopathological diagnosis of early gastric cancer must be traced back to MALLORY (1936). Its significance in Japanese medicine lies in the adoption of this technique as a clinical preoperative diagnosis. The "Research Society for Early Gastric Cancer" supervised by Prof. T. MURAKAMI, has published numerous findings in that field and has been playing a dominant role.

It is not rare in Japan that one doctor uses both x-ray and endoscopic diagnoses. It can be positively asserted that, besides being expert in each gastric speciality, mastery of and skill in the use of these two diagnostic techniques together will greatly and immediately enhance diagnostic capabilities. This is because each technique possesses specific characteristics, advantages and disadvantages of its own.

The present book was created in such an atmosphere and is a unified version, with revisions, of two different books published on different dates in Japanese: *Atlas of Gastric Protruded Lesions* (K. KAWAI) and *Atlas of Gastric Excavated Lesions* (H. TANAKA).

Usually doctors are trained in either roentgenological or endoscopic technique, but both techniques are essential in clinical practice. The authors both mastered endoscopy (flexible gastroscopy, gastrocamera examination, and gastrofiberscopy) during their medical training but acquired their knowledge of roentgenology through clinical practice. We hope this volume can help overcome the shortcomings of overspecialization by encouraging the use of each approach where it is most effective.

The authors are still young and feel the need for more experience, but we look forward to hearing both criticisms and advice from others concerned with this field. We hope this book will prove serviceable for the readers' daily diagnoses.

January, 1974

Authors

Contents

I. General Section

A. On the concepts of protruding and excavated lesions

What are protruding and excavated lesions?

In this book any lesion differing from the surrounding mucosa is treated either as a protruding type or an excavated type. With the development of radiologic and endoscopic diagnoses, small protrusions and excavations on the gastric mucosa which were not observable before can now be seen, making it more difficult to differentiate between benign and malignant lesions.

Several procedures must be followed to make correct diagnoses. It is necessary to understand the kinds of lesions characterized by a localized protrusion or excavation on the gastric wall. When the objects to be diagnosed are advanced gastric cancers or large, deep peptic ulcers, actual clinical diagnoses are not difficult. However, when gastric lesions are small, benign or malignant, especially early gastric cancers of a superficially elevated or depressed type, the concept of "protruding or excavated gastric lesions" becomes one of great interest.

1. The protruding type of gastric lesion

The term "the protruding type of gastric lesions" has only recently come into use. In 1965 YAMADA and FUKUTOMI first differentiated the protruding type of lesions from gastric polyps and polypous lesions. Polyps have a long history having been described since 1557 (Amatus Lusitanus). MORGAGNI described that in a 50 year old woman in 1769. OTTO described his autopsy findings on a 40 year old man in 1824.

The main reason why we are obliged to call this type of lesion a "protruding type" is that the pathological name "gastric polyp" includes a combined form of different qualities. As pointed out by BOCKUS and HENNING, "a polyp" is named only by the appearance of a tumor, not histopathologically. Among pathologists there is a difference of opinion on epithelial polyps as to whether they are congenital or caused by gastric inflammation. BORRMANN and KONJETZNY discussed the histological findings of gastric polyps. EVANS and MING used different pathological features for the technical term of adenomatous polyp. It must be recognized that the concepts of polyps are widely varied.

Recent improvements in the x-ray equipment, with the rotating anode tubes, allow a new approach for discovering minute features of lesions. The clinical application of gastrocameras and gastrofiberscopes has enabled us to make rapid advances in the diagnosis of "fine protruding lesions".

If all these lesions are included in the category of "gastric polyps", there is the possibility that "gastric polyps" should also include nonepithelial tumors.

Judging from a pathological standpoint, "a polyp" means "an epithelial protuberance". It is essential for clinicians to consider these lesions protruding from the surrounding mucosa as "protruding lesions of the stomach", to let x-ray and endoscopic examinations go further than mere diagnosis. However, the term "a protruding type of lesion" sounds too vague. It is, of course as has been stated previously, unreasonable to include "a nonepithelial, submucosal tumor" among "gastric polyps".

The final quality diagnosis should not rely only on x-ray or endoscopic diagnosis but on "histopathological diagnosis", including biopsy under direct vision. X-ray and endoscopic examinations to a certain extent make it possible to discern "nonepithelial tumors" (submucosal tumors), benign epithelial tumors (gastric polyps), and malignant epithelial tumors (protruding type of gastric cancers), while we fail to diagnose some cases by other methods. Yet, quite a number of clinicians think it adequate to use the expression "polypoid lesions".

This book will try to give an analytical explanation of the radiologic and endoscopic approach to these lesions, unifying them as the "protruding type" for a new start in diagnostic standards.

To give a clear definition of a "protruding lesion" we must be certain of the normal mucosa. It has already been histopathologically proven that a healthy membrane can exist, but there can not be such a thing as "a normal membrane". Clinically there is no need for having a ridgid definition. Yet ruggedness of the healthy gastric membrane and the comparatively smooth healthy gastric area must be used as standards to diagnose a protuberant lesion. Four pictures taken by double-contrast radiography are shown here.

Because of an adequate amount of air and hypotonic gastrography (Fig. 1), a rather uneven and fine granular shadow lying from the central to the angular region could be observed. These granular findings could also be observed on the lower part of the pictures, but the marginal areas were comparatively smooth with no ruggedness. Radiologically, the marginal areas observed from a tangential direction did not show ruggedness. These features could be used to identify those of a normal gastric membrane.

In Figure 2 of the antrum, granules almost identical in size were seen. The marginal areas looked comparatively smooth.

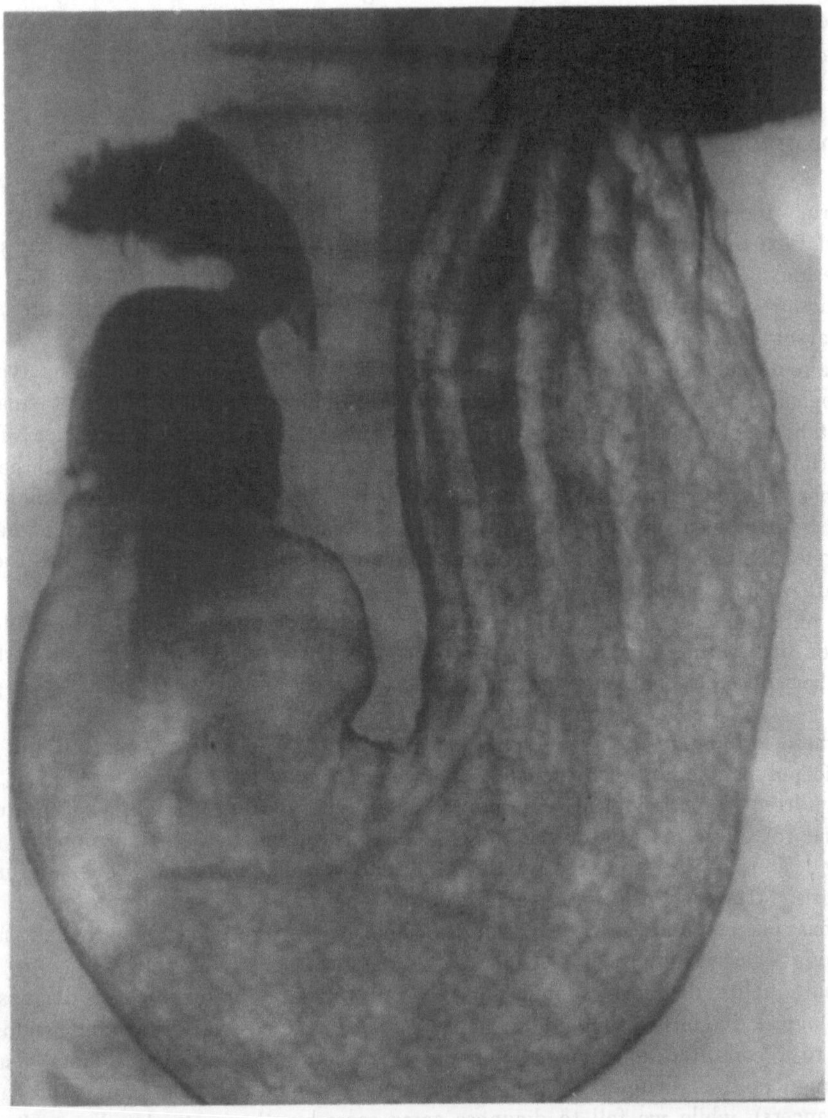

Fig. 1 Double-contrast study (Radiograph taken by the double-contrast method). A fine granular shadow can be observed from the gastric body to the angular region, but this finding may be that of a normal gastric mucosa.

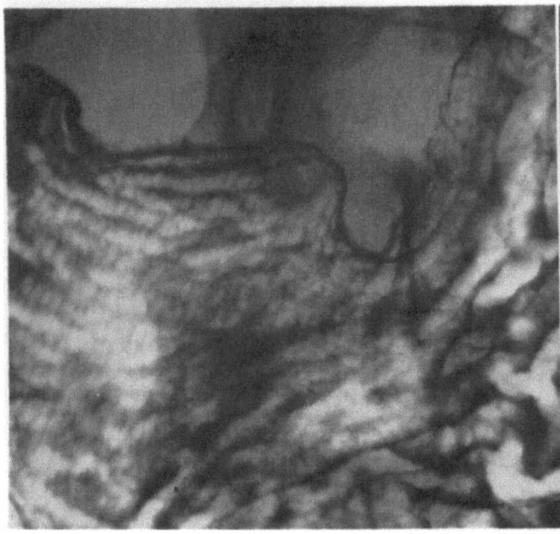

Fig. 2 Double-contrast study of the antrum. A uniform granular pattern is slightly visible.

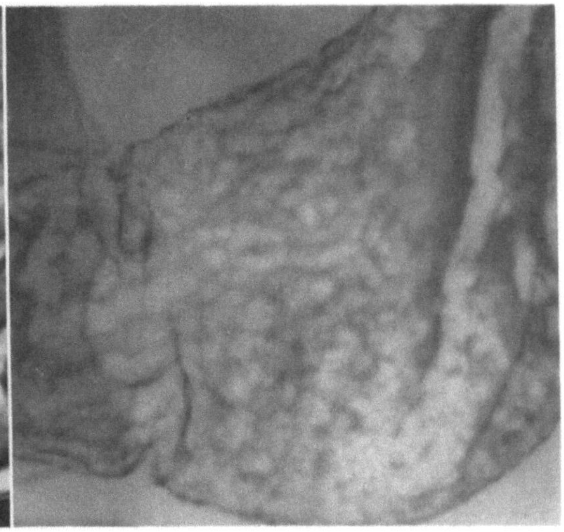

Fig. 3 Double-contrast study of the antrum. The granular change becomes rough and rugged with marked irregularity in the marginal areas.

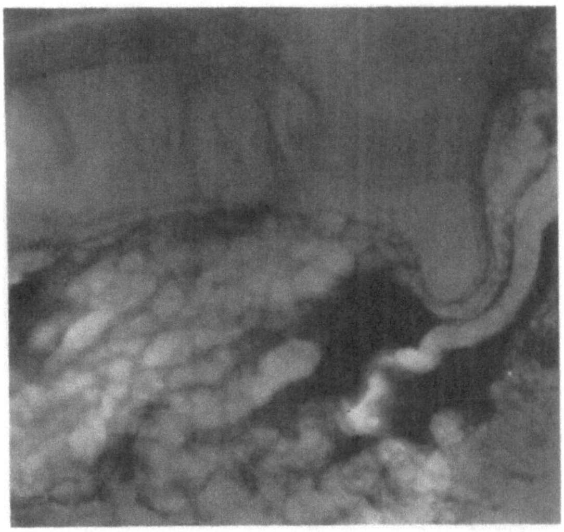

Fig. 4 Double-contrast study of the antrum. A rough gastric area can be observed, but these granules, generally uniform, may be considered a polypoid lesion.

Figure 3 is a different case showing more remarkable changes. Granules looked irregular and were not of the same size. A small, rough gastric pit was observed, and the marginal areas were more or less rugged.

In Figure 4 with less air, both frontal and marginal areas showed more irregularities.

In the resected stomach several granules were observed in a portion of the antral membrane (Fig. 5a). These findings could be regarded as multiple rough granules or small hemispheric filling defects.

As seen in these pictures (Fig. 5b, c), when a protuberance was discovered in the stomach standing out from the surrounding mucosa, we treated it as a "protruding lesion". Endoscopic examination also showed some scattered, low, reddened, protruding lesions (Fig. 5d). Pathologically

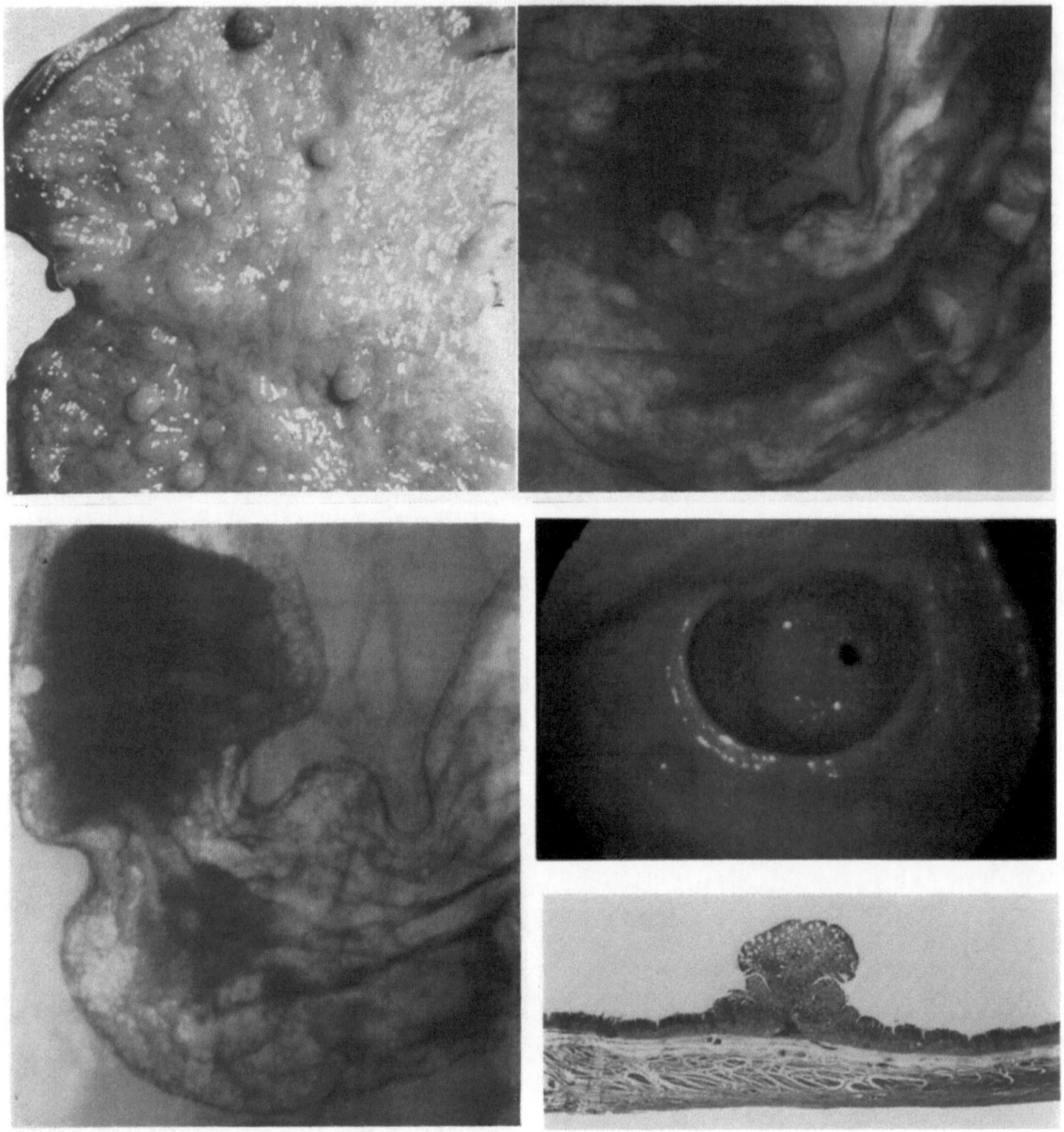

5a 5b 5c 5d 5e

Fig. 5

a. **Resected stomach.** Several clear protuberances can be observed in the antral region of the resected stomach.
b. **Double-contrast study in the supine position.** At the antrum, multiple rough granules or small hemispherical filling defects are visible.
c. **Double-contrast study.** Several filling defects are seen in the antrum appearing almost round in shape, but irregular in size. It is necessary to consider the existence of protruding lesions which have features comparable to rough gastric areas.
d. **Gastrofiberscopic picture.**
e. **Histological findings.** The relatively smooth gastric mucosa is abruptly elevated with findings of hyperplasia of the gastric epithelium and partial proliferation of the pyloric glands; however, elevation of the mucosal muscle can not be seen.

(Fig. 5e) this was a hyperplastic protuberance, not having developed the characteristics of an adenomatous polyp yet. As expected for such a typical adenomatous polyp, proliferation of the gastric epithelium, fusion and fountain-like proliferation of the mucosal muscle fiber were not seen in the resected stomach.

In Figure 6a, a mucosal protrusion was observed on the anterior wall of the borderline area.

6a
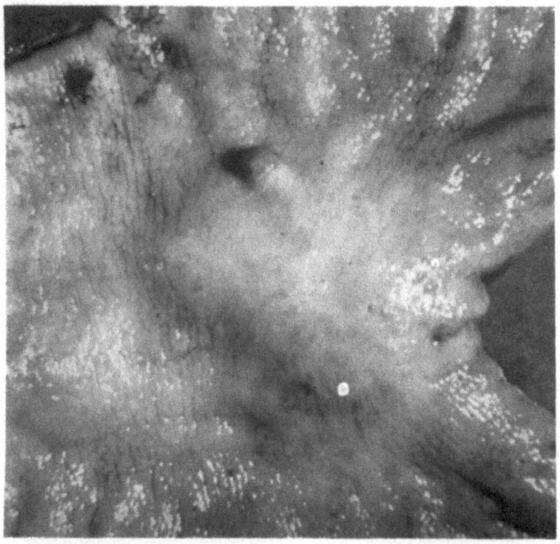

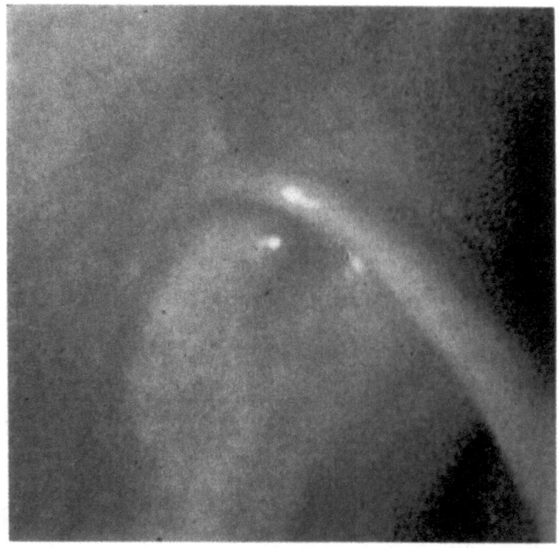
6b

6c
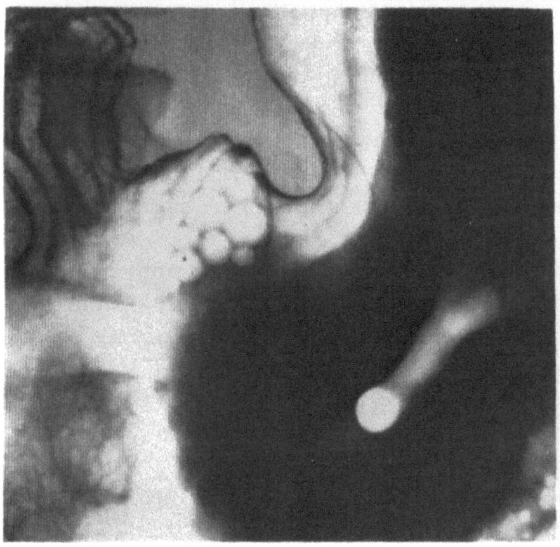

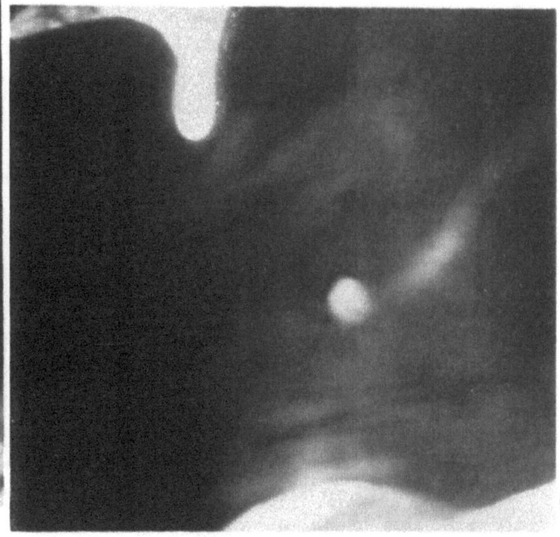
6d

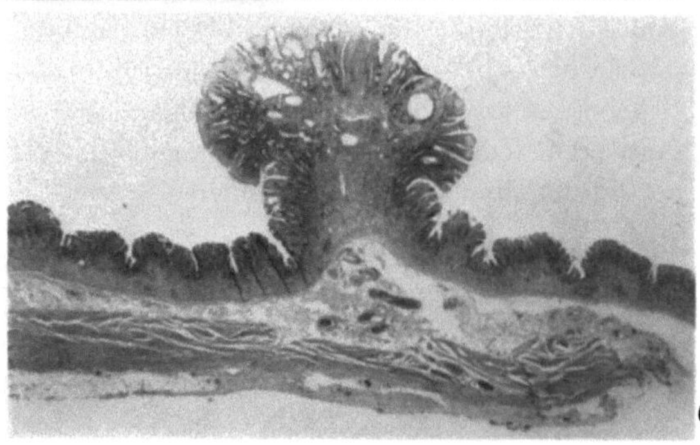
6e

Fig. 6
a. Resected stomach. A mucosal protrusion can be observed on the anterior wall of the antrum. The surrounding mucosa looks relatively smooth.
b. Endoscopic picture. A hemispherical protrusion sharply elevated from the surrounding mucosa can be observed on the anterior wall of the angular region fairly close to the antrum. The protrusion is accompanied by redness and light reflection which are considered to be findings of benign gastric polyps.
c. Double-contrast study. In the antrum, a small peanut-sized filling defect is seen in a thin barium layer.
d. Proper compression study. The round filling defect continues to the shadow of the mucosal folds running from the gastric body. Marginal irregularities or unevenness are not seen in this radiograph.
e. Cut surface of the specimen of Fig. 6a. Protrusion of the gastric epithelium is higher than the neighboring gastric mucosa and the elevation of the mucosal muscle is marked.

This finding was observed endoscopically as a reddened, low protrusion (Fig. 6b). This portion was apparently elevated from the surrounding mucosa, protruding into the stomach cavity. Histopathologically this was an adenomatous polyp with a short stem. Seen radiologically in a double-contrast study (Fig. 6c) and also in an adequate compression study (Fig. 6d), the lesion, shown here as a filling defect, looked as if it protruded from the surrounding mucosa. The size did not differ much from the rough protruding lesion mentioned in Figure 3.

2. The excavated type of gastric lesion

Excavated lesions are localized, concave lesions, depressed in the gastric mucosa. Those listed in Table 1 fall into this category. They are classified into two types, those with no gastric wall defects and those with defects. The former include diverticula and the relatively excavated portion of protruding lesions. The latter denote scars with no epithelial defects, peptic erosions, ulcers, and cancerous erosions. Rare diseases such as tuberculosis and syphilis are included in this category.

As for the diverticula, some are known to be congenital and some, postnatal. They naturally show different forms, the former having a narrow entrance and the latter being formed by an inflammation of the surrounding area or by adhesion. A diverticulum is a deformation or transformation and can hardly be called a gastric lesion; but, for convenience, it is classified in this book as an excavated lesion without any defect of the gastric wall. Both radiographically and endoscopically, it tends to be expressed as an excavation. Shadow flecks are observed radiologically because the contrast meal remains in the excavation between the elevated areas. Macroscopically the lesion is treated as an excavated lesion, and this classification is suggested for the convenience of reaching a diagnosis.

Both radiologic and endoscopic examinations should be based on a qualitative observation of the gastric mucosa, by which we are able to surmise lesions under the mucosa, regarding the activity and elasticity of the gastric wall. It is the authors' impression that diagnoses should begin with observations of defects of the mucosa. There are still many problems left in order to determine accurately the existence of defects of the mucosa. However, present x-ray examinations can reveal minute ruggedness, and with an endoscopic examination, defects of the mucosa can be found from precise observations of the coating of the stomach wall.

A defect of only the epithelium does not mean much, but it is possible to tell by examination whether the lesion on the gastric mucosa is an epithelial defect or not. In this sense, scars left after treatment of gastric ulcers are sometimes treated as excavated lesions without epithelial defects. It is convenient to follow MURAKAMI and KOIDE's classification of scars of gastric ulcers. Ulcer scars are classified into two types: those covered with only a mucosal layer, defined as scars with histologically open ulcers (incomplete scars), and those thickly covered with epithelium (complete scars) (Fig. 7 and page 211). The excavation seen in the healed area of an erosion should also be considered.

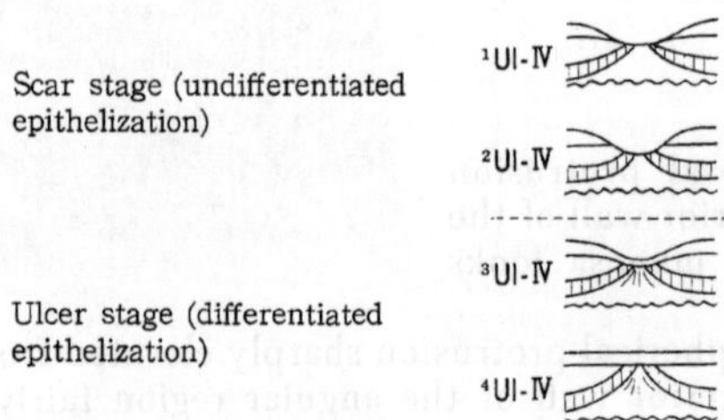

Fig. 7 Ulcer recovery stages (MURAKAMI, KOIDE).

Lesions with a defect of the mucosa and of the gastric wall are classified according to BORRMANN's classification of gastric cancer (Fig. 8), the early gastric cancer classification (Fig. 9), and MURAKAMI's ulcer classification (Fig. 10). At the annual meeting of the Japan Gastroenterological Endoscopy Society in 1962 and the Japanese Research Society for Gastric Cancer in 1963, this early gastric carcinoma was defined as a carcinoma of the stomach in which invasion was limited to the mucosa and submucosa.

Excavated lesions are classified roughly into two types, excavations with and without gastric wall defects. The former lesions are further classified into excavations with and without mucosal defects.

A little explanation should be added to MURAKAMI's ulcer depth classification (Fig. 10) and its practical application in actual cases. In Ul-II~IV, the depth does not indicate the numerical value of the depth measured from the gastric wall to the bottom of the excavation, but the depth according to the layer construction of the gastric wall affected by the lesion.

To verify the depth of the ulcer, changes of peristalsis caused by scar formation must be taken into consideration along with the actual depth of the ulcer. Concerning the real depth of the ulcer, there are still several points to be clarified. Ascertaining whether the excavation of

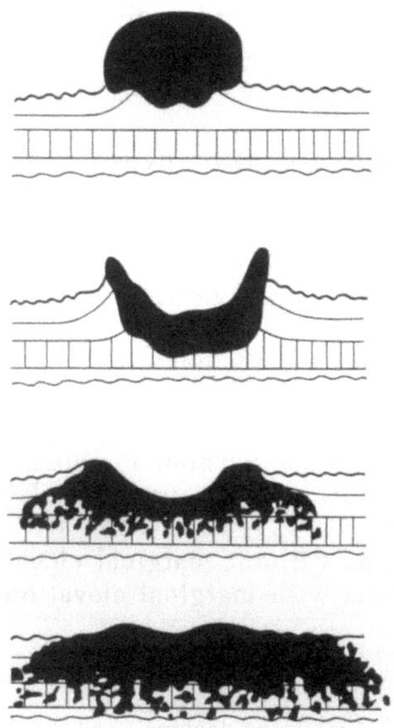

Fig. 8 Type of advanced gastric cancer.

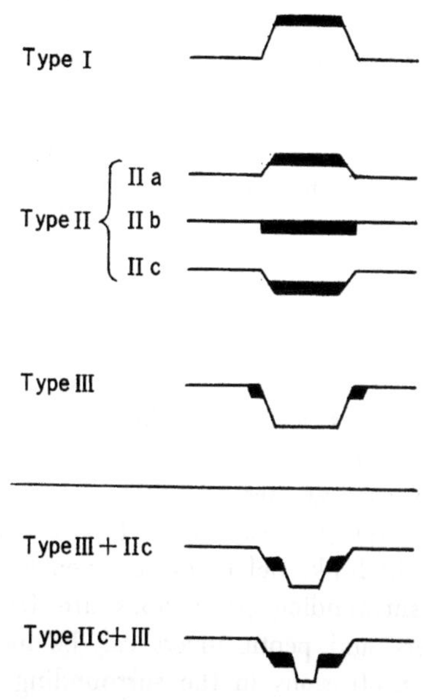

Type I (Protruded Type)
Protrusion into the gastric lumen is eminent.
Type II (Superficial Type)
Unevenness of the surface is inconspicuous. This is further divided into 3 subtypes, *i.e.*,
Type IIa (Elevated Type)
The surface is slightly elevated.
Type IIb (Flat Type)
Almost no recognizable elevation or depression from the surrounding mucosa can be seen.
Type IIc (Depressed Type)
The surface is slightly depressed.
Type III (Excavated Type)
An excavation in the gastric wall is prominent.

Fig. 9 Macroscopic classification of an early gastric carcinoma.

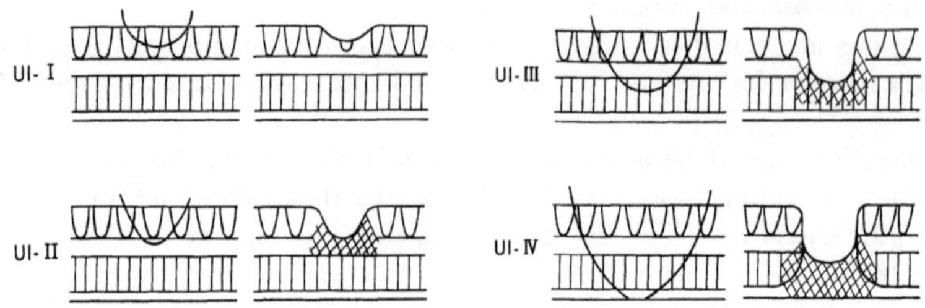

Fig. 10 Ul depth classification (MURAKAMI)

Table 1 Classification of excavated gastric lesion

I. Excavation without gastric wall defect.
  1. Malformation and Deformity
    1) Diverticulum
    2) Areas of excavation caused by hyperextension
  2. Comparative excavations
     Low areas surrounded by mucosal elevations
II. Excavations with gastric wall defects.
  1. Excavations without mucosal defects
    1) Ulcer scar
    2) Regenerated regions of erosions
  2. Excavations with mucosal defects
    1) Superficial excavations
      a) Superficial excavations without marginal elevation
      b) Superficial excavations with marginal elevation
    2) Deep excavations
      a) Deep excavations without marginal elevation
      b) Deep excavations with marginal elevation

Table 2 Classification of excavated lesions, and gastric disease

1. Apparent excavation: (defect of wall (−))	Diverticula, deformities, Meandering polypoid lesions.
2. Superficial excavation	
Mucosal defect (−):	Ulcer scars, regenerated erosions, congenital malformations.
Mucosal defect (+):	Early cancer (IIc, IIa+IIc), erosions, gastric ulcers (Ul-II~IV), advanced cancer classified by BORRMANN, and various gastric diseases with erosions.
3. Profound excavation:	Gastric ulcer (Ul-III, IV), Gastric cancer (BORRMANN II, III, IV), Early cancer (IIc+III, III+IIc), and various gastric diseases with ulcer formation.
4. Minute excavation on flat surfaces:	Advanced cancer (BORRMANN IV) Gastritis and other infiltrating gastric diseases.

the lesion is deep or shallow should be the first step toward reaching a diagnosis. Table 1 and 2 show the excavated lesion and its relation to the gastric lesion.

A shallow defect is of the IIc type early gastric cancer which is clearly defined (macroscopically) as a superficial type excavation, in contrast to deep excavations which are expressed by a ditch-like defect on an even gastric area. That is, lesions with superficial defects without any surrounding protrusions are IIc erosions, or Ul-II type ulcers. Advanced cancers, early cancers, and peptic ulcers can be included under profound excavations. Superficial excavations with protrusions in the surrounding area, type IIa+IIc early cancers, are sometimes included in this classification.

As for excavated lesions, we must develop our diagnostic technique and improve our understanding of whether they are superficial or deep excavations. We will didactically explain each case, considering each stage of the diagnosis.

B. The fundamentals of an x-ray diagnosis

First, a basic explanation of our radiographic technique of distinguishing protruding and excavated lesions in the stomach will be demonstrated.

1. General remarks on the technique of x-ray diagnosis

X-ray diagnosis of gastric lesions has almost been settled with improvement of x-ray equipment and advancement of the technique. The advantages are as follows; the first is that x-ray examinations allow observations of the extent of submucosal, intramural, and subserosal lesions, while endoscopic examinations deal only with the surface of mucosa. The second is that an endoscopic examination tends to show localized lesions, failing to observe whole lesions stereoscopically. The third is that there are no blind areas in an x-ray examination. Blind areas are the result of faulty technique.

A combination of any of the four methods among the six listed below will allow satisfactory x-ray pictures of gastric lesions; however, the advantages and disadvantages of each method must be understood.

1. Filling study
2. Mucosal-pattern study
3. Double-contrast study
4. Adequate-compression study
5. Polysography
6. Double-contrast study with pneumoperitoneum for gastroparietography

a. Filling study

In this study, there are four main photographs, according to the different directions of the patient's position, that is, radiographs taken in the standing position, right and left oblique positions, and prone position (Fig. 11).

Advantages

1) Marginal changes of the stomach are well presented. Deformation of the stomach is easily detected.

2) Neither gastric juices nor barium meals have much influence on the picture.

3) The examination itself is easy and there is not much difference in the picture, regardless of who takes them. Pictures can be reproduced.

Disadvantages

1) When the lesion is located away from the lesser and greater curvature, it may be in a blind area.

2) This method cannot be solely depended on for diagnosis of minute lesions and quality diagnosis, unless the lesion is located at the margin.

b. Mucosal-pattern study

In this study, there are two main photographs, that is, radiographs taken in the supine and prone positions (Fig. 12).

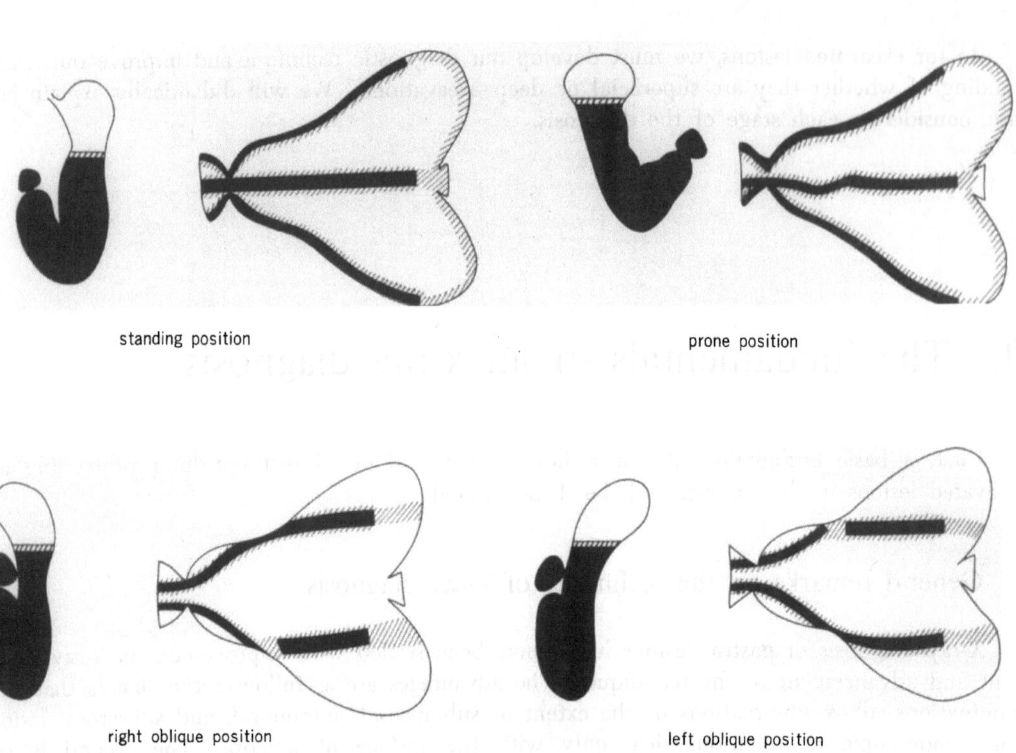

Barium-filled study

■ shows the area where the lesion can be described unequivocally on the x-ray film in this position and with this method.

▩ shows the area where the lesion can usually be described correctly on the x-ray film in this position and with this method.

□ shows the area where the lesion cannot be described on the x-ray film in this position and with this method.

Fig. 11 Diagnostic ability of x-ray photographs.

Advantages

Changes in the gastric membrane are observed in this picture. The area of the membrane that appears in the mucosal-pattern study is wider than that of the double-contrast study. It helps to diagnose minute lesions in addition to giving a description of the gastric area.

Disadvantages

1) It requires good technique to take good mucosal patterns and results are affected by the presence of gastric juices.

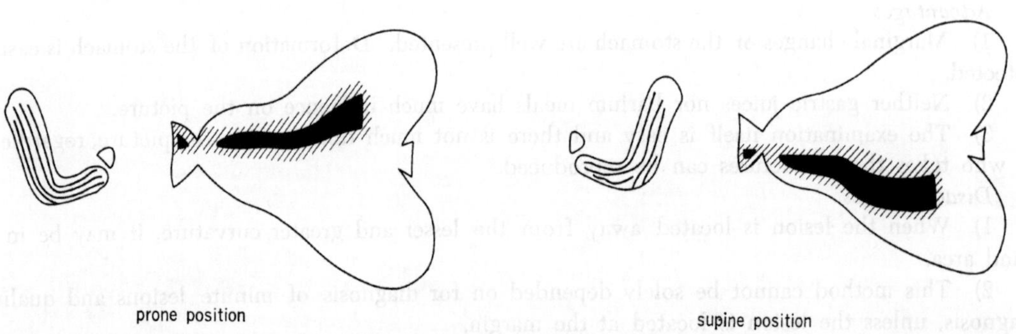

■ shows the area where the lesion can be described unequivocally on the x-ray film in this position and with this method.

▩ shows the area where the lesion can usually be described correctly on the x-ray film in this position and with this method.

□ shows the area where the lesion cannot be described on the x-ray film in this position and with this method

Fig. 12 Mucosal study.

2) They are difficult to read.

3) It is difficult to reach a diagnosis when a lesion is seen in marginal areas.

c. Double-contrast study

In this study, there are four main photographs, that is, radiographs taken in the supine position, right oblique supine position, left oblique half-standing position, and prone position (Fig. 13).

Clinically two to three hundred ml of barium are used depending on the type and location of the lesion. Too little barium will not adequately coat the mucosal surface while too much distorts the minimal lesion by overdistending the gastric wall. The barium should be non-flocculating and have the proper viscosity in order to coat the mucosa optimally.

The patient is first examined in the erect position to see how much air is present in the fundus. If the amount is insufficient (about 250 ml is optimum), additional air is added, either via a nasogastric tube or by an effervescent drug. Palpation, compression, and abdominal breathing are used to distribute the air.

Advantages

1) The minute lesions on the posterior wall of the stomach are observable in a wide area extending from the gastric corpus to the pyloric ring. Almost any part of the stomach can be observed.

2) Deformations of the stomach and marginal granules can be observed, and these findings can be reproduced.

3) The picture is not affected much by either the gastric juice or adherent mucus.

4) The technique is comparatively easy only for experienced personnel.

Disadvantages

1) At least 200 ml of air is needed for a double-contrast picture.

2) It is difficult to grasp the findings if the shadow of the intestine or of the spinal column falls on the picture.

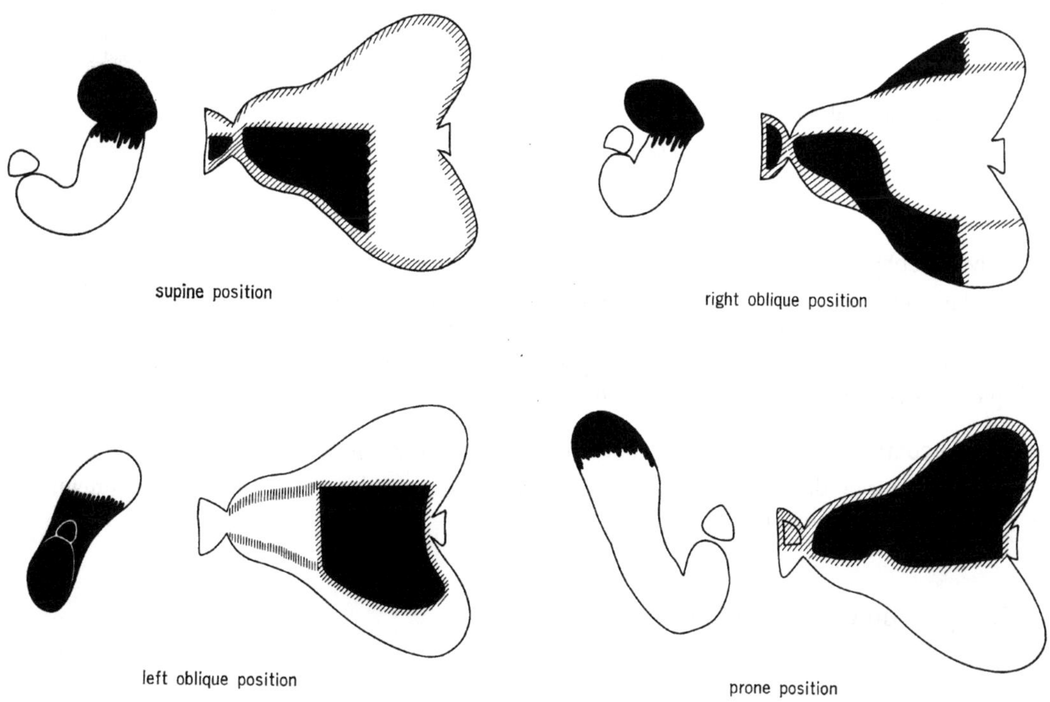

■ shows the area where the lesion can be described unequivocally on the x-ray film in this position and with this method.
▩ shows the area where the lesion can usually be described correctly on the x-ray film in this position and with this method.
□ shows the area where the lesion cannot be described on the x-ray film in this position and with this method.

Fig. 13 Double-contrast method.

d. Adequate-compression study

In this study, we can compress any location in any position in any direction, except for the subcardiac region (Fig. 14).

Advantage

It allows a diagnosis of minute changes of lesions.

Disadvantages

1) It requires a technician with long experience who has a good sense of x-ray examinations.
2) The area that can be read at one time is limited.
3) No observation can be made under the costal ribs because of blind areas.

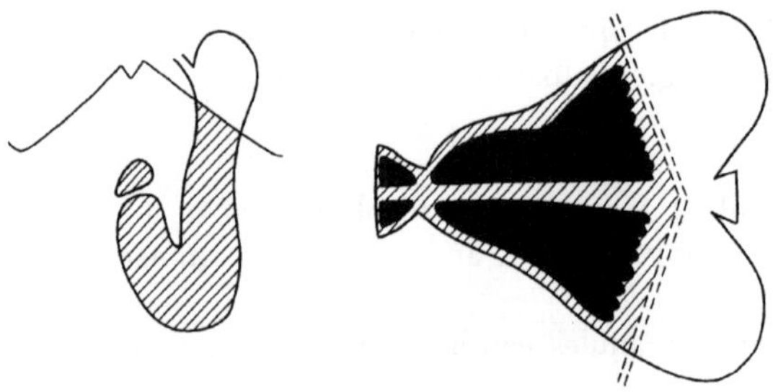

standing position

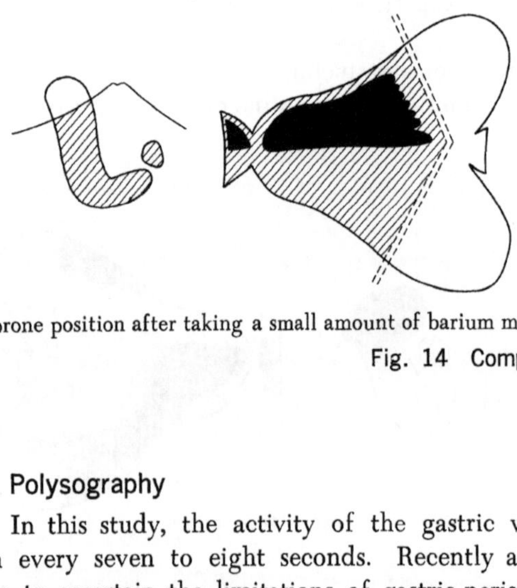

■ shows the area where the lesion can be described unequivocally on the x-ray film in this position and method.
▒ shows the area where the lesion can usually be described correctly on the x-ray film in this position and method.
□ shows the area where the lesion can not be described on the x-ray film in this position and method.

prone position after taking a small amount of barium meal

Fig. 14 Compression study.

e. Polysography

In this study, the activity of the gastric wall can be viewed by repeatedly exposing one film every seven to eight seconds. Recently a method has been developed by which it is possible to ascertain the limitations of gastric peristalsis or the stiffness of the gastric wall by reading multiple radiographs taken in the same position.

f. Double-contrast with pneumoperitoneum for gastroparietography

This study is a double-contrast radiograph of the stomach with a pneumoperitoneum for the diagnosis of an exogastric tumor.

2. X-ray findings on examination

a. Protruding lesions

Characteristics of photographic technique have been mentioned previously. More basic knowledge is required to find protruding lesions when a quality diagnosis is in greater demand than a superficial diagnosis.

We must produce a realistic picture on the x-ray film, making the most of the skillful techniques

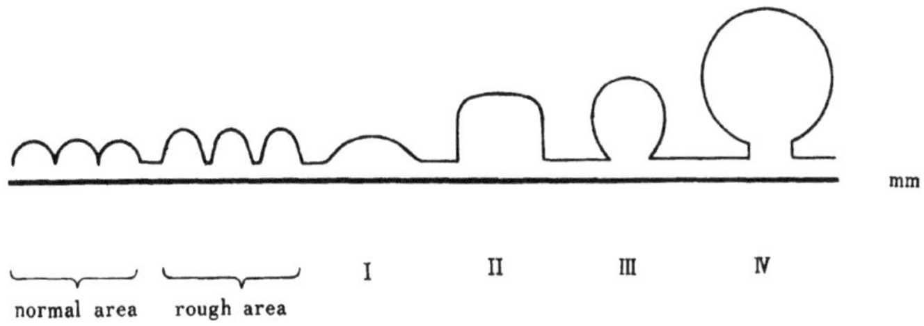

Fig. 15 Diagram of gastric protruding lesions (YAMADA).
Type I: Lesions smoothly elevated with no definite border at their bases.
Type II: Lesions which have definite borders at their bases, but no definite collars.
Type III: Lesions which have collars at their bases but no stalks.
Type IV: Lesions with stalks.

and characteristics of photography. After such basic knowledge of the x-ray technique has been acquired, the process of diagnosis can be fairly well standardized.

Let us study the characteristics of the technique in an actual case. The object in the first case study was a protruding type II gastric lesion using YAMADA's classification (Fig. 15), broad based, 5mm in diameter, and seen on the anterior wall of the antrum (Fig. 16a, b, c).

Figure 16d is a barium-filled radiograph of a resected stomach. Unless the lesion appeared in the margin, small protrusions tended to be hidden under the barium layer in a barium-filled stomach.

Figure 16e is an x-ray picture with a thin barium layer. In Figure 16d mucosal findings were increased to quite a large extent after this barium was pushed away. However, in a mucosal picture with a small amount of barium, both the anterior and posterior walls were folded together, and it was difficult to point out polypoid lesions unless the proper amount of barium was used. In this relief picture the foldings of both the anterior and posterior walls look superimposed, making it difficult to determine on which wall the lesion was to be found. The protrusion of a polyp was pointed out by the arrow, but an exact diagnosis could not be made. A mucosal study with only a small amount of barium meal would make it difficult to read the picture, as the picture would be affected by the presence of gastric juices. An indistinct mucosal picture is not of much diagnostic value.

Figure 16f is a double-contrast radiograph taken from a dorso-ventral view. After the previous mucosal picture was taken, about 100ml of air was insufflated into the stomach. Because of the air, a very fine, regular gastric pit was clearly expressed together with the folds. But the lesion was localized on the anterior wall, and the protrusion was not revealed in the routine double-contrast study since only areas of the posterior wall were exposed. In order to expose this lesion on the anterior wall by the double-contrast method, the picture had to be taken from a ventrodorsal exposure. Clinically, it must be a double-contrast study in the prone position.

A good picture could not be taken unless a relatively large amount of air was insufflated into the stomach with a small or adequate amount of barium. The patient should assume the Trendelenburg position and the right hip should be lightly flexed so that the air in the stomach could extend the antrum.

A resected stomach could be photographed from the opposite direction as seen in Figure 16f. In Figure 16g, a hemispherical mucosal protuberance was revealed, which possessed quite a different feature from the regular surroundings, shown by the arrow in Figure 16g.

Figure 16h is a picture of a barium filled stomach with the proper amount of compression. It revealed a protuberance clearly circumscribed from the surrounding area, near the pyloric ring. Generally in pictures taken with the proper amount of compression, it is desirable to be able to observe as much of the surrounding mucosal area as possible. Small protruding lesions on the anterior wall are demonstrated only by the double-contrast method and by observations with the proper amount of compression.

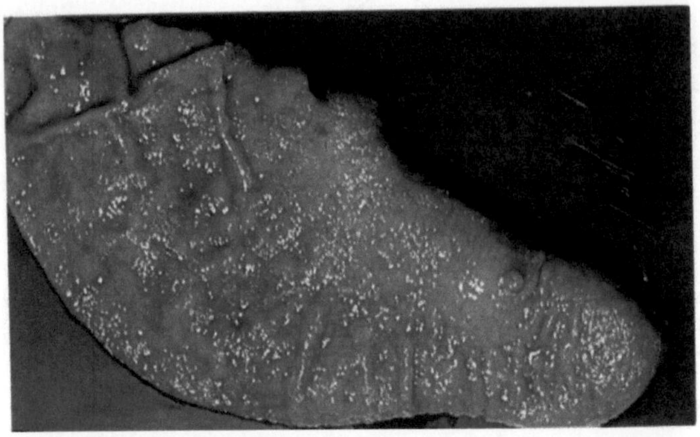

Fig. 16a Resected stomach. A polypoid lesion can be seen on the posterior wall of the antrum. It is hemispherical in form and almost the same color as the surrounding gastric mucosa. The surface of the lesion is almost smooth.

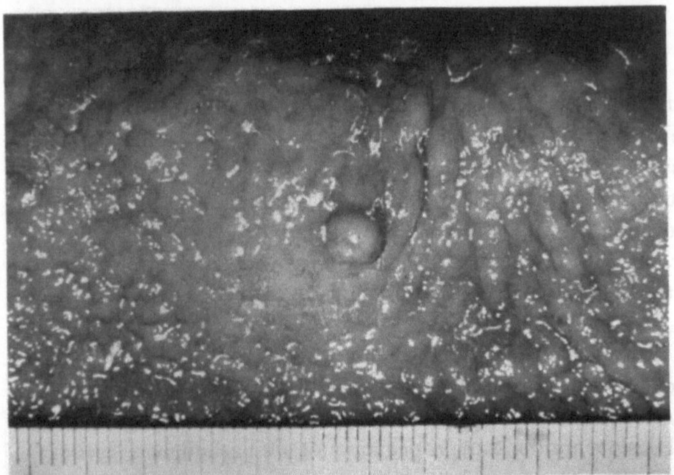

Fig. 16b Lesion in a resected stomach. 5 mm ×5 mm in diameter. The top of the polypoid lesion is slightly depressed. The surrounding mucosa shows fine granular change.

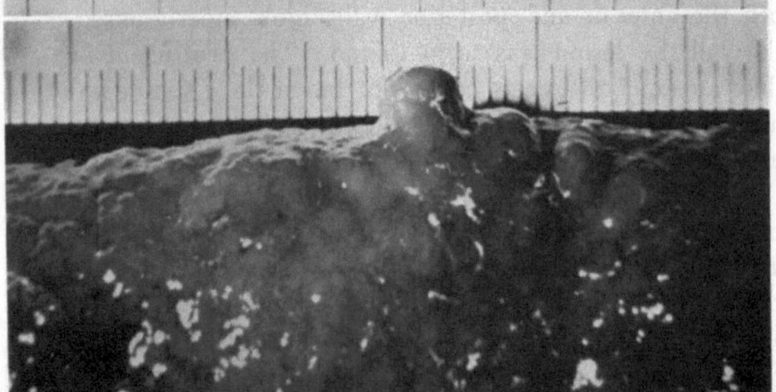

Fig. 16c The height of the lesion is approximately 4 mm. The neck is indistinct at its base. The uneven surrounding mucosa can be clearly observed.

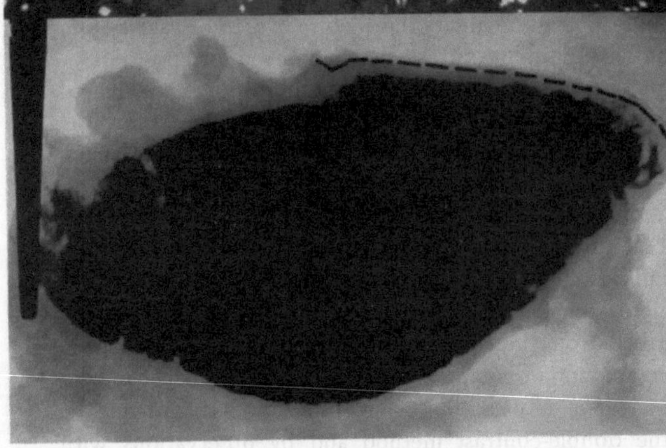

Fig. 16d Barium-filled resected stomach. It is difficult to point out the lesion from this radiograph.

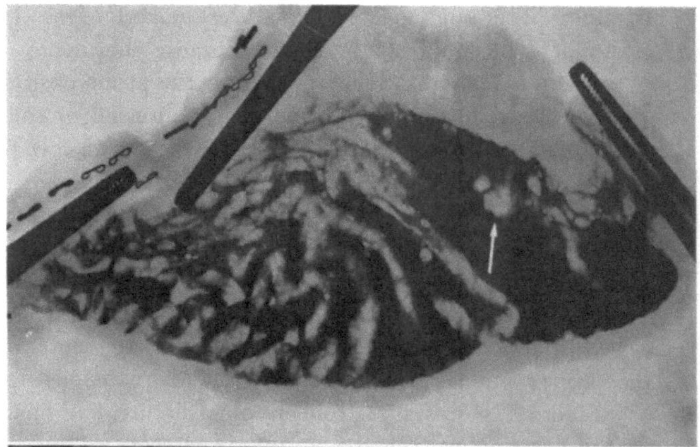

Fig. 16e Relief pattern of a resected stomach. The stomach is not well distended. The lesion is detectable, but its shape is not clearly defined.

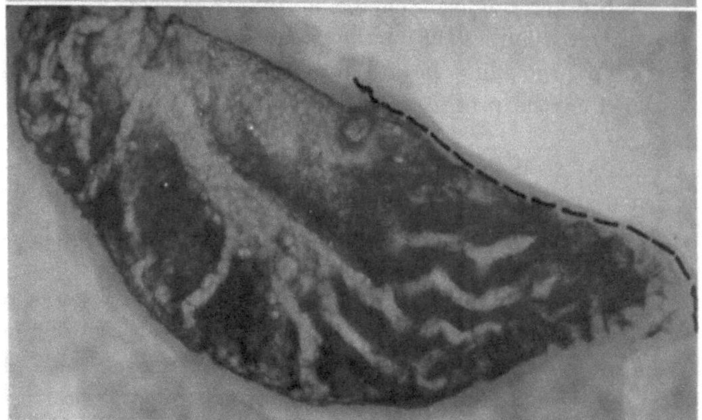

Fig. 16f Double-contrast study of a resected stomach (posterior wall). The mucosal folds and mucosal patterns are very clear. A fine granular mucosa can be observed. The lesion is not seen in this radiograph because it is located on the opposite wall of the stomach.

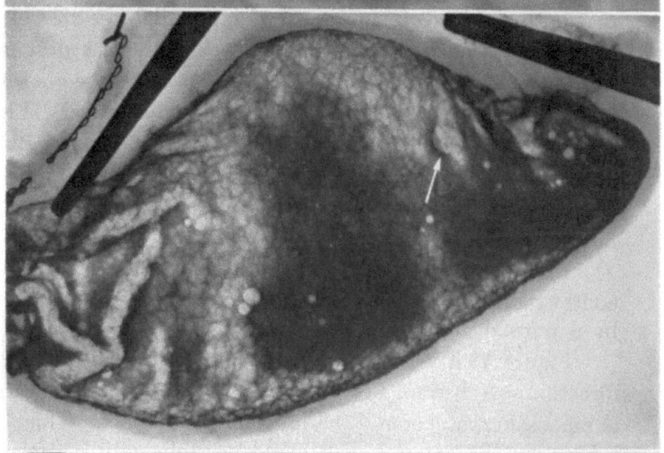

Fig. 16g Double-contrast study of a resected stomach (anterior wall). The stomach is well distended with a suitable amount of air. The size of the lesion (arrow) and mucosal pattern are well defined.

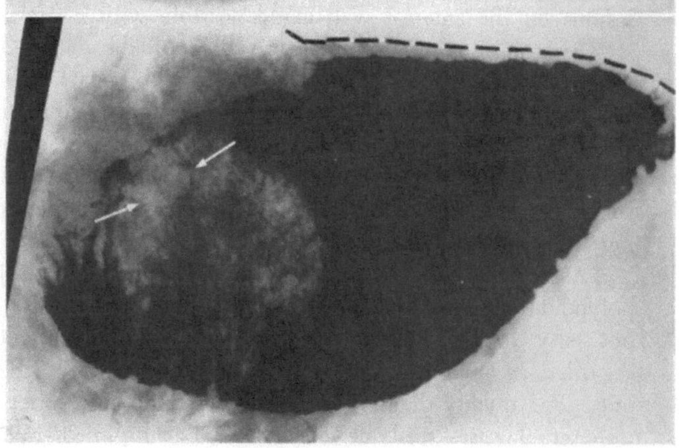

Fig. 16h Compression study of a resected stomach. The lesion is seen in the region indicated by the arrows (↗), but is lacking in definition.

Figure 17a was a preoperative, upright filled study of this actual case (Fig. 16). The margins of both lesser and greater curvatures looked even. Lesions located either on the anterior or posterior wall could not be shown because they were covered with a thick layer of barium.

Figure 17b was a relief picture in the prone position. The lesion on the anterior wall should be recognized in this picture, but only a normal or somewhat rugged mucosa was observed. As mentioned previously, in the position with which this picture was taken, it was difficult to detect lesions smaller than the width of a fold when hidden among the folds.

In Figure 17c, a double-contrast study in the supine position, the area of the posterior wall of the antrum was well exposed as seen in the resected stomach. No polyp was seen on the anterior wall.

Figure 17 d was a compression study. With pressure enough to express the surrounding area, a hemispherical protuberance was seen on the anterior wall. This showed the significance of the proper amount of compression for adequate pictures.

Figure 17e was a gastrofiberscopic picture. A small reddened polyp was readily noticeable on the anterior wall of the antrum. As seen in this case, an endoscopic examination made it easier to find lesions on the anterior wall. It was important to be able to diagnose the reddened polyp protruding inward into the stomach as of epithelial origin, before making a decision whether the protrusion was benign or malignant.

As seen in the resected stomach (Fig. 18a), there was a flat-shaped mucosal polyp of 1 cm in diameter on the posterior wall of the border area. It was a spherical polypoid, nonpedunculated, II–III type lesion. If diagnosed according to the later mentioned program, it could be a cancer.

In the filled study (Fig. 18b), no abnormalities were seen in the marginal area. As shown in the double-contrast study, Figures 18 c–g, a different area was presented depending on the position with which the picture was taken even with identical amounts of air.

Figure 18 c presented an abnormal mucosal protrusion, whose height was not clear because of the thick layer of barium. In Figure 18 d, the size of the protrusion was clearly shown because it was surrounded by barium, but the height was obscure. Figures 18 d and e demonstrated the thin layer method; barium was more or less the height of the protrusion into the stomach, which was estimated by the thickness of the barium layer. Flecks surrounding the protrusion could be observed by the effect of the thin layer of barium. But as shown in Figure 18 d, if the amount of barium was increased slightly, the protrusion became hidden under the shadow of the barium. The fact that the protrusion was hidden even by the thin layer seen in Figure 18 e indicated how low the mucosal polypoids were.

In Figures 18 f and g, the protrusion was beautifully demonstrated by the effect of double-contrast radiography. Low protuberances or groups of rough granules were exposed surrounded by a normal area.

Figure 18 h was a picture radiographed by the double-contrast method from the opposite direction. A barium fleck was seen on top of the elevation, and at a glance the picture presented a mucosal protuberance with a central defect. This indicated the kinds of x-ray findings of lesions on the anterior wall made possible with x-ray exposure from the opposite direction.

Even lesions on the anterior wall could be detected clearly by double-contrast radiography, if barium adhered sufficiently. In this case a dark shadow fleck was revealed in the center of the protuberance caused by a drop of barium. In Figures 18 i–k, the degree of the compression was varied. To diagnose such protruding lesions, several pictures were indispensable to show the surrounding mucosa and its height. As seen in Figure 18 i, the picture showed only the surface of the protruding lesion. Combinations of pictures to allow visualization of the surrounding mucosal areas are desirable.

As seen in this case, the protruding lesion, 1 cm in diameter, was a spherical, nonpedunculated polypoid and was diagnosed as epithelial in origin by the x-ray examination. However, it was not easy to tell whether it was benign or malignant because x-ray examinations should be regarded as an indirect diagnostic method. Actually the problem of differentiation is a frequent one. For quality diagnosis, a biopsy or cytology under direct vision is necessary.

Actual cases will be discussed. Barium-filled radiographs (radiographs of a barim filled stomach) in the upright and prone positions are shown in Figures 18 l and m. No abnormal

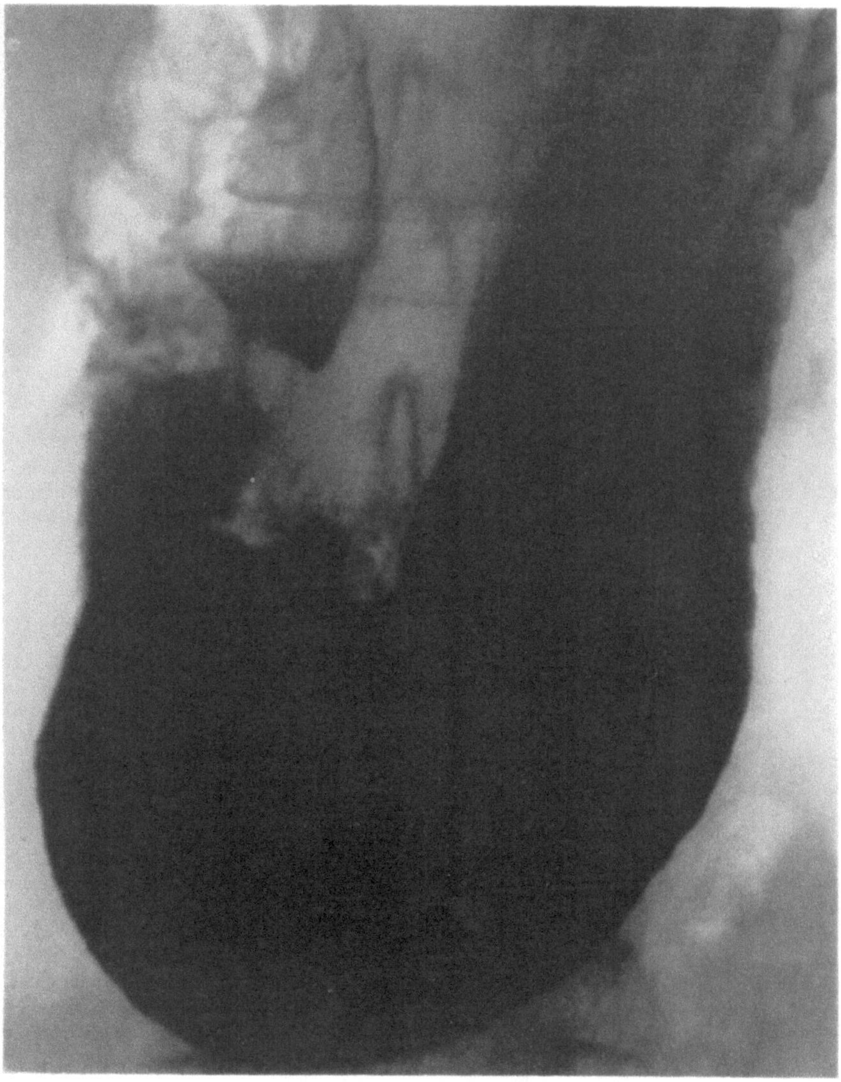

Fig. 17a Barium-filled radiograph (Radiograph of the barium filled stomach) in the upright position. An irregular contraction is observed at the lesser curvature of the antrum, although overlapping with the shadow of the duodenum. The filling defect, which is suspicious of a polypoid lesion, cannot be found in this picture.

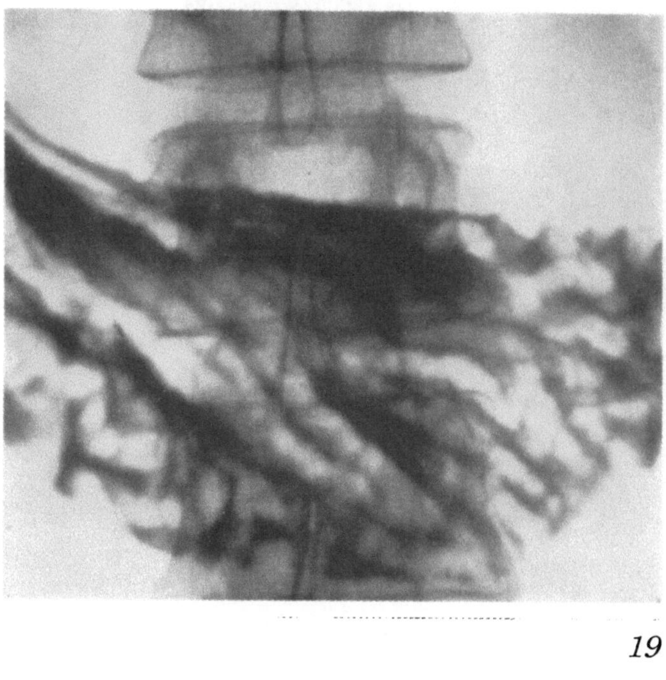

Fig. 17b Relief pattern in the prone position. Mucosal folds are extending from the gastric body and thicken at the anterior wall of the antrum. The existence of a polypoid lesion may be suspected, but cannot be affirmed.

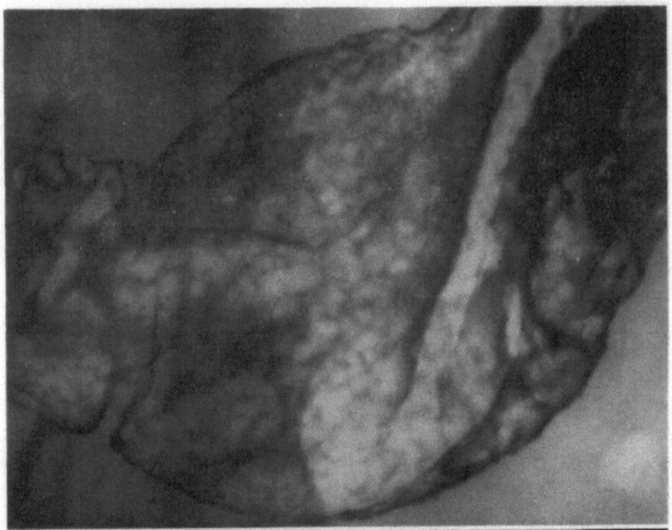

Fig. 17c Double-contrast study in the supine position. A large number of fine granular shadows considered to be hyperplastic changes are present.

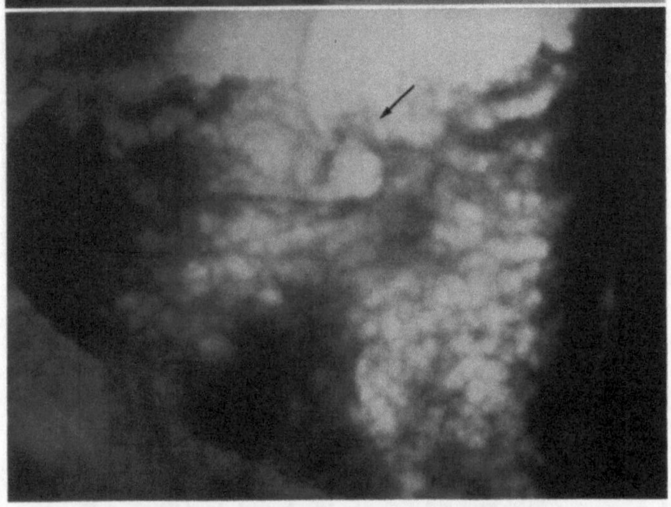

Fig. 17d Compression study in the supine position. A round-shaped shadow defect pointed out by the arrow is observed in the compression study. Note the differences in comparison with hyperplastic change.

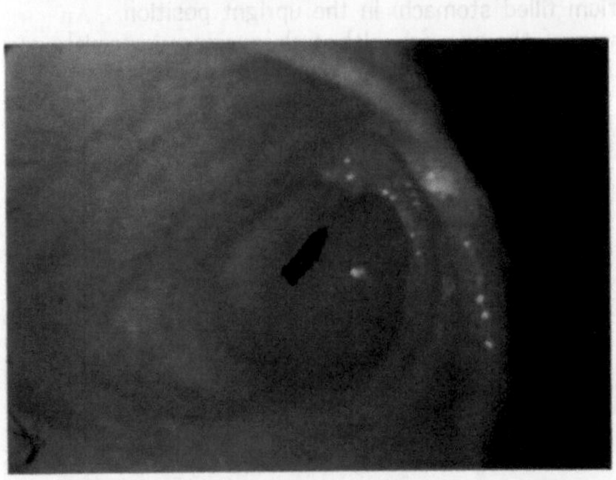

Fig. 17e Gastrofiberscopic picture. A mucosal elevation protruding clearly from the surrounding mucosa is observed on the anterior wall of the antrum (indicated by the arrow). The surface of the mucosal elevation is relatively smooth.

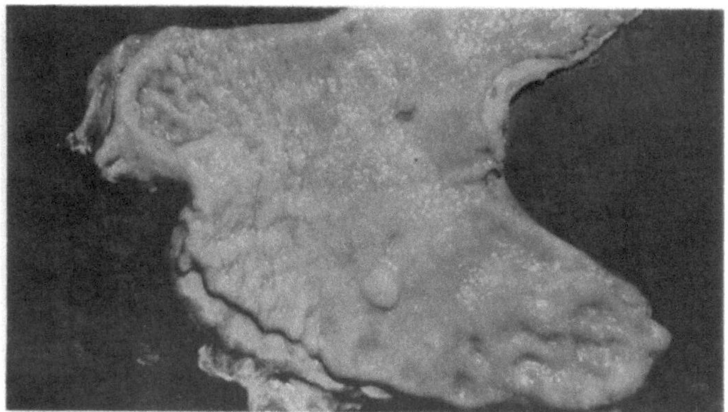

Fig. 18a Resected stomach. A flat-type protrusion measuring 1×1 cm in diameter is seen on the posterior wall of the borderline region.

Fig. 18b Barium-filling effect in a resected stomach. The tumor is hidden in the barium layer.

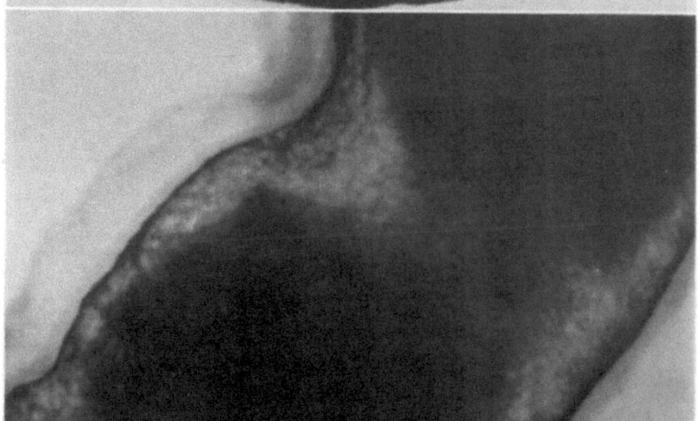

Fig. 18c Radiograph of a resected stomach using a moderately large amount of barium. A flat protrusion is hidden in the barium layer.

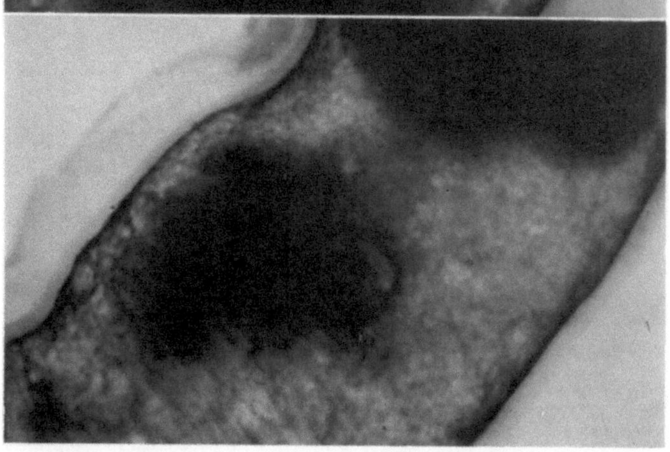

Fig. 18d Effects of a thin barium layer. This picture does not sufficiently reveal the lesion, because barium still remains in the region of the lesion.

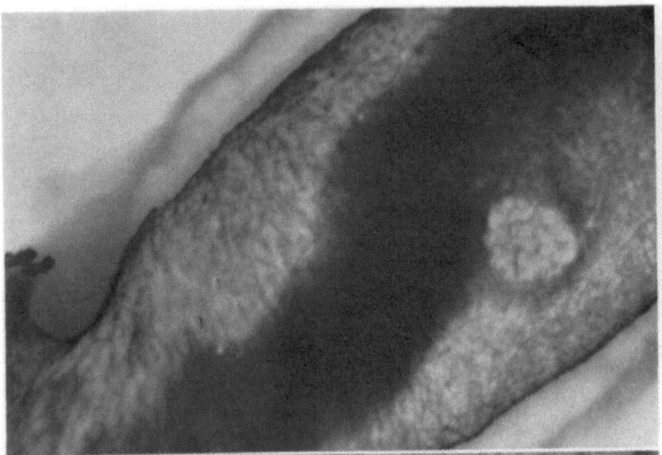

Fig. 18e Effects of a thinner barium layer. The grade of protrusion into the gastric cavity is estimated by collecting the barium around the lesion.

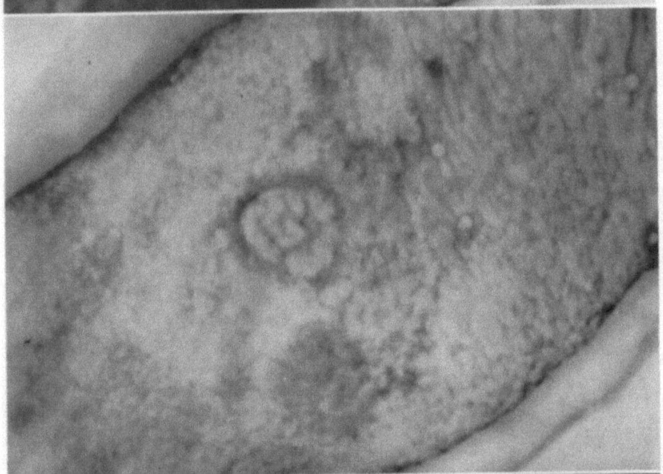

Fig. 18f Double-contrast effect. A rough area is seen on the surface of the low protrusion.

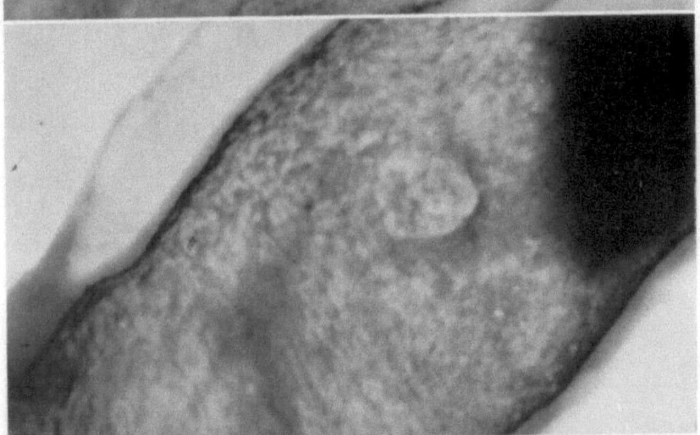

Fig. 18g Double-contrast effect. A low mucosal elevation is observed surrounded by regular gastric areas.

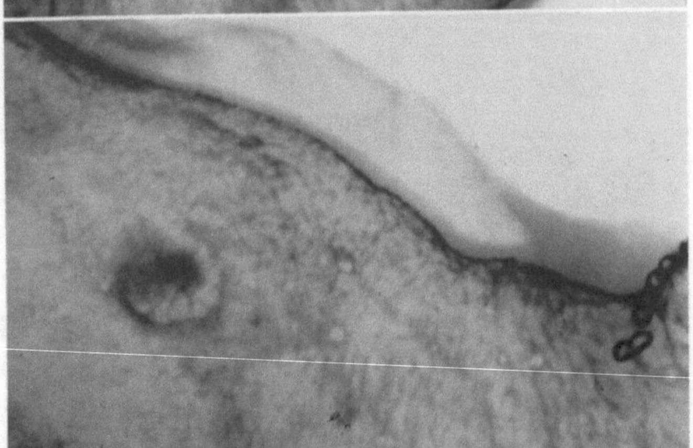

Fig. 18h Double-contrast study of the opposite wall. A drop of barium is seen in the center of the tumor surface.

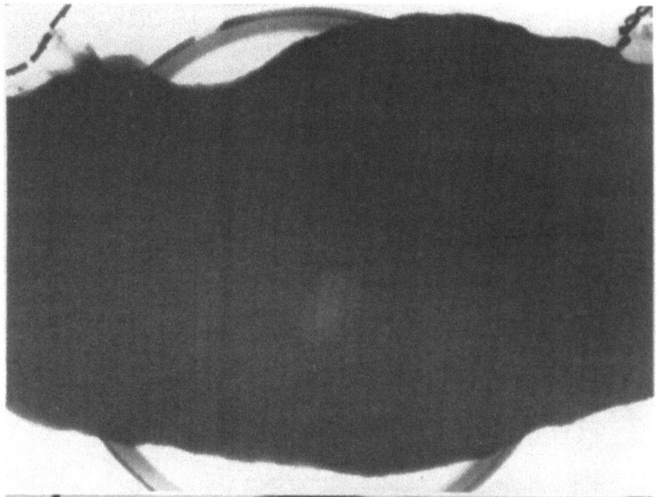

Fig. 18i Slight-compression study. Only the top of the protuberance is seen.

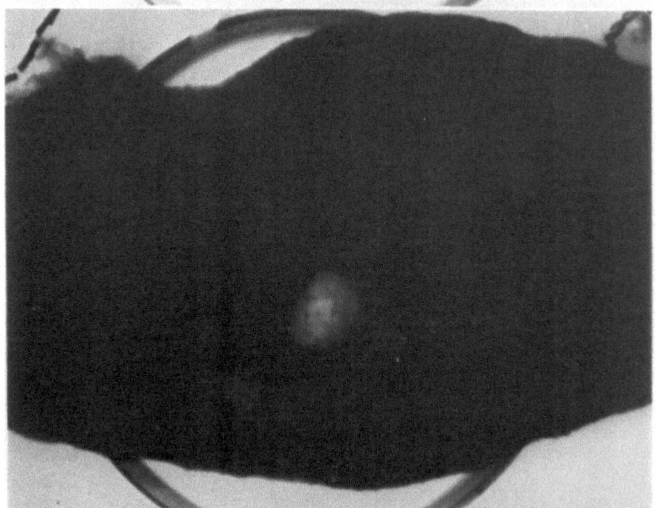

Fig. 18j Slight-compression study. The whole pattern can be seen with a firm compression.

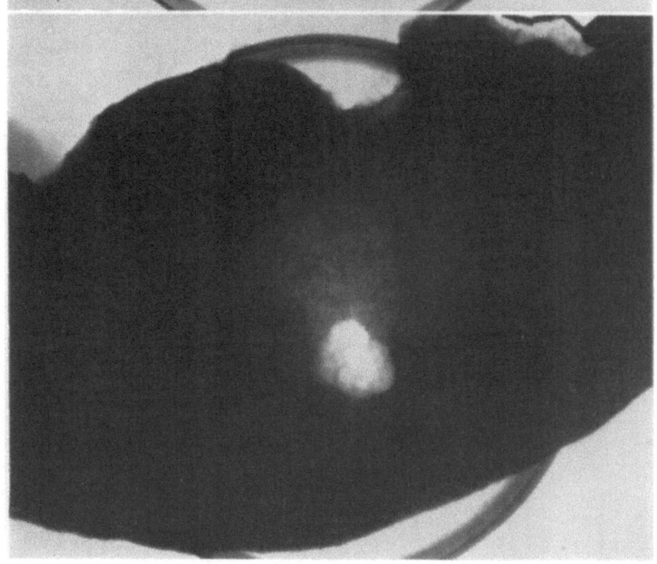

Fig. 18k Adequate-compression study. Optimal compression allows the area of the surrounding membrane to be seen. The surface is a granulated Grade 2 (Fig. 48), and it may be diagnosed as benign, though nonpedunculated.

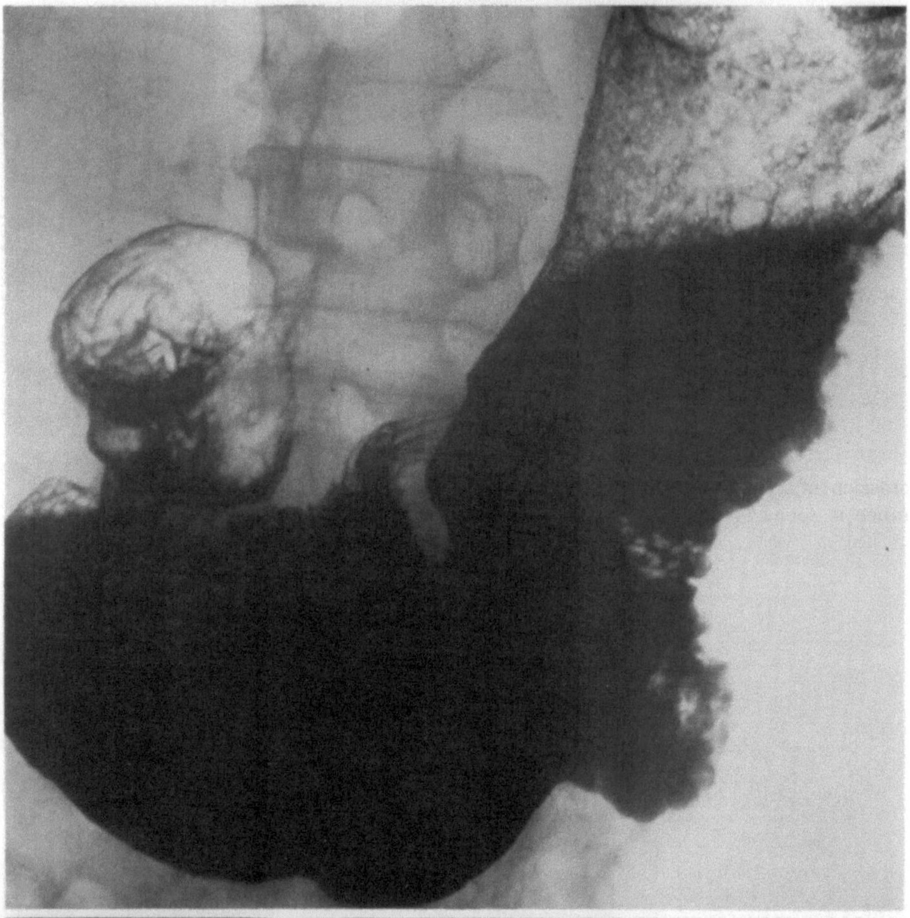

18l

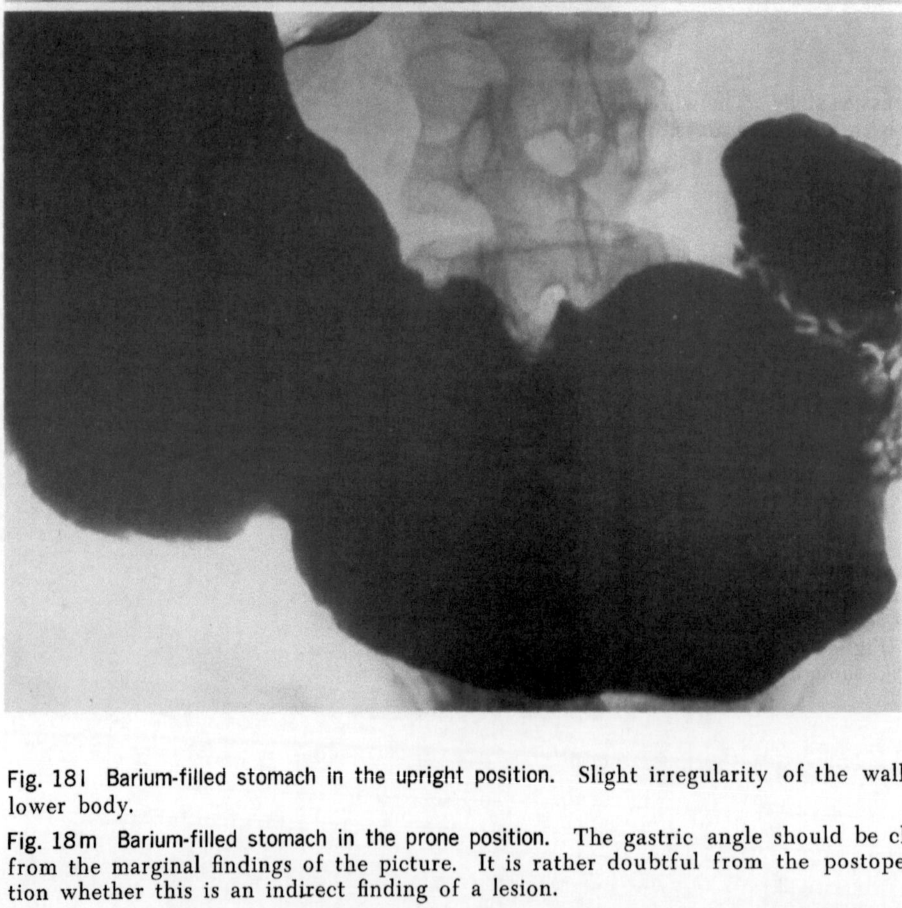

18m

Fig. 18l Barium-filled stomach in the upright position. Slight irregularity of the wall is seen in the lower body.

Fig. 18m Barium-filled stomach in the prone position. The gastric angle should be checked, judging from the marginal findings of the picture. It is rather doubtful from the postoperative examination whether this is an indirect finding of a lesion.

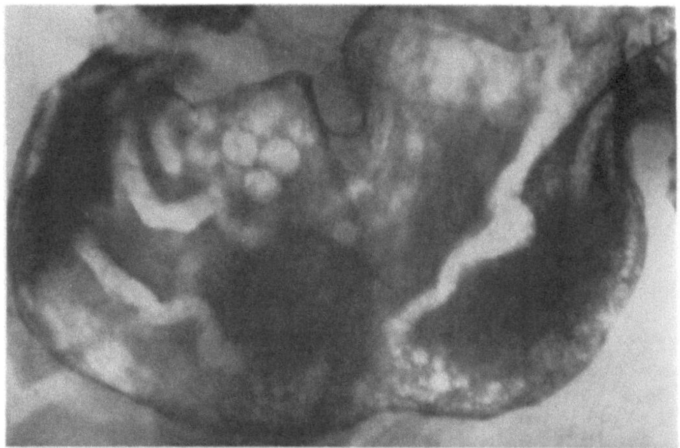

Fig. 18n Double-contrast study in the supine position. The double-contrast method is not always effective with a small amount of air.

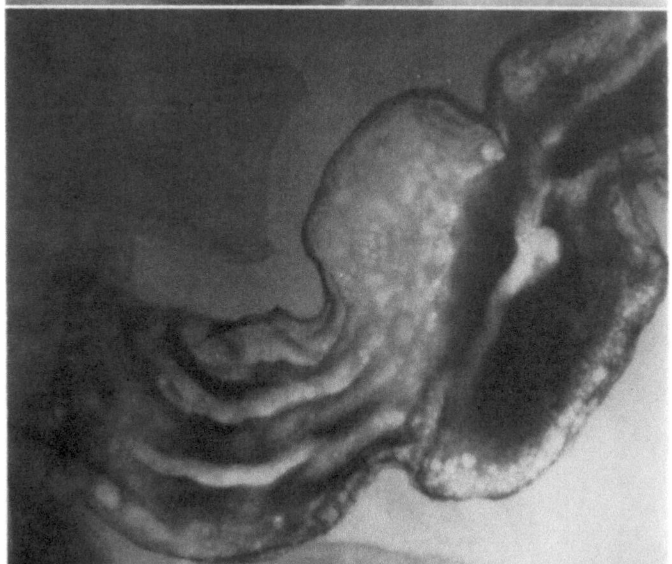

Fig. 18o Double-air-contrast study. One of the mucosal folds at the posterior wall of the gastric angle looks as if it is broken and bent. It is due to inadequate description with a small amount of air.

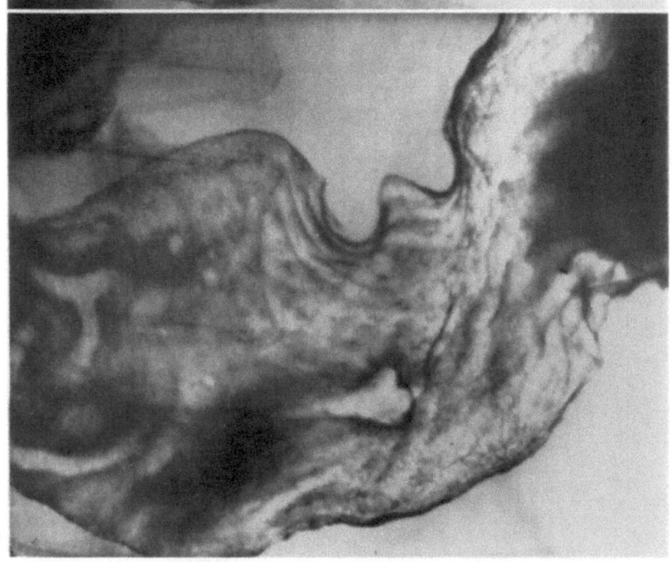

Fig. 18p Double-air-contrast study with a moderate amount of air. When the amount of air is increased, the shadows of unnecessary folds disappear.

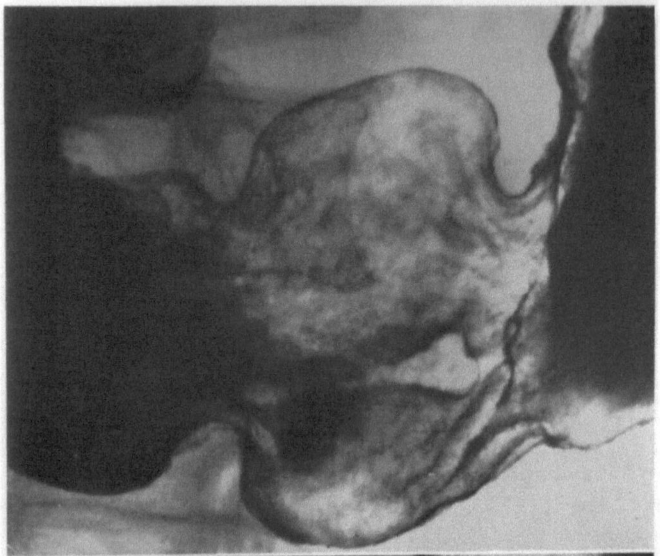

Fig. 18q Double-contrast study with a moderate amount of air. The top of the protuberance is irregular in shape with an uneven, granular formation on its surface.

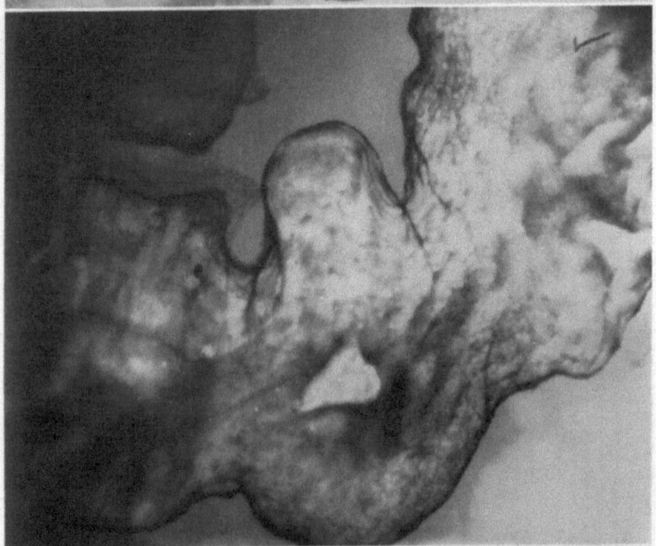

Fig. 18r Double-contrast study. Good double air contrast pictures are not always taken with the same amount of air. It is necessary to change the amount depending on the case.

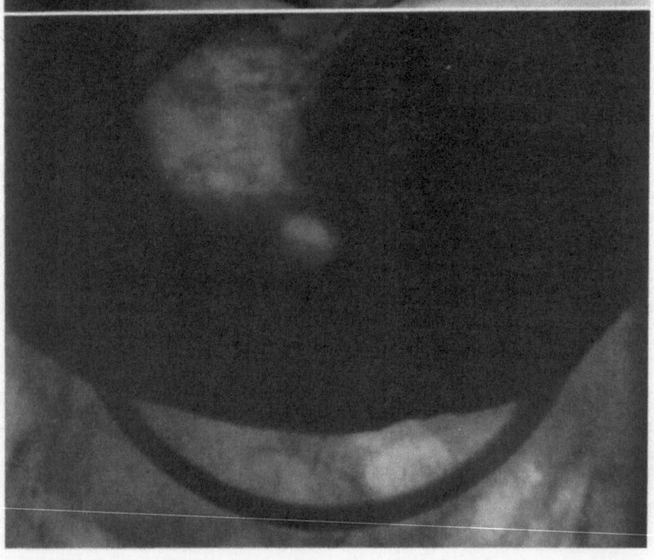

Fig. 18s Compression study. A granular pattern can be observed on the surface of the protuberance by compression. This finding is unusual in a submucosal tumor.

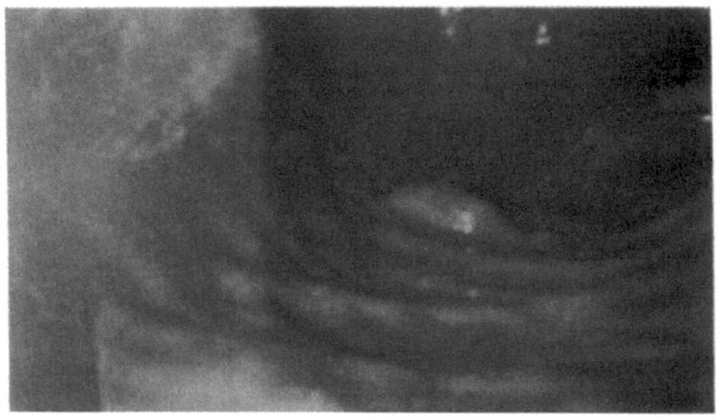

18t

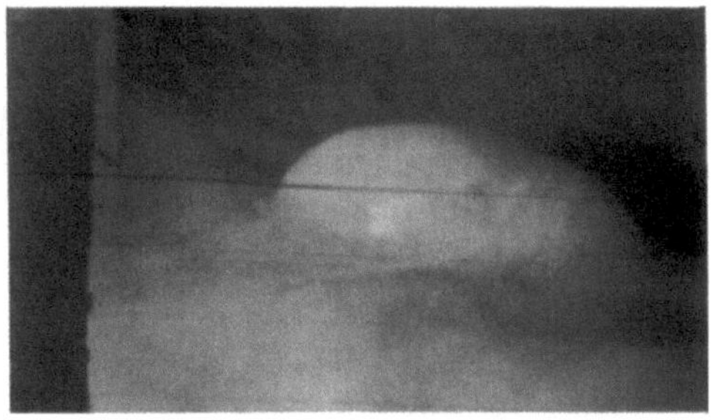

18u

Fig. 18t Distant endoscopic pattern. The surface is smooth and not reddened, but the phyma protrudes at a sharp angle into the stomach.

Fig. 18u Close-up endoscopic pattern. No hemorrhage or erosion on the surface is seen.

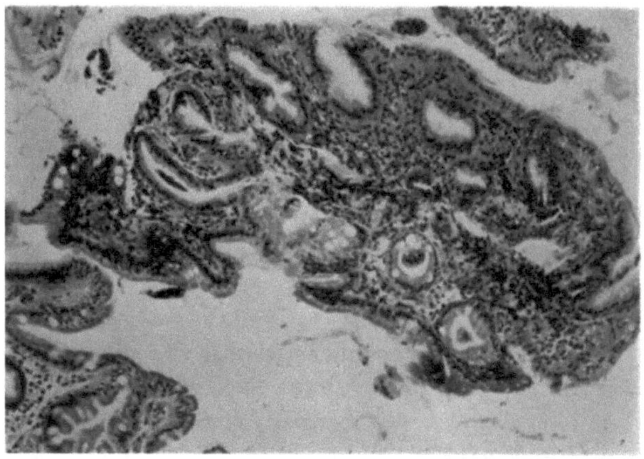

Fig. 18v Gastric biopsy observations. Abnormal columnar cells having irregular nuclei and cytoplasms are hyperstained with HE stains. It was diagnosed as an atypical epithelium.

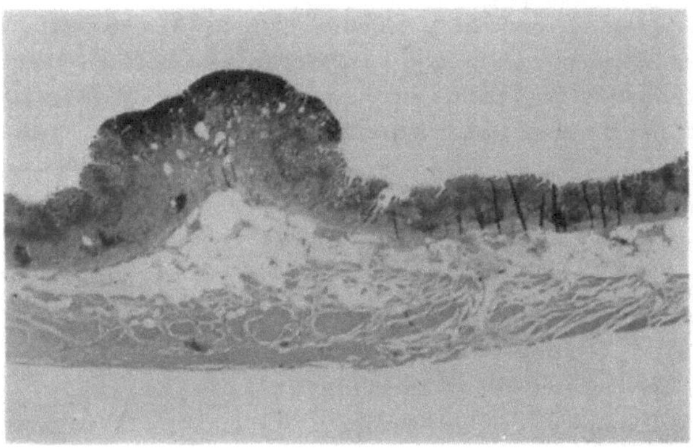

18w

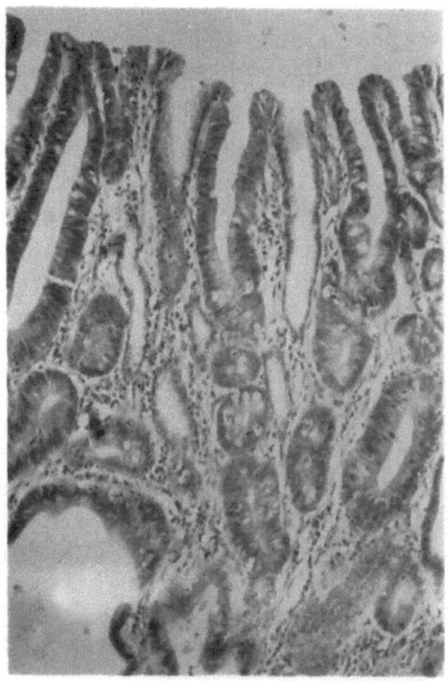

18x

Fig. 18w Histopathological observations.

Fig. 18x Histopathological observations. At the top of the protuberance, the slight disturbance of a partially formed cyst was observed in the duct structure. However, since the nuclei were aligned on the basal membrane, it could not be diagnosed as malignant.

changes were observed in the marginal areas except an irregular wall in the lower part of the stomach.

The angular region of the posterior wall was the area best depicted by double-contrast radiography. But in Figures 18 n and o, this area was revealed to have distorted folds on the posterior wall. In a double-contrast study with a little more air (Figs. 18 p, q, r), the flat, broad-based, protruding lesion covered with a rough area could be observed.

In the upright compression picture (Fig. 18 s), low protuberances, which had been diagnosed as epithelial polypoid lesions, could be observed.

Figure 18 t was a picture taken during an endoscopic examination from a comparative distance and Figure 18 u was a picture taken close-up.

In actual cases, an excavated lesion could readily be seen as a lateral projection or a borderline deformation in the radiographs of barium filled stomachs. Accordingly, the presence of an excavation was detected chiefly by filling radiography. In other words, by referring to the frontal exposure of a depression on x-ray pictures together with lateral exposures, the lesion was outlined macroscopically, and on the basis of characteristic observations of the lesion outlined, a definitive diagnosis was made.

b. Excavated lesions

In Figure 19, a resected stomach on a plate after fixation, covered with a thin layer of barium on the extended gastric wall, was shown by means of an experimental x-ray with softex.

Figure 19a was an open ulcer of Ul–IV. Figure 19b was also an open ulcer of Ul–IV, but a partial regeneration was noticed from the margin to the surface of the defect by the regenerated epithelium. Figure 19c was an ulcer scar corresponding to MURAKAMI's [2]Ul–III, *i.e.*, an incomplete type scar. Figure 19d was a [3]Ul–IV, *i.e.*, a complete-type scar (Fig. 7). Figure 19e disclosed shallow mucosal defects in connection with gastric erosions.

These photographs indicated that the slightest depression of the gastric wall was sufficiently outlined by x-ray; and that the approximate depth of the depression in reference to the mucous membrane could be estimated in connection with the surrounding areas. With the gastric wall in a fixed condition, the ruggedness of the wall was distinctly observed by means of the concentration of barium with the concurrent evaporation of moisture and shrinkage of the mucous membrane. Thus, if similar conditions were selected in actual x-ray examinations, patterns of the gastric inner wall (gastric small sections) might be adequately seen.

Compare Figures 19a and b (Ul-IV open) with Figure 19e (erosion). In respect to the concentrations of barium, spots deposited in depressions were expressed in similar shades. Regarding the mucous membrane around the depression, the ruggedness was intensified in the former because of the thin barium layer, while in the latter there existed a rather thick barium layer. With respect to the bordering areas, in the former, the border was distinct and shadow spots were formed independently of the ruggedness of the surrounding mucous membrane; while in the latter, the border was not distinct and appeared to be surrounded by a fine, convex-surfaced mucous membrane. In other words, discrimination between shallow and deep depressions would be possible from the x-ray picture alone, if the following two points were taken into consideration: the thickness of the surrounding barium layer and the state of the surrounding wall of the depression.

Furthermore, experimental x-ray photographs of scars as shown in Figures 19c and d showed that in depressions (Figs. 19a, b) with mucosal defects, patternless and homogeneous shadow spots could be observed, such as depressed surfaces covered by epithelium as seen in scars. This proves that when clear x-ray pictures of a depression are obtained, the presence or absence of defects in the epithelium can be judged through an analysis of shadow spots, supported by the above observations. This is applicable to both double-contrast and compression radiography, and the diagnosis of depressed areas by x-ray is based on these findings.

There are two ways to demonstrate these depressions radiologically, lateral and frontal patterns. The former is a profile niche and the latter, a frontal view niche. There may be a transient pattern (oblique pattern) between them according to the angle of observation, making it necessary to obtain frontal and lateral exposures correctly. The possible existence of an affected part unsuitable for x-ray examination in either the front or lateral area should not be discounted. The final diagnosis depends entirely on how the front pattern, or frontal view niche, is expressed;

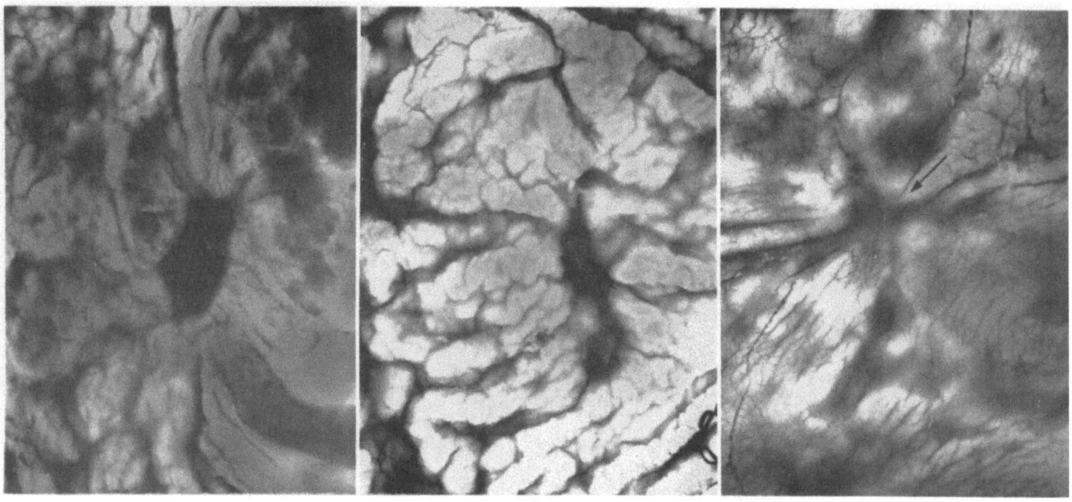

a. Ul-IV b. Ul-IV c. ^{2}Ul-III

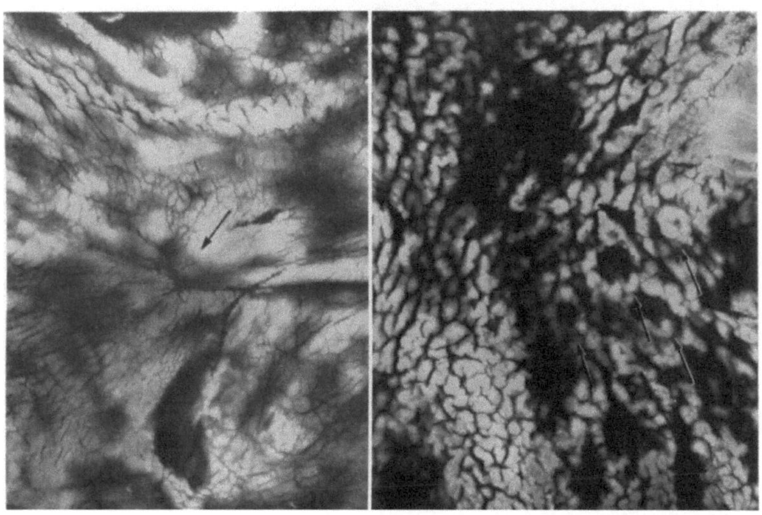

d. ^{3}Ul-IV e. Ul-I

Fig. 19 Experimental x-ray pictures of excavated lesions using softex. Note the definition of shadow spots, especially the contrast with surrounding mucous membranes, shape of the shadow spots, clearness of the borders, and characteristics of the marginal and surrounding parts of the depressions.

because size, shape, and distribution of ruggedness of a depression can be accurately judged from the frontal exposure, and diagnosis of the depth of the depression is possible by a comparison with the surrounding barium layer.

Therefore, the final x-ray diagnosis of depressed lesions depends on the frontal exposure, making it necessary to use both the double-contrast and compression methods varying the patient's position and the amounts of barium and air. Nowadays it has become possible to demonstrate fine and minute changes of the mucosa, as the technical problems have largely been resolved.

1) Defects of the gastric wall

In depressed lesions without defects of the gastric wall, as in gastric diverticula (Figs. 20 a, b) or extensive depressed lesions, smoothness on the bottoms of the depressions and their edges are

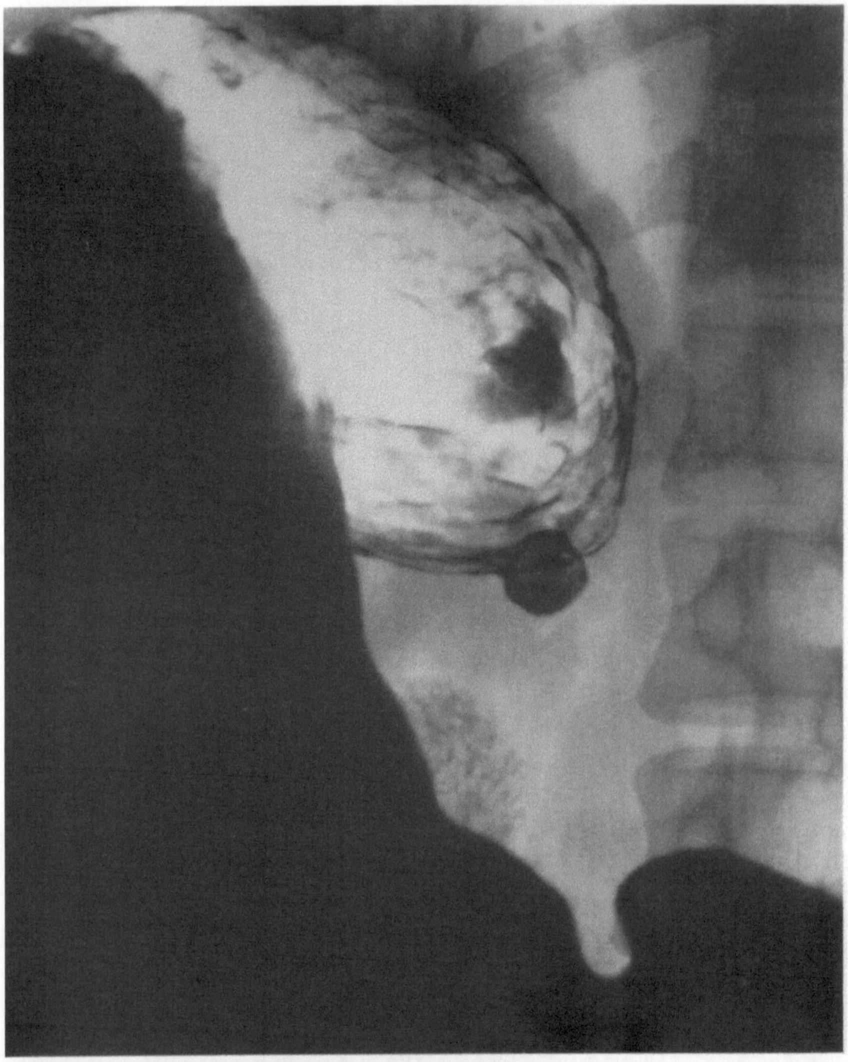

20a

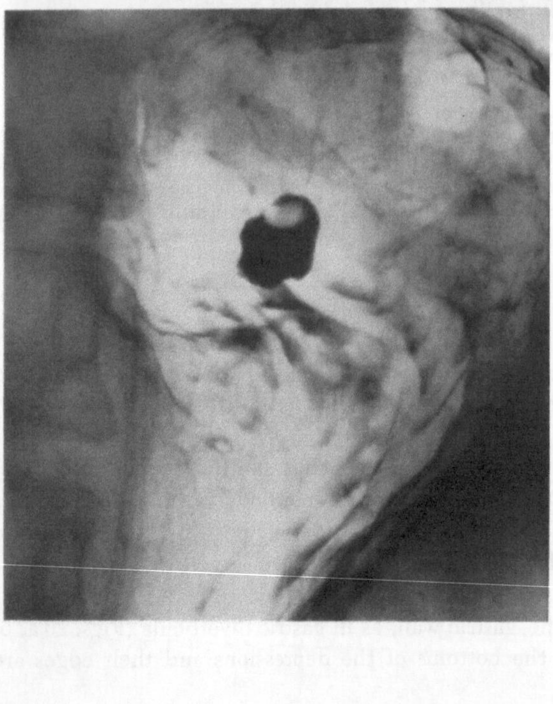

20b

Fig. 20 X-ray photographs of a depression without a defect of the gastric wall.

a. Gastric diverticulum (prone filled picture).

b. Gastric diverticulum (upright double-contrast picture).

characteristically observed by air insufflation. On the other hand, in other depressed lesions with defects of the gastric walls, such as gastric ulcers (Fig. 21), irregularly depressed bottoms or differences in contrasts of the barium are found. Fibrous tissues are histologically observed in the submucosal or muscular layers of resulting scars from gastric ulcers, and then surfaces are not smooth. Therefore, radiographs of ulcer scars are presumed to show an intermediate picture of the former and the latter.

2) Shallow and deep depressions

It is difficult to diagnose the true depth of a depression from a profile view of the niche. As Eschbach and Kumakura, et al. have already reported, radiographic depressions generally seem to be deeper than they actual are. Referring to our radiographic experience, we have roentgenologically classified gastric depressions into shallow and deep types.

Figure 21 a was a resected specimen of a gastric ulcer on the lesser curvature of the gastric body, which was resected after hospitalized treatment lasting two months. In this picture, there was a long linear scar along the lesser curvature. Changes in the profile view of the niche with the passage of time will be presented in Figures 21 b–d. Two niches could be seen situated along the lesser curvature upon admission (Fig. 21 b), and these niches were surrounded by depressions with smooth surfaces and mucosal prominences. This was a profile picture of a deep type of depression with surrounding mucosal prominences. After two weeks, these two gastric ulcers were endoscopically observed to coalesce into one long oval ulcer and gradually to decrease in size. After one month, this ulcer was radiographically seen to become linear (Fig. 21 c). In this picture, the surrounding mucosal prominences had almost disappeared, and from the profile picture, the depth of the ulcer was estimated to be 1 or 2 mm. After two months (Fig. 21 d), the niche could not be found, and only the rigidity and irregularity of the gastric wall could be observed.

Profile pictures of depressed lesions were presented in Figures 21 b–d. Their longitudinal circumferences and depths were easily discernible; however, the widths of the depressed lesion could not be established. Therefore, the double-contrast and/or the compression method should be used to correctly visualize the total circumference of the lesion. Not only the circumference of the lesion, but also the irregularity of the margin, the uneveness of the bottom, and the depth of the depression must be observed. When diagnosing a depressed lesion, the characteristics of the depressed surface must be kept in mind; in addition, an attempt should be made to demonstrate the surrounding mucosa or the mucosal folds around the lesion.

A deep depression (Fig. 22) and a shallow cancerous ulcer (Fig. 23) were presented in their frontal view. From the contrast, we could easily diagnose the former as a depression of the deep type and the latter as a shallow type with mucosal prominences around the lesion. We should take careful note of the differences in the density of the barium on the lesion and the surrounding mucosa. In the deep-type depression (Fig. 22), we could observe the dark barium fleck in the lesion, even if the density of the barium was not appropriate. On the other hand, in the shallow type (Fig. 23), we could not observe marked differences due to the density of the barium on the lesion and the surrounding mucosa. On the basis of this point, this lesion could be diagnosed as shallow. After that, we should try to read the total picture of the depressed lesion accurately.

3) Noteworthy profile niche

A depression on a cancer, which is usually an ulcer produced on the mucosal elevation, presents an x-ray finding of a niche or filling defect, *i.e.*, "Schattenplus im Schattenminus". But this does not always mean that a niche projecting from the gastric wall is not a cancer. When the cancer is an early one, the filling defect is slight as a profile finding because the prominence of the gastric mucosa is slight. Thus, it is important to observe the shape, the edge of the niche, and the surrounding mucosa in detail.

i) Niche en castre: This niche is observed as a small "Schattenplus im Schattenminus", or a niche in the depressed surface of the gastric wall, and extreme cases may be niches on the level floor. Therefore, depressed lesions which have this finding in profile represent ulcers on the mucosal elevation and they are mostly small cancerous depressions. For differential diagnosis of these niches, an acute ulcer with edematous marginal swelling and a chronic ulcer with marked fibrosis in the surrounding mucosa must be kept in mind.

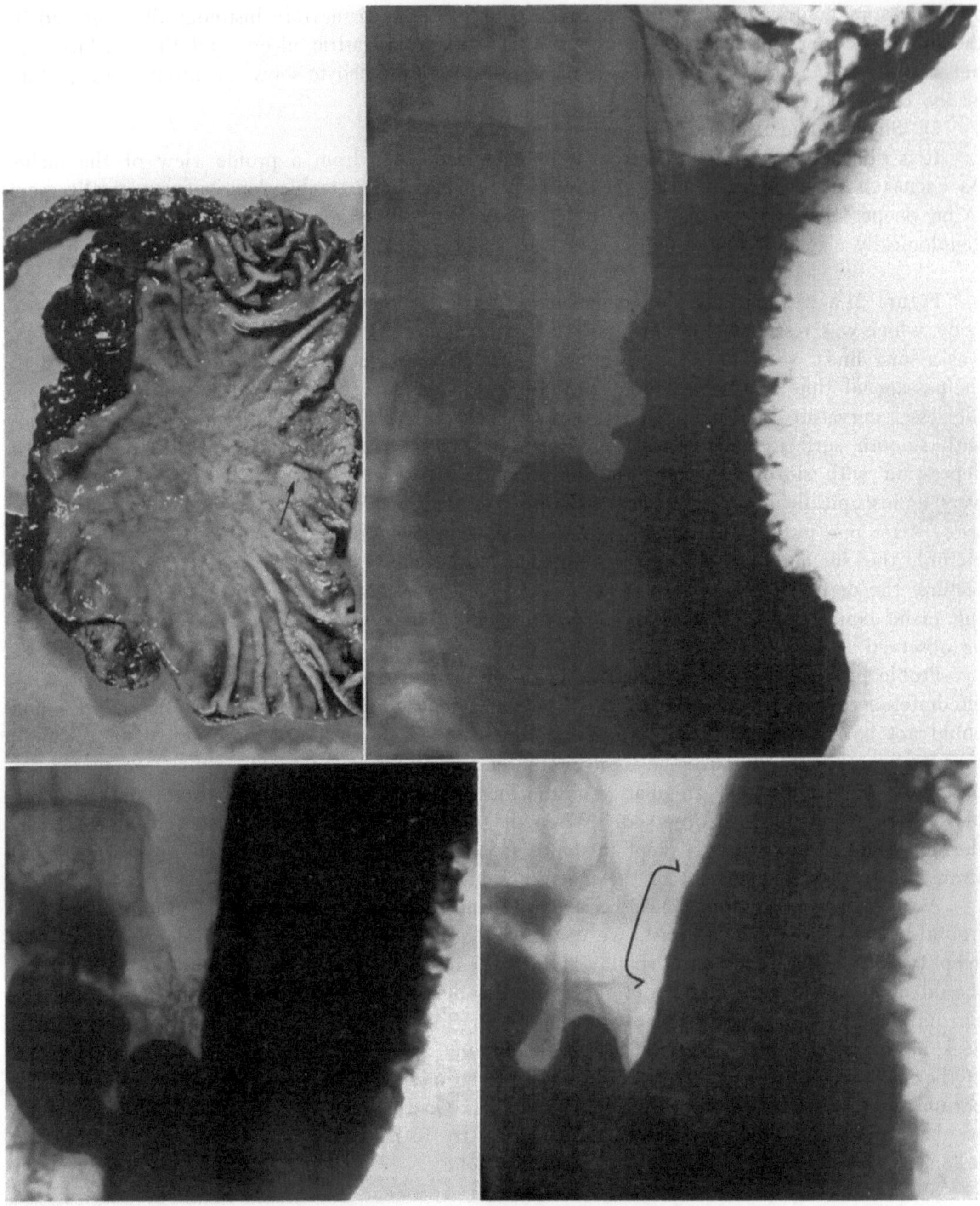

21a 21b

21c 21d

Fig. 21 X-ray photographs of deep and shallow depressions.

a. Resected stomach showing a linear scar at the lesser curvature of the body.
b. Two deep niches at first.
c. X-ray photograph, one month after Fig. 21 b.
d. X-ray photograph, two months after Fig. 21 c.

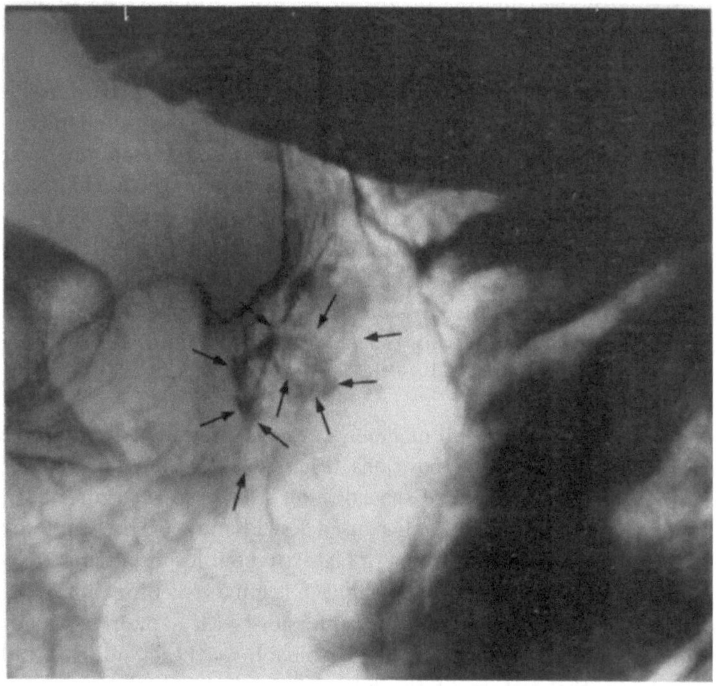

Fig. 22 Deep type of depression.

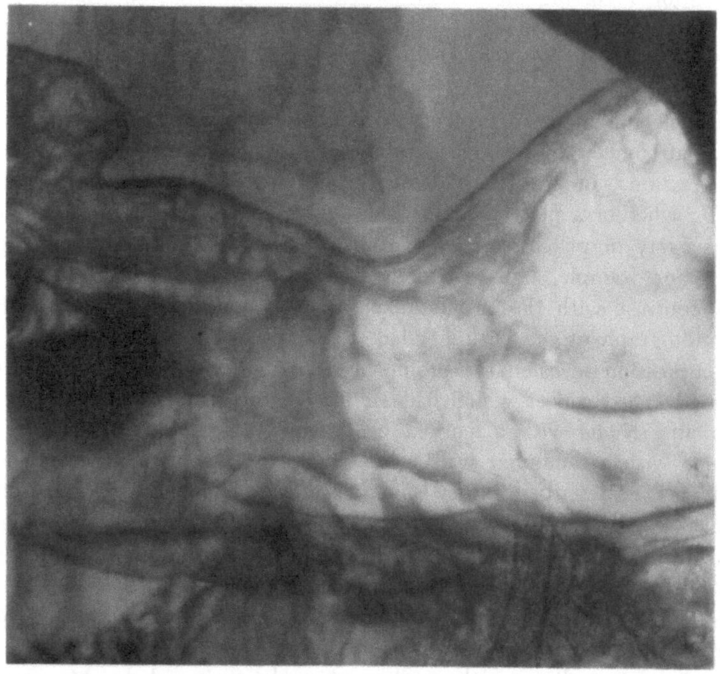

Fig. 23 Shallow type of depression (advanced gastric cancer just like an early gastric one).

We must read the peripheral changes of profile views of niches in detail, so it is necessary to take adequate photographs of barium filled stomachs. With inadequate exposures, it is not rare to interpret profile views as benign in the presence of cancerous ulcers. It may be useful to take a profile picture under slight compression of a barium filled stomach in the right or left oblique position. It is extremely important to obtain good pictures of barium filled stomachs.

One case is presented here. A niche was detected on the gastric angle (Fig. 24 a). Poor extension and irregularity on the distal margin of the niche was noticed on careful observation. From the compression study (Fig. 24 b) and the resected stomach (Fig. 24 c), this lesion was judged as a gastric cancer of the Borrmann III type. Nodular elevations were well described around the niche in the compression study. These were undoubtedly "Schattenplus im Schattenminus" or niche en castre. Thus, when a cancerous ulcer is not accompanied by a remarkable mucosal elevation as in this case, it may be diagnosed as a benign ulcer niche, especially in a stomach insufficiently filled with barium (Fig. 24 a). The slight changes around a niche may sometimes be overlooked.

Another case of a small niche en castre is presented in Figure 25. The barium filled stomach in the upright and prone positions (Figs. 25 a, b) showed a small finger-sized niche with a slight concavity on its margin. Especially on the anal margin of the niche, the rigidity with an irregularity of the gastric wall caused a widening of the angle and the rigidity extended to the lesser curvature of the antrum. This excavated lesion with an ulcer-like niche could be regarded as a lesion accompanied by a slight marginal swelling and a rigid zone which inhibited the extension of the gastric wall. A depression with a poorly extending zone of the wall shown in the radiograph of the barium filled stomach in the standing position (Fig. 25 a) was represented correctly in the picture of the filled stomach in the prone position (Fig. 25 b) or the double-contrast study (Fig. 25 c). This case was macroscopically diagnosed as a II c+III type early gastric cancer, as shown in the resected stomach (Fig. 25 d), however, the cancerous infiltration had already reached the muscle layer proper in the center of the lesion.

Thus, a demonstration of the change around a niche is necessary in a well-filled barium situation involving the site of the lesion. And it is important to investigate all of the following minutiae: slight depressions, irregularities, poor extension and rigidity of the gastric wall surrounding the niches.

ii) Niche en plateau: A shallow depression with a slight marginal swelling usually appears as a plateau niche in profile. A roentgenological profile of a fine depression is described as a plateau niche, an irregular finding of the gastric margin, and a flat lesion, sometimes a fine depression. In shallower plateau niches, irregular margins with poor extensions are seen. Therefore, whether a plateau niche or a slightly depressed lesion is hidden or not must be determined. Discovery of plateau niches requires a skilled technique in radiology.

For example, a plateau niche was seen on the lesser curvature of the gastric body (Fig. 26 a). In contrast with the profile taken by the compression method (Fig. 26 b), a plateau niche in a radiograph of the barium filled stomach exhibited the profile of a depressed lesion accurately. Compression revealed the profile of an irregular, slight depression (Figs. 26 c, d). This case was an advanced cancer which had IIc-like features macroscopically.

iii) Niche with a marked ulcer wall: This finding is called a "Meniscus sign", that is, a niche with a semilunar wall means the existence of a mucosal elevation around the excavation which was described earlier under "Excavated niches". These niches were shown in Figure 27, a Borrmann III advanced cancer, and Figure 28, a schirrhus. This type of niche should be expressed as the so-called "Schattenplus im Schattenminus" or excavated niches. However, there is a problem in differential diagnosis concerning ulcer niches in the pyloric antrum, because this niche is not always a sign malignancy. Few findings requiring special attention when reading profile shadows of excavated lesions have been discussed above.

Recent studies on the malignant cycle proposed by Murakami have also been applied to clinical data, that is, peptic ulcers may occur on cancerous as well as noncancerous mucosa and will scar like ordinary peptic ulcers (Fig. 29).

Furthermore, it is possible to say that peptic ulcers on the IIc or IIb, early gastric cancer can be observed. Applying this point to the evaluation of profile niches, the surrounding mucosa of ulcer niches which are rarely considered to be cancer may possibly be cancer. Therefore even if a radiograph shows a very common ulcer niche, since we cannot rule out gastric cancers

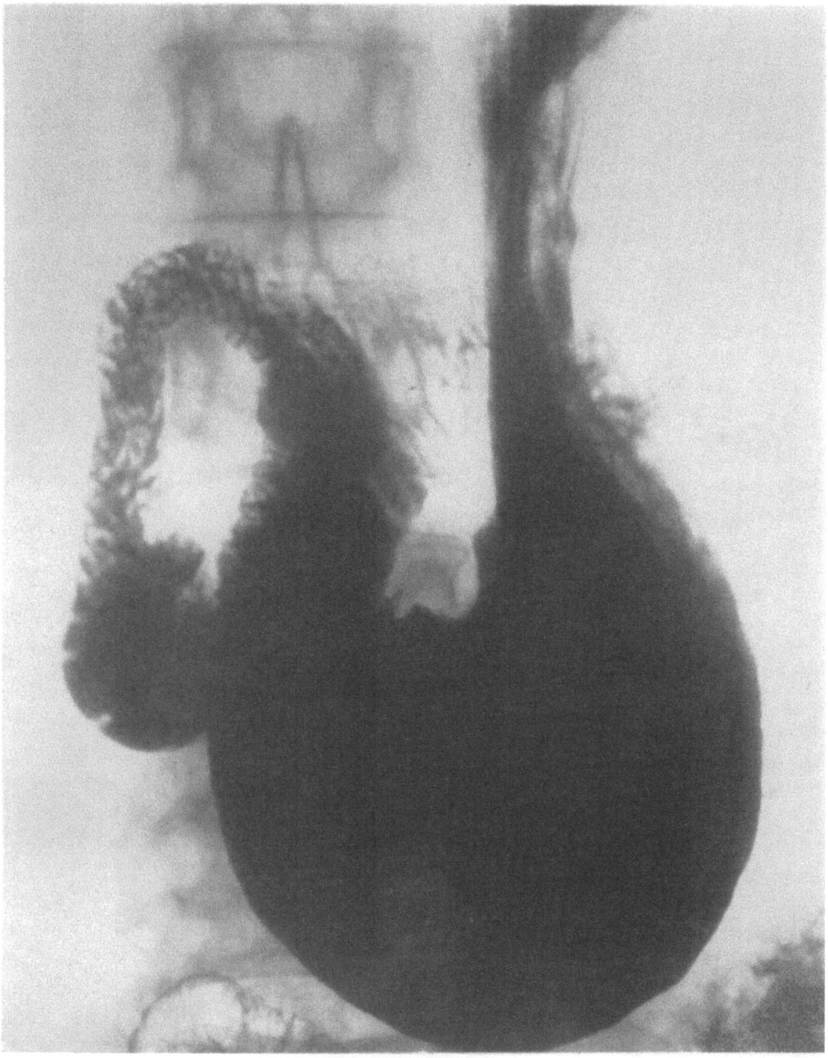

24 a

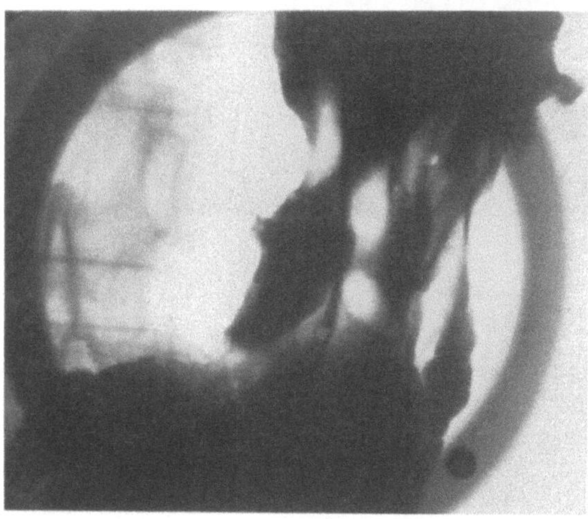

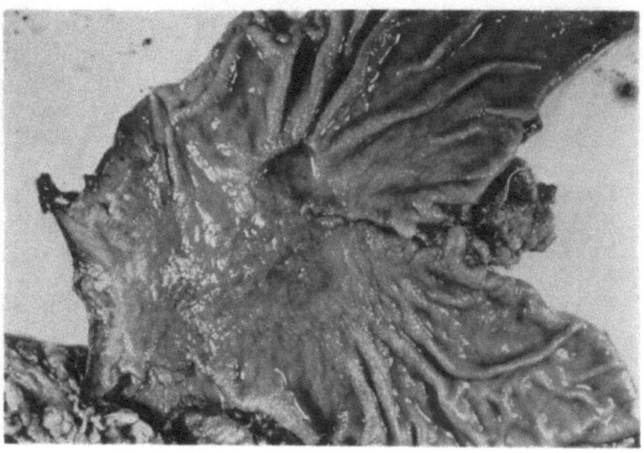

24 b

24 c

Fig. 24 Niche en castre. The region surrounding the niche must be carefully interpreted, and it is important not to neglect even a slight change in the gastric wall.

a. Barium filled stomach in the upright position. The niche above the gastric angle looks like a benign ulcer.

b. Compression study. Niche en castre is well represented.

c. Resected stomach. Cancer has infiltrated the bundle layer of the muscle proper.

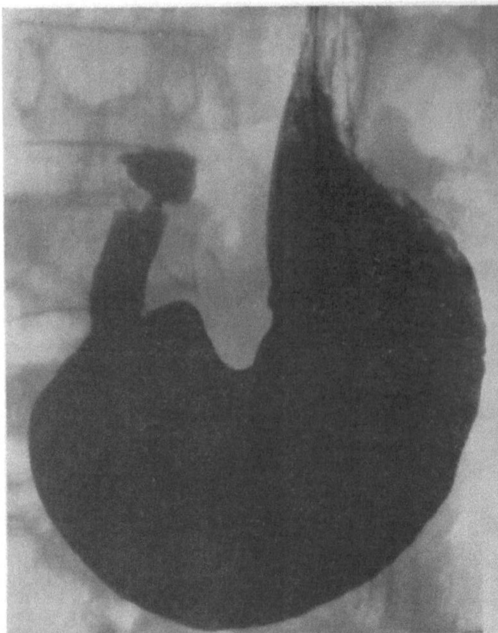

25a

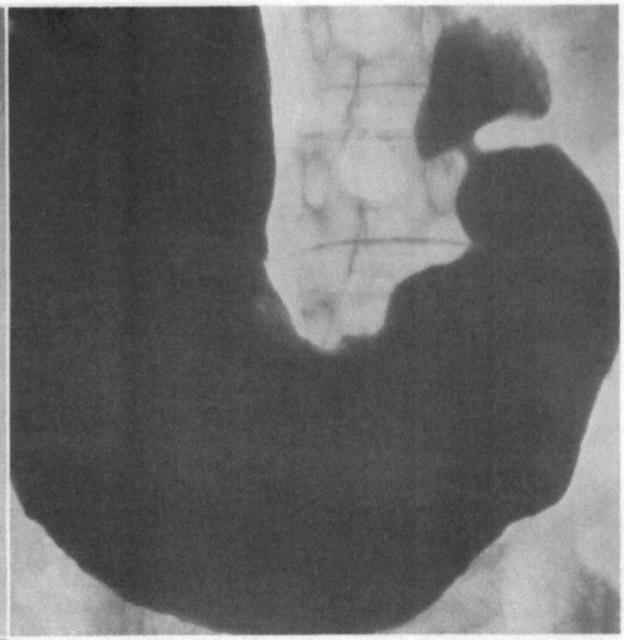

2

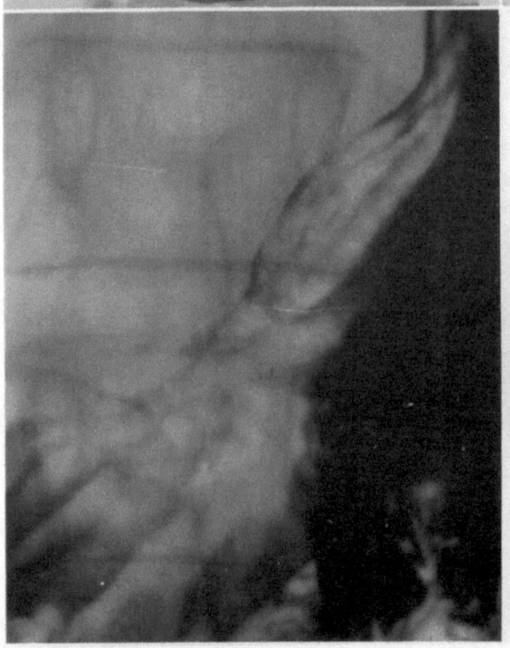

25c

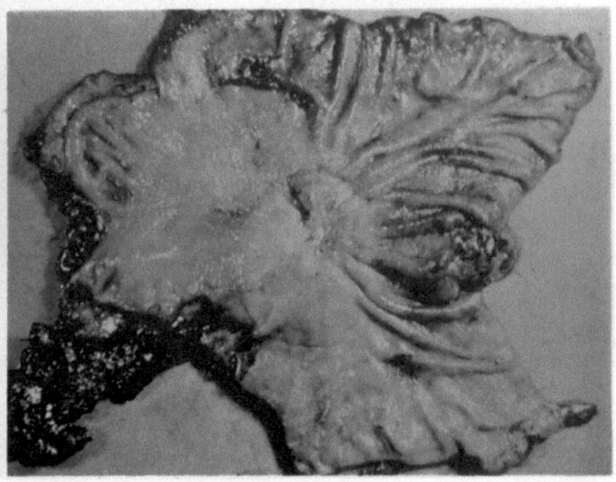

2

Fig. 25 Niche en castre.
a. Barium filled stomach in the upright position.
b. Barium filled stomach in the prone position.
c. Double-contrast study.
d. Resected stomach. Advanced cancer like the IIc+III type of an early gastric cancer (cancerous infiltration to the bundle layers of the muscle proper).

26a 26b 26c 26d

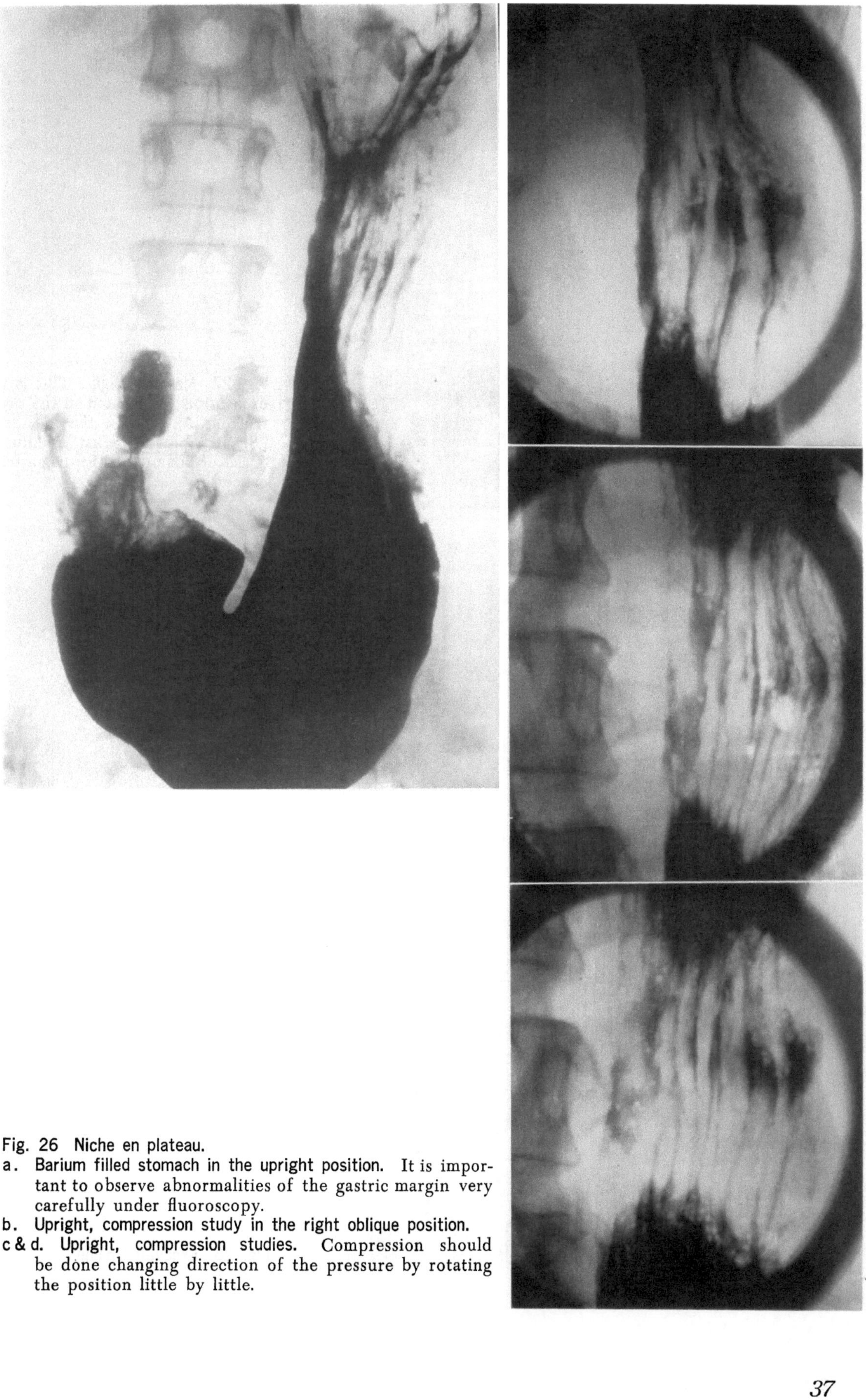

Fig. 26 Niche en plateau.
a. Barium filled stomach in the upright position. It is important to observe abnormalities of the gastric margin very carefully under fluoroscopy.
b. Upright, compression study in the right oblique position.
c & d. Upright, compression studies. Compression should be done changing direction of the pressure by rotating the position little by little.

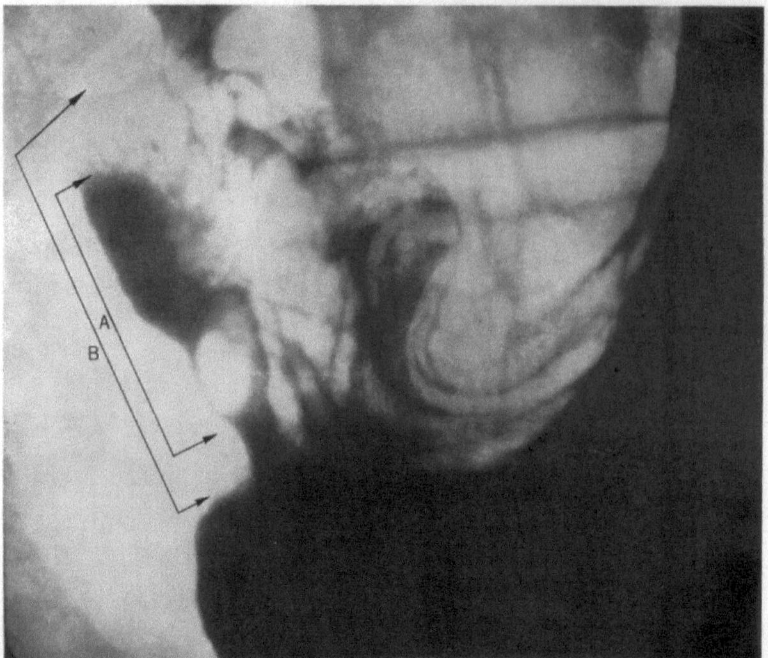

Fig. 27 Meniscus sign. This is an excavation (A) located in the protrusion (B), that is, the so-called "Schattenplus im Schattenminus". (Case of BORRMANN III type gastric cancer).

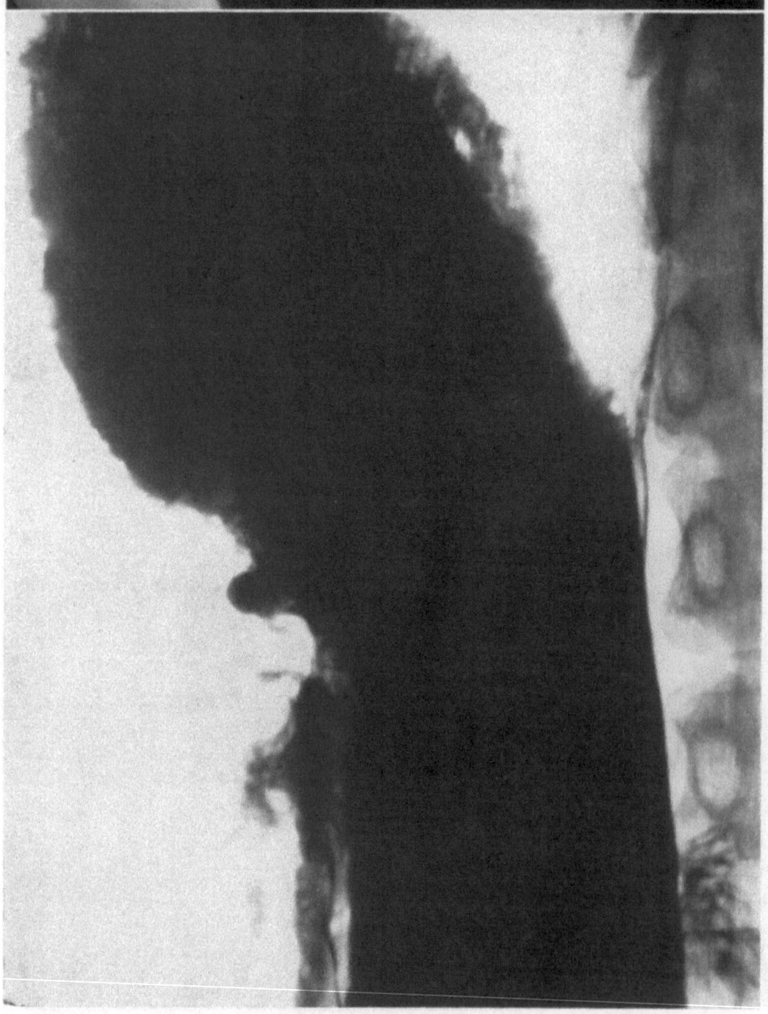

Fig. 28 Excavated niche.

unless we can photograph a niche from a frontal view, not only in a profile view, it should not be diagnosed as a benign ulcer with only profile views.

When frontal views of a niche are unavailable, it is necessary to make a diagnosis after demonstrating the uneveness of the surrounding a mucosa by a relief pattern or the compression method. In such cases it is better to refer to the endoscopic findings of the lesion.

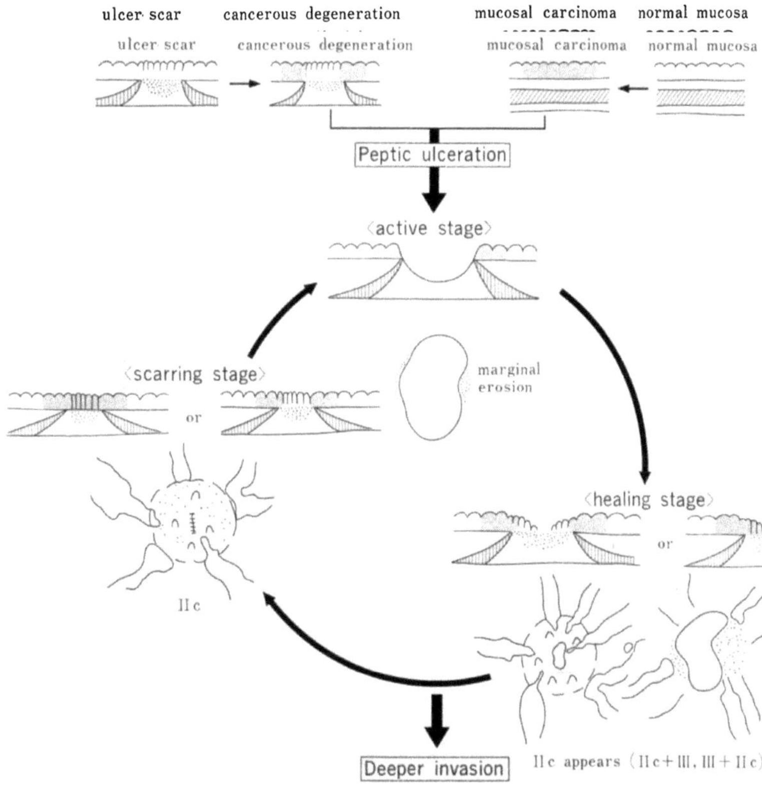

Fig. 29 Malignant Cycle (Life cycle of malignant ulcer)
It is clear that an ulcer of the excavated type of early gastric cancer changes its size and depth in its process of development, exhibiting almost the same healing process as a benign one. Initially, a malignant ulcer may begin as an ulceration in the area of a mucosal carcinoma or in a malignant degenerative mucosa of a benign ulcer scar. In the active stage, the ulcer in a mucosal carcinoma is sometimes difficult to differentiate from a benign one. MURAKAMI has confirmed the existence of a nonmalignant regenerating mucosa in the center of an ulcer scar. Malignant invasion of the scar occurs, and finally a fresh ulceration again develops. Temporary reduction or disappearance of ulcers is no proof of benignancy. Life cycle of a malignant ulcer is frequently found in superficial cancers.

30 a

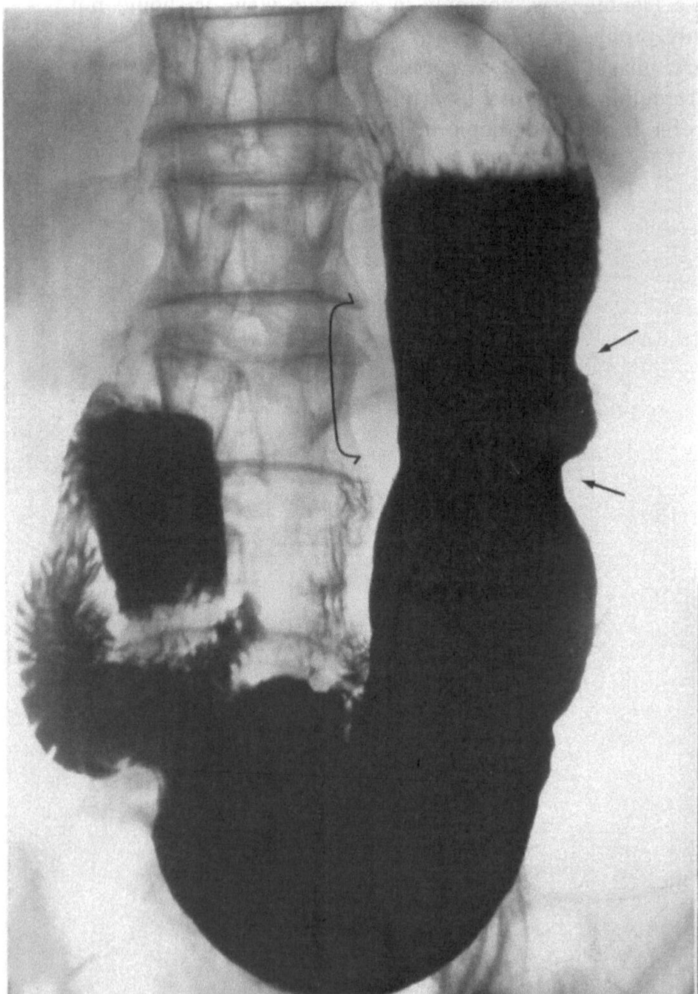

30 b

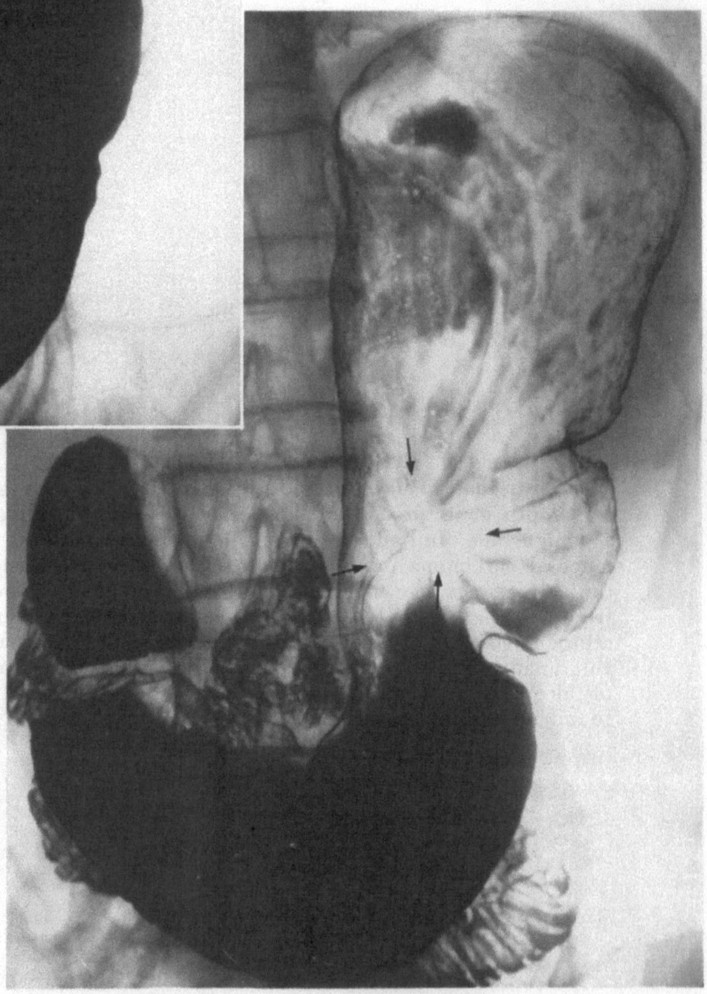

Fig. 30

a. **Barium filled stomach in the upright position.** Marginal deformities of the lesser and greater curvatures are demonstrated.

b. **Double-contrast study of the upper corpus.** This picture clearly shows marginal deformities and a IIc pattern (↗) on the posterior wall of the gastric body. Histological examination showed this to be an advanced cancer, infiltrating to the bundle layers of the muscle proper.

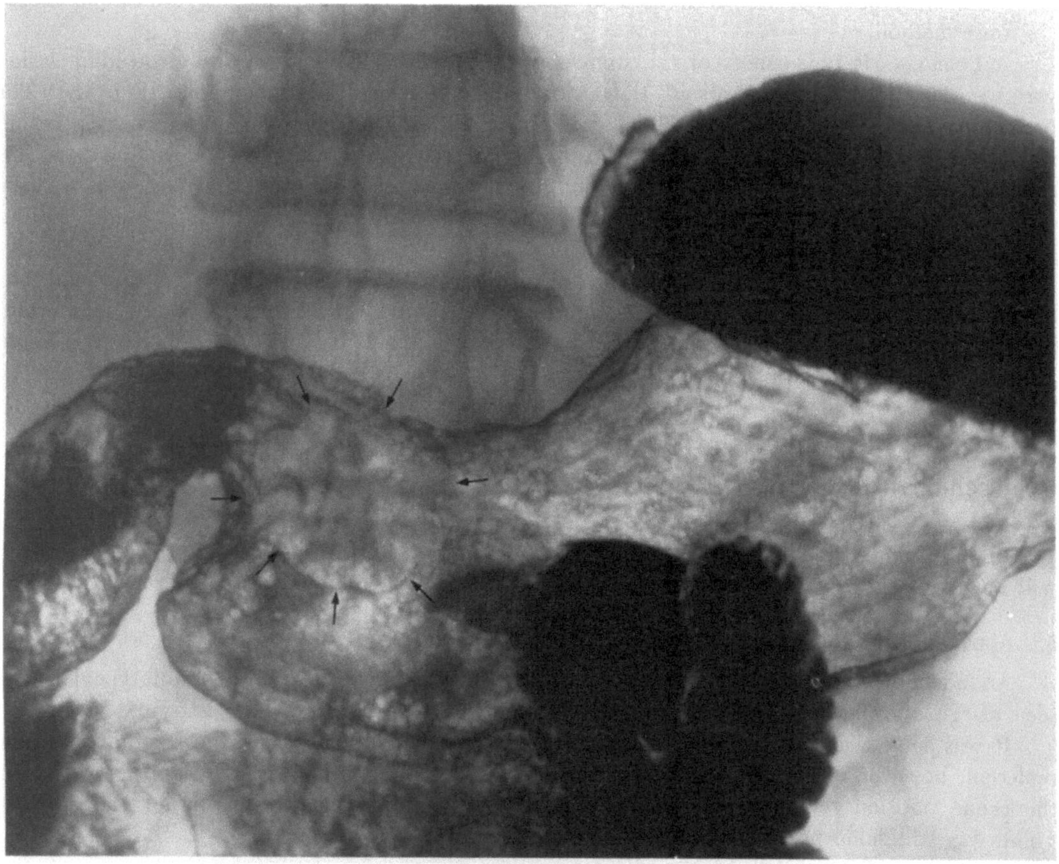

Fig. 31 Double-contrast study of a protruding lesion containing an excavated lesion. A protruding lesion with a distinct circular line is clearly bordered (↗↗), and a gentle slope towards the central portion is demonstrated. The barium flecks in the center of the protruding lesion indicate an excavation.

iv) Depressions which are not revealed at the margin of the stomach: As for depressions of the central portion of the stomach, profiles can be radiographed in the oblique and supine positions.

When depressed lesions cannot be demonstrated as profile findings due to their location, the abnormalities of the gastric wall, which are caused by fibrotic deformations in the gastric wall, appear to be marginal findings.

Figures 30 a and b showed definite findings of the gastric wall. The straight rigidity of the lesser curvature of the upper corpus, which seems to be a flat niche, or the profile niche of the greater curvature is expressed as marginal findings. Depressed lesions superimposed on protruding lesions of the gastric wall are demonstrated as marginal changes in radiographs when the lesions are not located on the greater or lesser curvature of the stomach.

Therefore, depressed lesions which have no fibrosis on the gastric wall cannot be expressed as a change in the contour of the stomach when they are located on the posterior or anterior wall. Shallow mucosal defects especially erosion, acute ulcers with shallow defects, or IIc without scarring are included in this category. Thus it is necessary to observe the shallow depressions with the double-contrast method and compression studies, even if there are no profile niches and marginal changes.

If we find depressions at the center of the stomach fluoroscopically, we may fail to notice almost all shallow depressions. We must take pictures of all parts of the stomach by contrast radiography and try not to overlook lesions which are present in the margin of the stomach.

4) Protruding lesions superimposed by excavated lesions photographed by the double contrast method.

A Borrmann II type cancer of the stomach with a comparatively small, low protruding lesion was seen on the posterior wall of the antrum by double-contrast radiography (Fig. 31). The protruding lesion was shown as a filling defect and the excavated lesion was shown as a barium shadow in the defect. In this picture, the margin of the defect was rather clear and was surrounded with light barium flecks. These findings demonstrated the protruding lesion as a sharp cliff, thus the indistinctly bordered defect should be considered a protruding lesion with a gentle slope.

Excavations in protruding lesions and excavations with protruding parts in the total circumference can be found easily by the compression technique. A compression study is important in order to describe this lesion more precisely on x-ray film and to know the extent of the lesion and the shape of the excavation in the lesion.

3. Technical details of x-ray examinations

In this chapter, technical problems of x-ray examinations for demonstrating protruding lesions will be discussed.

a. Application of the prone position double-contrast method

An adenomatous polyp (Fig. 32 a), 1.5×1.0×1.4 cm in area, of a protuberant type III was seen marginally on the anterior wall of the greater curvature in the pyloric antrum.

It was somewhat difficult to demonstrate these polypoid lesions using the standing position repletion, however, a circular transparent pattern with clear margins was noticed (Fig. 32 b). In the prone position repletion, no distinct hardening was found at the margin of the antrum. There was still some possibility of the presence of protuberant lesions (Fig. 32 c).

Hardening of the wall in the ulcerous parts are nothing but x-ray expressions of the accompanying proliferations of connective tissue. This suggested that observations such as the hardening of the wall could not be used as clues for the diagnosis of protuberant lesions (Fig. 32 c).

In the prone position, a relief picture in which about 50 ml of barium was used (Fig. 32d), a hemispherical shadow defect was readily detected because of the compression of the vertebra. The usefulness of thin-layer barium diagnosis for protuberant lesions has been proved. In a double-contrast study with first a small (Fig. 32 e), then a moderate amount of air (Fig. 32 f), an almost globular tumor was noticed at a short distance from the greater curvature. In the radiograph of the barium filled stomach in the prone position, it was seen as an apparent hemisphere, but in the double-contrast study the origin was expressed as a double shape. Probably because the affected part was hanging in the stomach from the anterior wall, the original part might be shown as a separate shape within the margin of a polyp. The compression in Figure 32 g exhibited a hemispherical tumor with clear margins, but the characteristics of the original part could not be analyzed by this alone. Subsequently, through photographing the high pelvis in the right anterior oblique projection and the prone position, a projecting hemispherical protuberance with a short peduncle was clearly observed in the collected air of the pyloric antrum (Fig. 32 h). Apart from the routine work, such prone position double-contrast studies are desirable.

Figure 33 was another case. A clearly bordered circular shape was noticed in the antrum, together with a faint twilight pattern in the center. This was a typical x-ray observation of a protuberance (polyp) on the anterior wall. The polyp on the anterior wall hung into the stomach in the supine position. Moreover, at its top (at the lowest part, as the polyp hung dorsally) a barium drop was accumulating, making the twilight pattern.

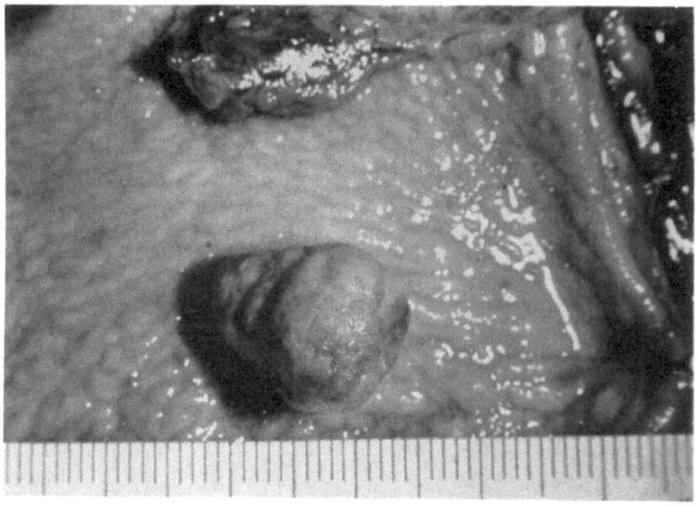

Fig. 32a A large polyp 1.2 cm in diameter projecting from the mucous membrane of the stomach on the greater curvature of the antrum. Because of the approximately upright photography, the presence of a peduncle is not clear, but a little irregularity of its head is noticed in the mucous membrane. Its properties are clearly different from the surrounding mucosa, having characteristics of an epithelial tumor.

32b

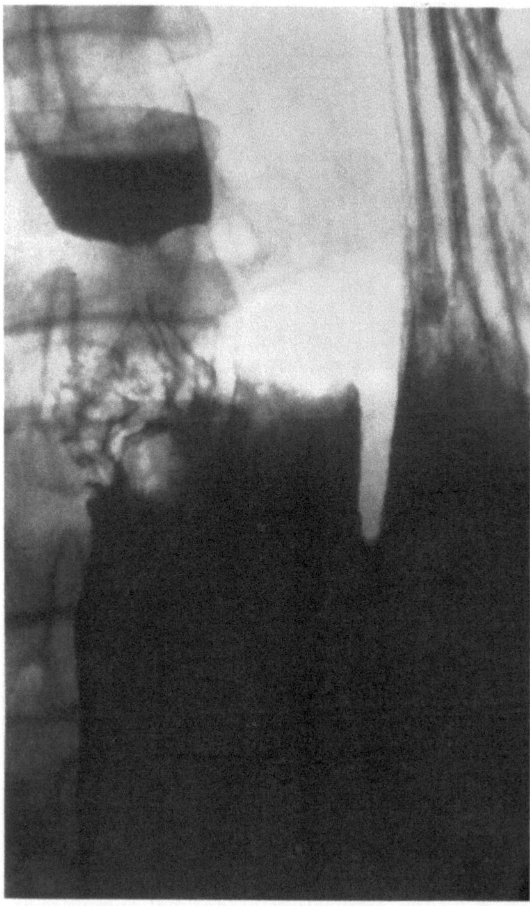

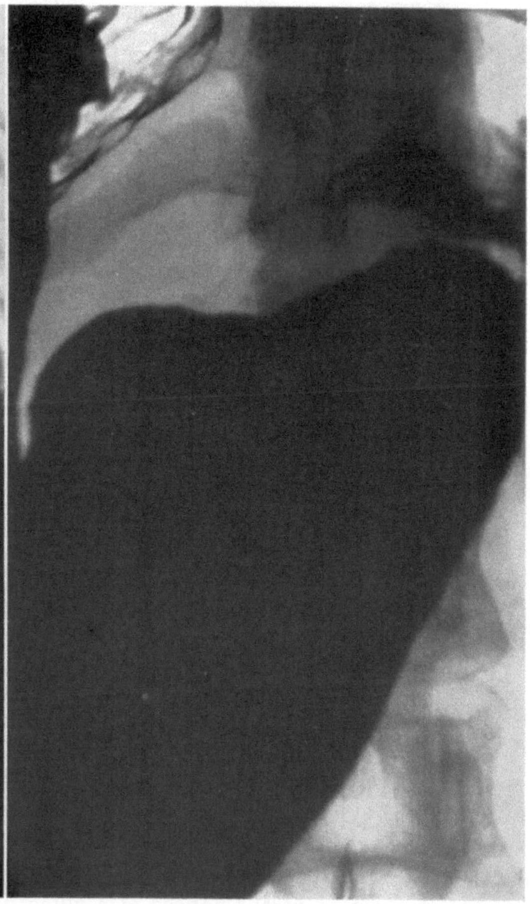

32c

Fig. 32b Barium filled stomach in the upright position. This is a filling photograph with a rather small amount of barium in which an almost round filling defect can be seen at the greater curvature of the antrum. The lesion can be considered a relatively circumscribed one, judging from the scarce findings at its margin.

Fig. 32c Barium filled stomach in the prone position. This is a stomach completely filled with barium. The existence of the lesion observed in Fig. 32b can not be suspected from this picture.

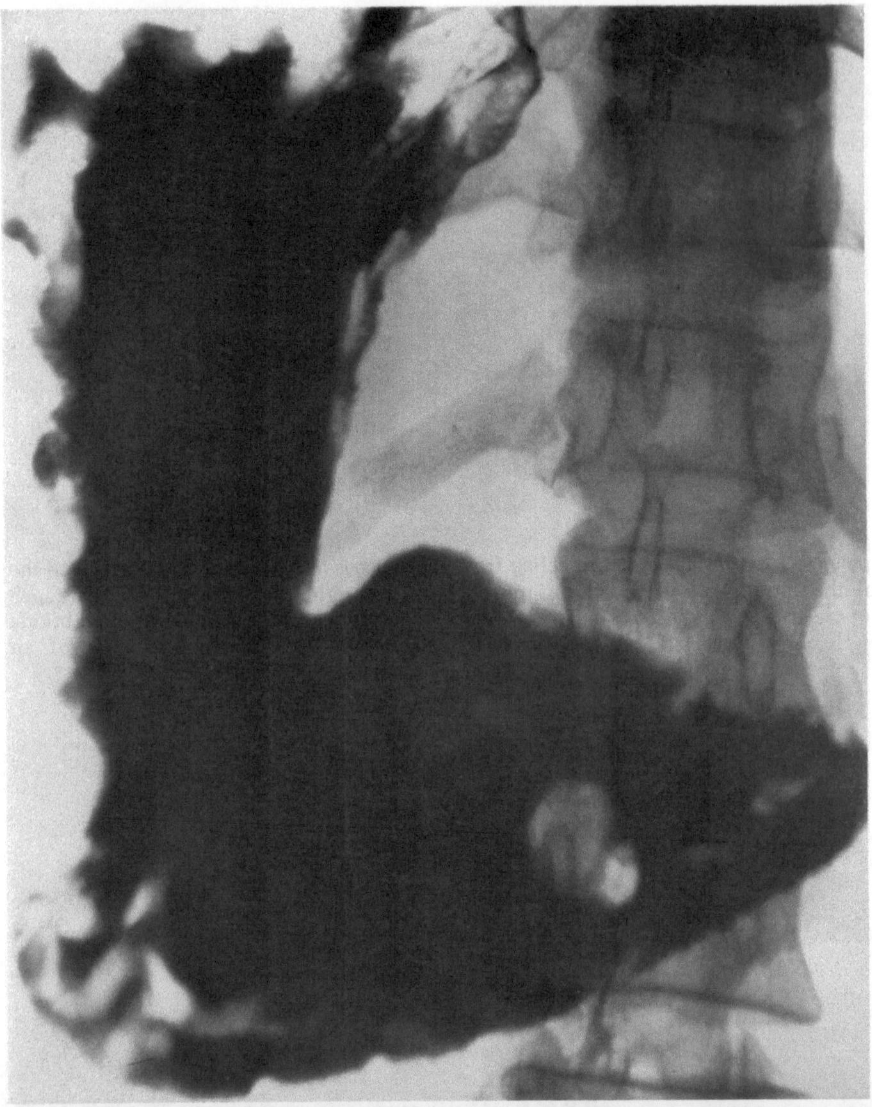

32 d

32e

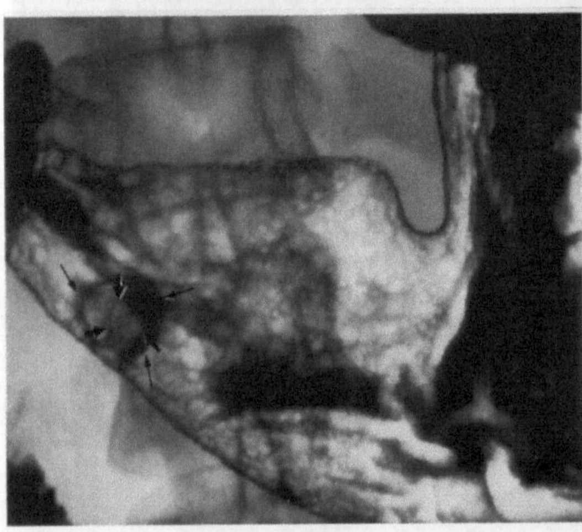

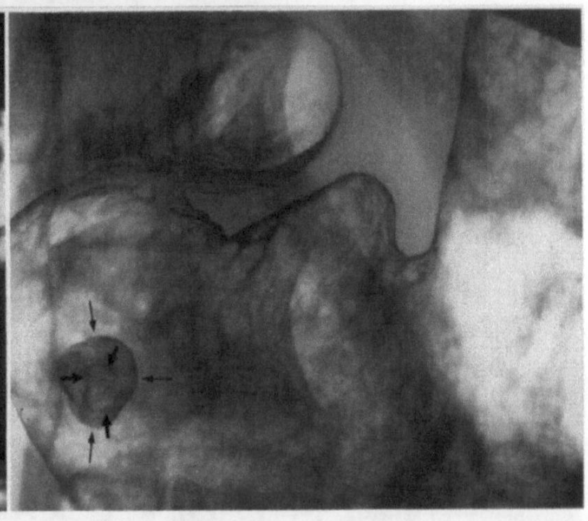

32 f

Fig. 32 d Prone position, relief study. This is a relief pattern with a rather large amount of barium, but the protuberant part is noticed as a filling defect by the application of optimal compression.

Fig. 32 e Supine, double-contrast study. The protuberance on the greater curvature of the antrum is evident, but because of the inadequate air, the surface property and the amount of protrusion remains obscure.

Fig. 32 f Double-contrast study. Not only the protuberance (↗) but also the stem can be observed (↗), by double contrast using the proper volume of air. As mentioned later, a diagnosis of an epithelial, benign tumor was readily made.

32g

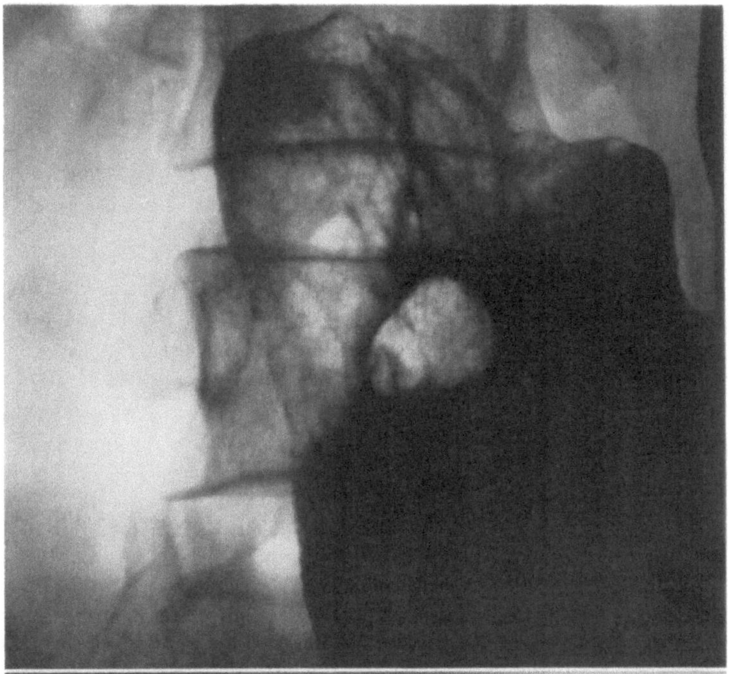

32h

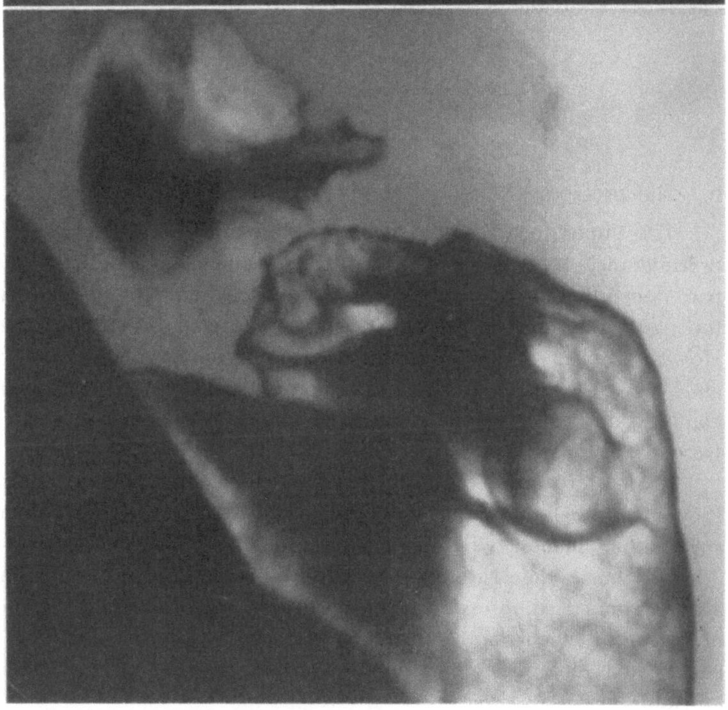

Fig. 32g **Compression study.** By means of compressing towards the vertebra, the shape of the protuberance is excellently demonstrated and the surface is more easily discernible.

Fig. 32h **Double-contrast study in the supine position.** In the prone position with the pelvis high, the protuberance from the anterior wall shows clearly. This is a useful method to make an affected part of the anterior wall observable.

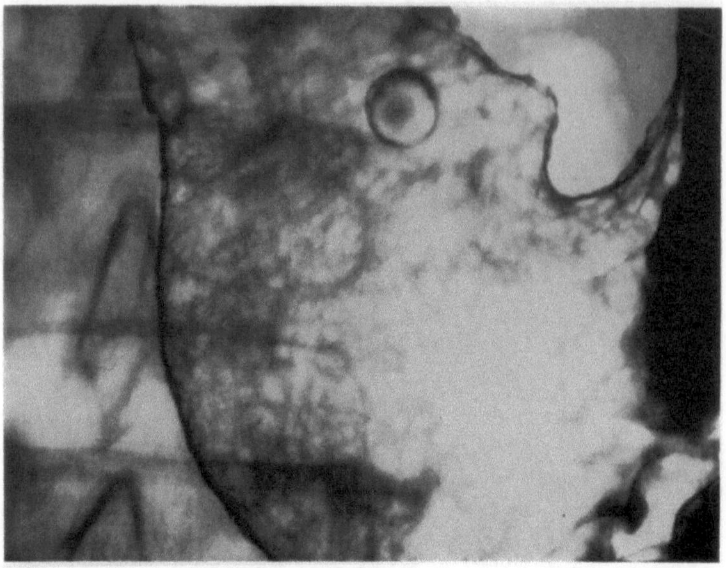

Fig. 33 Supine, double-contrast study. A small protuberance 7 mm in diameter is noticed on the antrum. Because of the sharp barium outline at the margin of the protuberance and the thin barium layer in the central part of the protuberance, it appears to be located on the anterior wall.

b. The problem of optimal compression

The importance of optimal compression will be stated below. The present case was a so-called protuberance type II. A considerable difference was noticed in the appearance of the affected part depending on the intensity of the compression. In extreme cases, when the compression was too weak, the affected part could not be detected because of the amount of barium (Fig. 34 a). However, when the compression was too intense, it could not be observed as a protuberance and it was revealed in the x-ray picture solely as a white part (Fig. 34 b). Under optimal compression as shown in Figures 34 c and d, the characteristics of the type II protuberance were readily observed.

In order to observe an affected part sufficiently, several photographs are desirable; however, they must be taken from the optimal positions in which the mucosal folds and areas of the surrounding mucosa will best be exposed.

Of course there are lesions where compression cannot be applied, but in such cases the author applied compression using a cushion in a half-standing position with a medium amount of barium. When photos are taken in a standing position with a large amount of barium, much effort yields but little effect in most cases because of the thick barium layer in the pyloric antrum.

c. Direction of the compression

In the following case of a IV type protuberance (Fig. 35 a), the difficulty in deciding the direction of the compression was the result of insufficient compression. Figures 35 b and c were regarded to be almost optimal since the surface area of the protuberance could be seen. But, as shown in the double-contrast photographs of Figure 35 d, this protuberance had a short peduncle which could not be observed in a frontal exposure with compression. The state of the granulated surface of the protuberance was excellently and homogeneously seen, allowing the case to be diagnosed by x-ray as an epithelial protuberance. Adequate observations, however, could not be made unless not only the top of the protuberance but the peduncle were photographed by changing the direction of the compression. Now this could be diagnosed as a benign epithelial protuberance.

34a 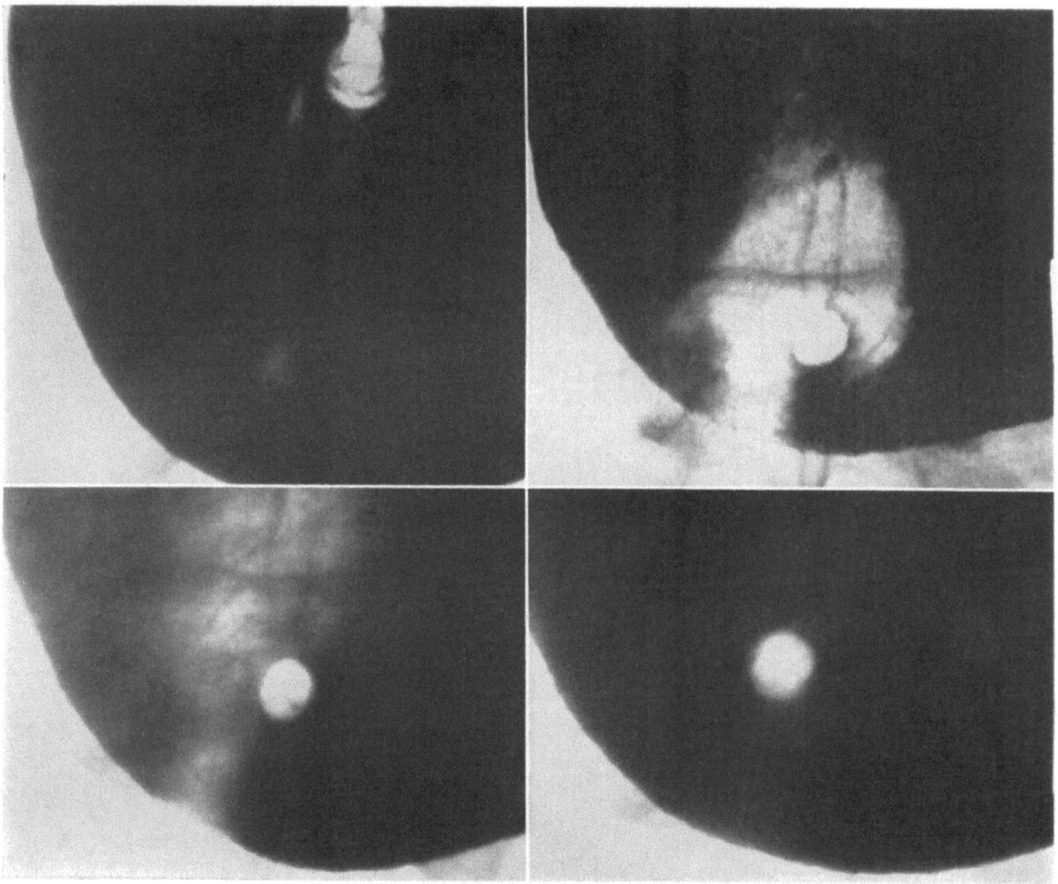 34b

34c 34d

Fig. 34a Radiograph taken under weak compression. In photographing the mucous membrane of the stomach, compression is an excellent method but requires considerable technique to photograph the affected part properly by using the optimal compression. This picture shows a slightly transparent portion at the greater curvature in the pyloric antrum caused by a weak compression.

Fig. 34b Radiograph taken under strong compression. No fine observation of the surrounding mucous membrane is possible because of the intense compression.

Fig. 34c Radiograph taken under optimal compression. The shape of the protuberant lesion is observable and the surrounding mucous membrane can be judged.

Fig. 34d Radiograph taken under optimal compression. This somewhat weaker compression than that in Fig. 34c seems to be acceptable for an observation of fine changes in the protuberant surface.

Of course, it is difficult to obtain such pictures consistently. Repeated and detailed examinations with the aid of endoscopic observations as well as the desire to obtain satisfactory photographs enable us to acquire pictures almost identical with macroscopic observations.

d. Compression phase and stage

In actual cases, sometimes a mere change in intensity and/or direction of the compression cannot give sufficient information. Compression should be applied during the resting stage of peristalsis. When compression was applied during the peristaltic stage as shown in Figures 36a and b, the affected part was shaded by longitudinal mucosal folds. Figures 36c and d were insufficient on the whole because of inadequate compression.

If optimal compression was used during the resting stage of peristalsis, a pedunculated protuberance with branched surfaces and rough areas could be recognized (Figs. 36e, f). On the contrary, if improper compression was applied from an unsuitable position during the peristaltic

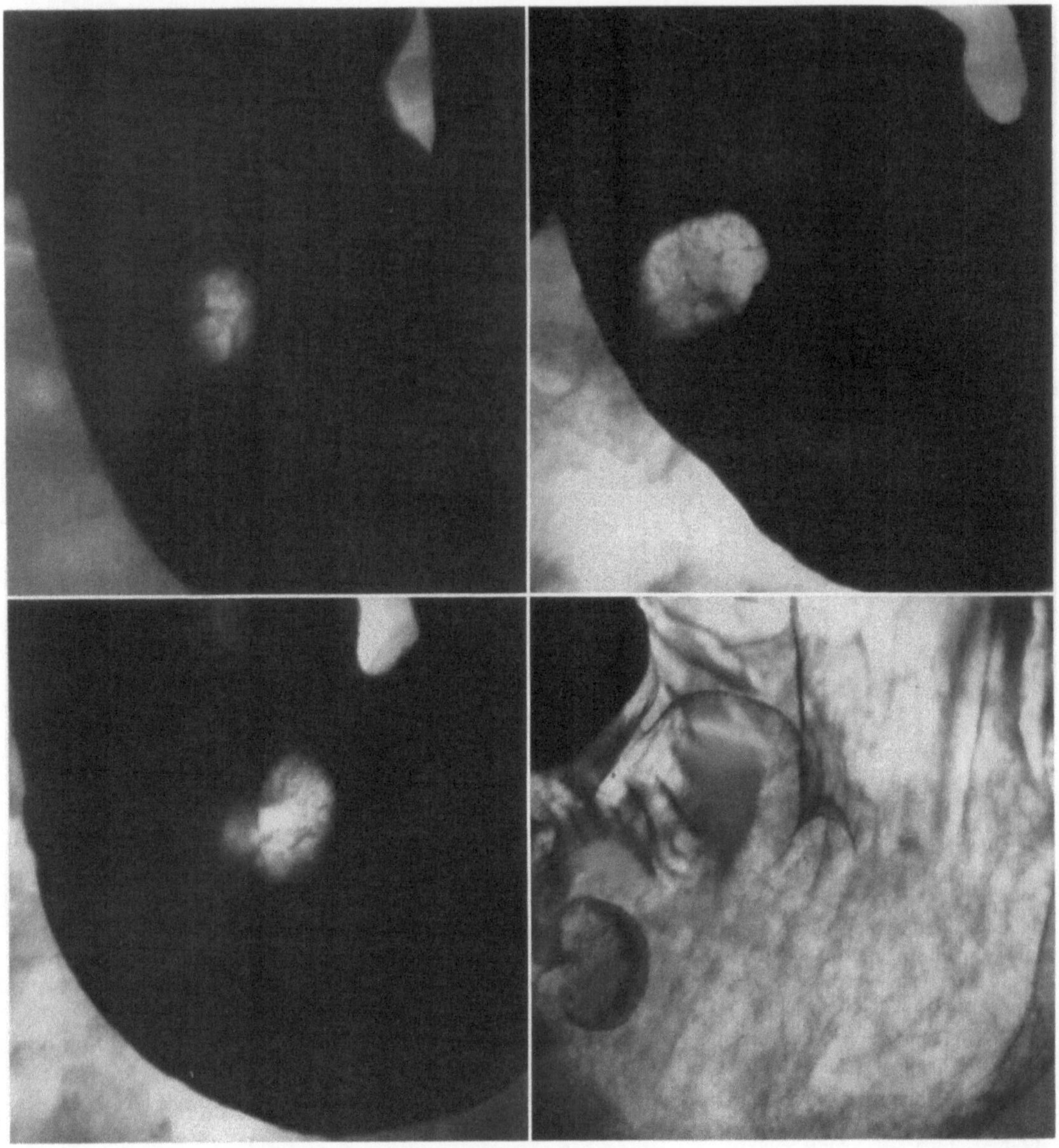

35a 35b 35c 35d

Fig. 35a Compression study. A transparent part is recognized at the pyloric antrum, but the whole pattern of the affected part cannot be observed because of the weak compression.

Fig. 35b Optimal compression study. This is an optimal compression study in which the clear margin of the protuberant lesion as well as the fine surface ruggedness can be observed.

Fig. 35c Compression study. This radiograph shows not only a fine granulated head of the polyp, but a short stem. Compression is regarded to be optimal as in the case of Fig. 35b. The difference in position from that of Fig. 35b is probably due to a difference in the direction of the compression.

Fig. 35d Double-contrast study in the supine position. Even the basal part of the lesion found in the compression studies of Figs. 35a–c is demonstrated more clearly with an adequate amount of air and barium.

36a

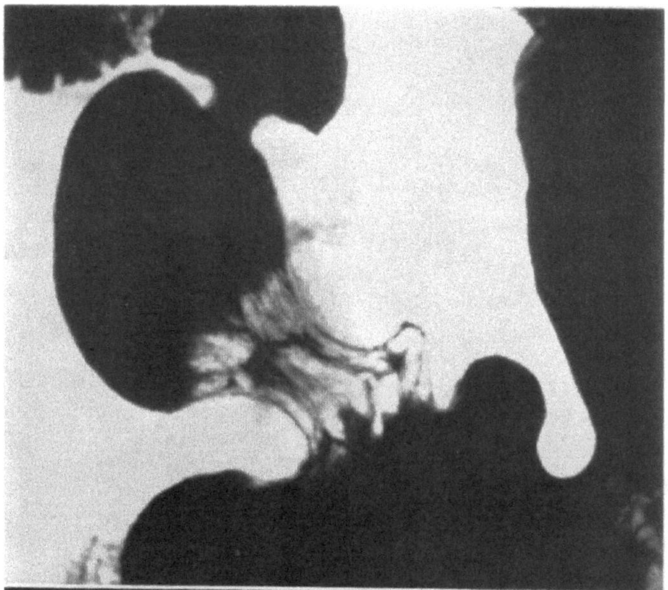

Fig. 36 a Compression study. A long, affected part protruding from the anterior cardiac portion of the stomach is seen. As the photograph was taken during the peristaltic stage, the mucous membrane is poorly extended and the shape of the protuberance is slightly deformed.

36b

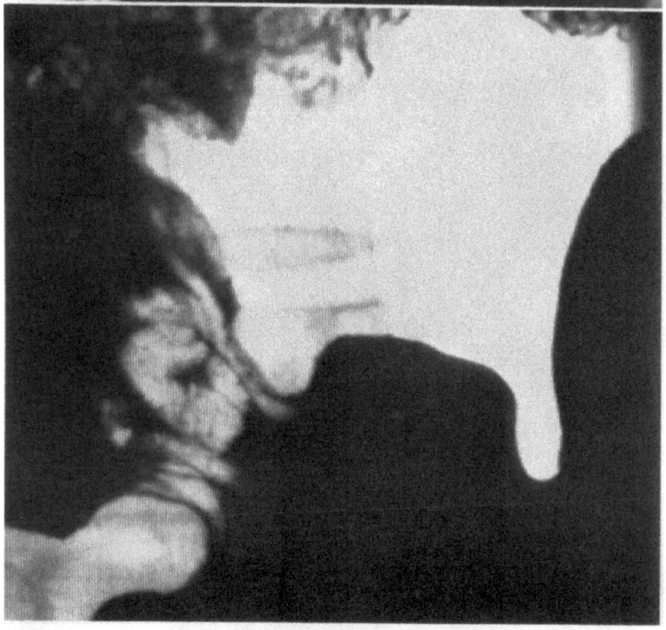

Fig. 36 b Compression study. Compared with Fig. 36 a, the shape and surfaces are well photographed. The presence of a central depression may be suspected from this picture, but it is difficult to obtain exact information from photographs taken during peristalsis.

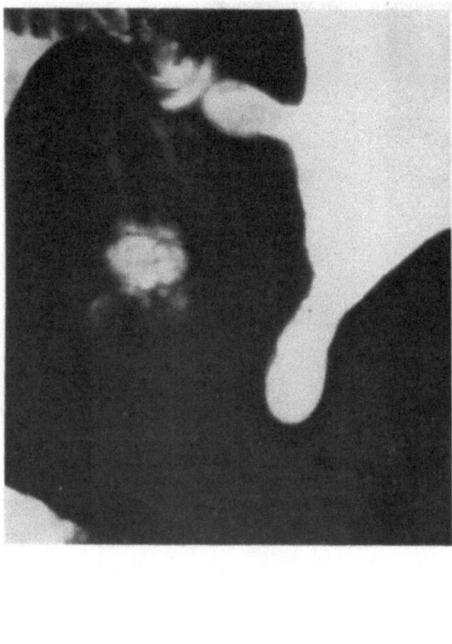

36c

Fig. 36 c Compression study. Peristalsis is not observed at the affected part, and the mucous membrane is well extended with sufficient barium. Only a part of the affected portion can be noticed because of the weak compression.

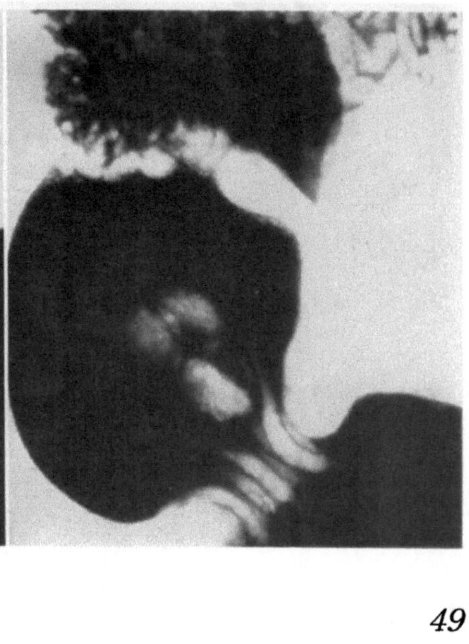

36d

Fig. 36 d Compression study. A little stronger compression was used than that of Fig. 36 c. The affected part becomes clearer, but the margin remains vague because of insufficient compression.

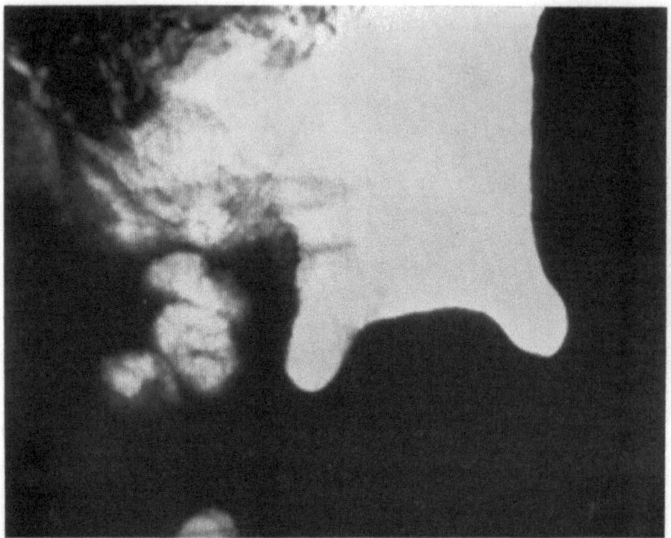

36e

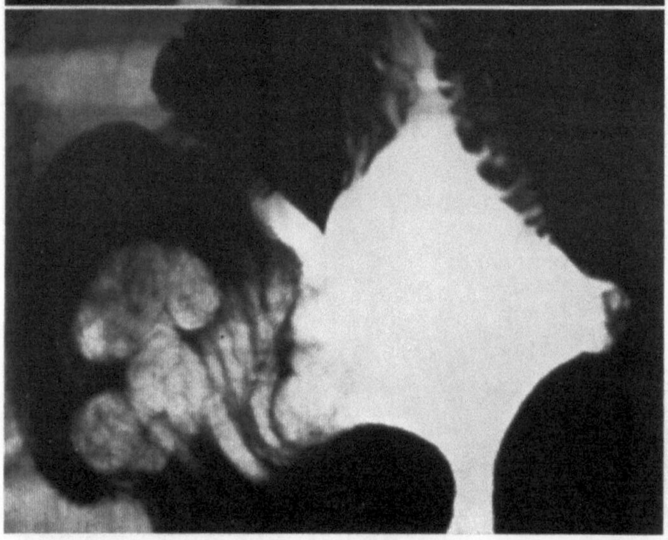

36f

Fig. 36e Compression study. An approximately suitable compression. The entire surrounding area of the knotted, protuberant lesion can be seen, but the surrounding mucous membrane has not been clearly photographed. Therefore, it is doubtful whether this picture shows the tumor adequately.

Fig. 36f The affected part photographed under optimal compression. The affected part is found to be composed of three large knots and a peduncle. Granulated changes of the surface are also observed distinctly.

Fig. 36g Resected stomach. Knotted protuberant lesions are found on the anterior wall of the antrum.

Fig. 36h Endoscopic picture. Only two knotted protuberances on the anterior wall of the antrum are noticed from this direction, but a short peduncle can be seen.

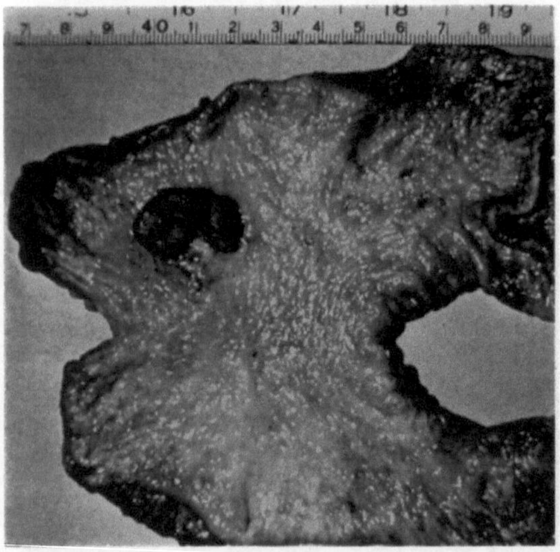

36g

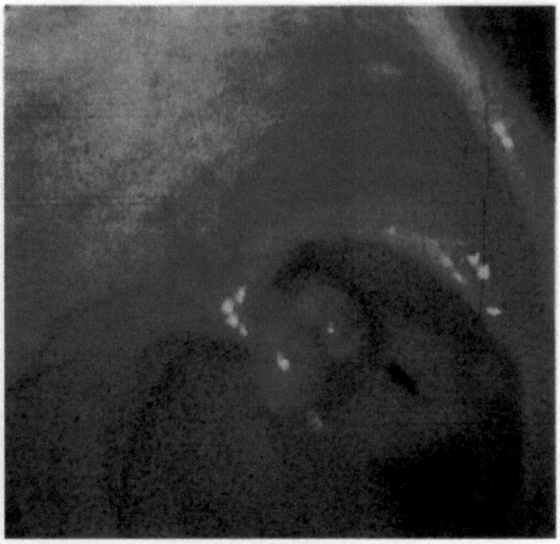

36h

phase, a flower bed-like mucous protuberance with a central depression was observed, as in Figure 36 b, leading to an incorrect diagnosis of early cancer of the type II a+II c. From Figure 35 f, however, the reddened epithelial polyp of type IV on the anterior wall of the antrum, as seen in the resected stomach of Figure 36 g or in the gastrocamera photograph, could be readily diagnosed.

e. Application of respiration

Respiration can be added to the diagnostic techniques for protuberant lesions in the stomach, as with common gastric disorders. In the supine position, the bottom of the stomach extends on inspiration and shrinks on expiration. The stomach approaches a position parallel to the view plate during inspiration and separates on expiration, accompanied by foldings and shrinkage, thus being unsuitable for photographing the entire affected part. In x-ray photography, it is important to take sufficient photographs with the subject relaxed and respiring easily.

Protuberant lesions in the stomach, including not only mucosal or submucosal protuberances but protuberances due to external compression, must be considered. The stomach is in contact with a number of surrounding organs through its serous membrane (Fig. 37). Consequently, with exogastric tumors, they sometimes appear in the stomach as a protuberance making a discrimination from submucous gastric tumors difficult.

For instance, in Figure 38 a, a wide shadow defect was noticed in the lower part of the stomach. The surface, however, was not very irregular. It seemed to be a tumor developing in the gastric cavity or by compression outside the stomach. In Figure 38 b, which was photographed in a slightly right, anterior-oblique position, the shadow defect extended to the lesser curvature of the pyloric antrum.

For a tumor developing within the gastric wall, no difference would be noticed. Figure 37 c was taken during expiration, and when the pyloric antrum was sufficiently filled with air, the shadow defect extended only to the gastric angle. In Figure 38 d, in spite of an almost identical position and respiratory condition, the lower part of the stomach extended straight forward and showed no indication of hardening. The lack of uniformity in observations suggested that the compression of adjacent organs, such as the liver or pancreas, caused the impressions rather than the presence of a gastric tumor.

Figure 38 e of the prone, relief position demonstrated that the mucosal folds of the mucous membrane extended regularly from the lower part of the stomach to the pyloric area. In Figure 38 f which was a compression study in a semi-standing position, little change was noticed on the surface of the mucous membranes. Multiple photographs in different positions are necessary.

Through laparoscopy, the compression on the lesser curvature of the stomach wall proved to be due to a hypertrophy of the liver and was also verified by x-ray photographs. The addition of the respiratory activity facilitated discrimination from a submucous gastric tumor.

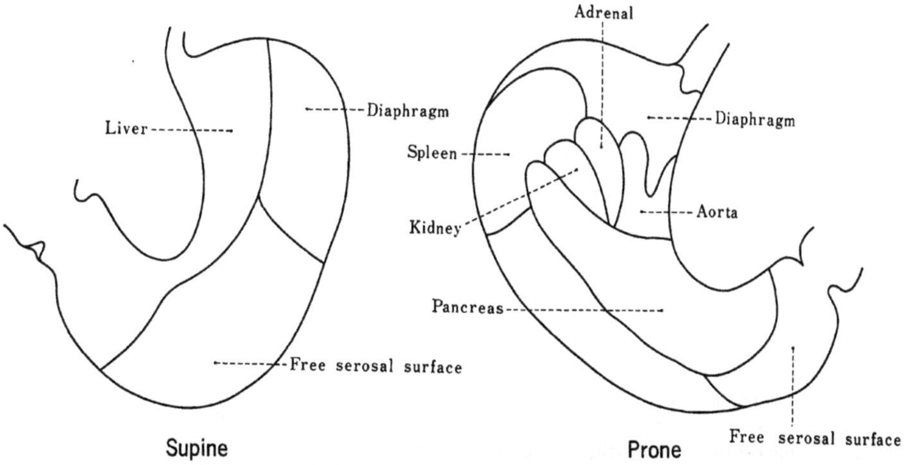

Fig. 37 Relationship of the stomach with the surrounding organs.

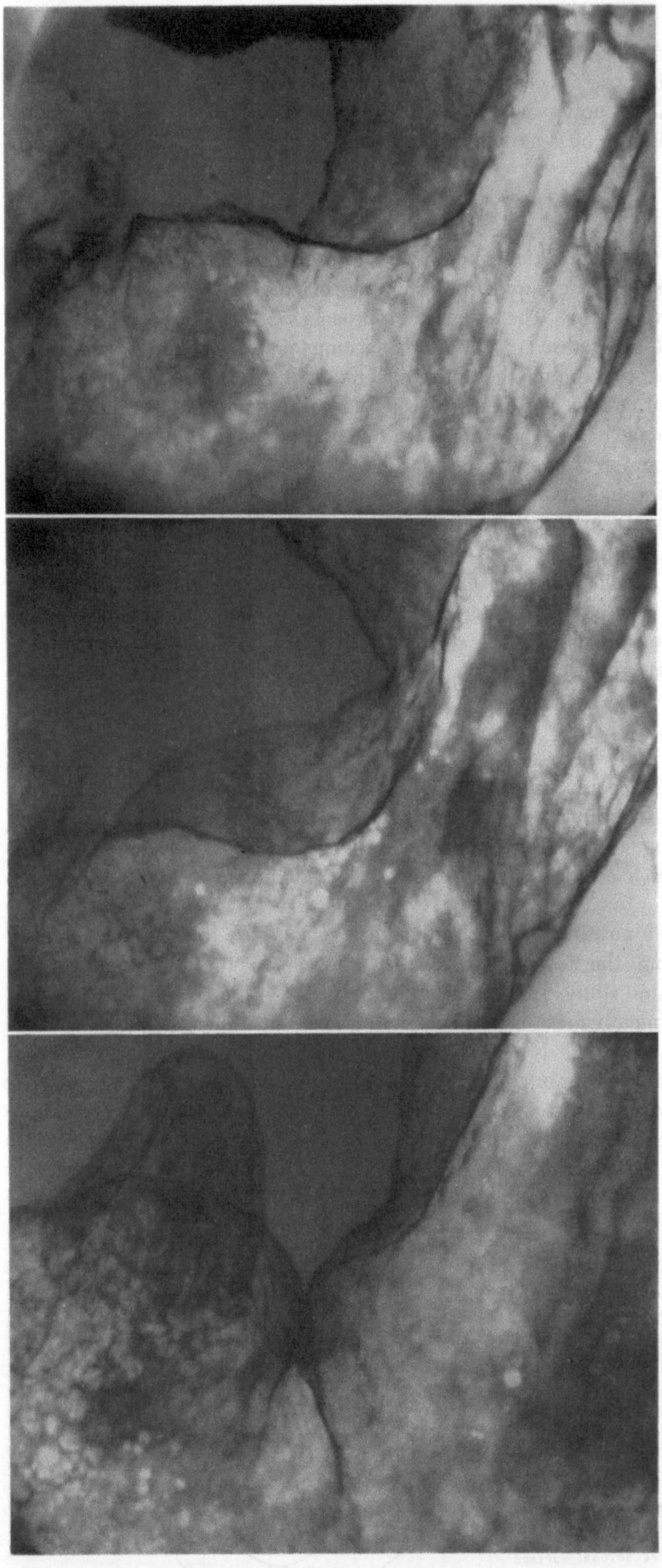

38 a

38 b

38 c

Figs. 38 a–d Supine, double-contrast studies. A shadow defect-like observation suggesting a widespread tumor is seen centered in the upper part of the stomach. The margin is slightly rigid, but the mucous membrane is smooth, being devoid of the characteristics of protuberant lesions. Furthermore, changes in the position as in Figs. 38 b, c, and d, verified the size and the location. Thus, the protuberance should not be regarded as an endogastric disorder but as a compression by exogastric structures.

38 d

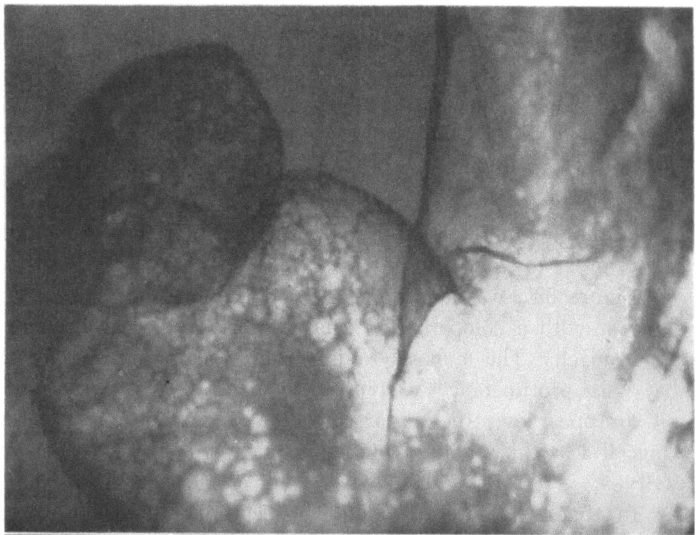

38 e

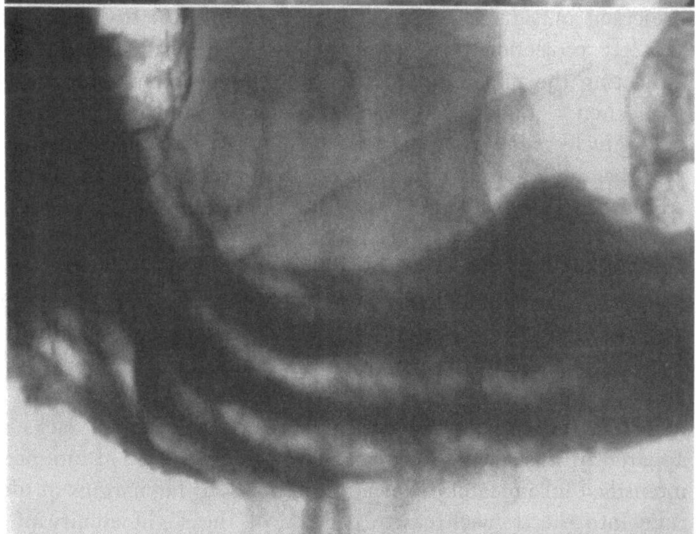

38 f

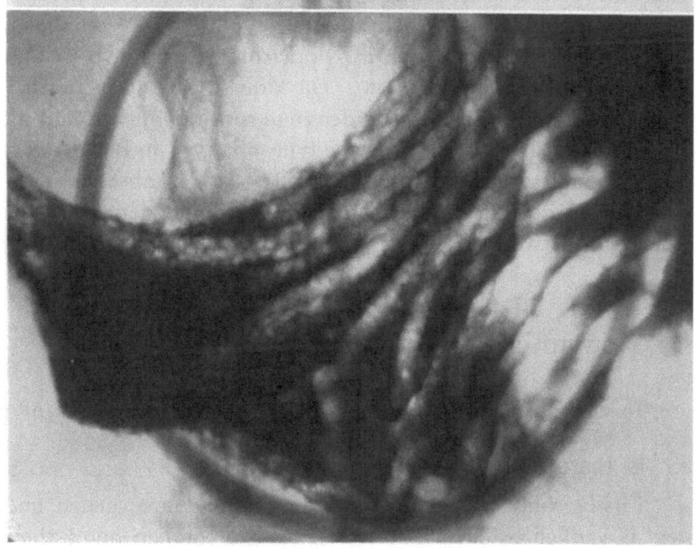

Fig. 38 e Prone position, relief picture. A tumor-like shadow defect found in the supine double-contrast study is not seen. This is a frequently encountered observation due to compression by the liver.

Fig. 38 f Compression study. In spite of an optimal compression, no abnormality was noticed in the mucosa, clearly indicating that the tumor-like shadow defect was exogastric.

f. Conversion of the position

Care should be taken so that x-ray photographs show not only the endogastric features but all the organs in the near vicinity. When an affected structure exists outside the stomach and the x-ray is positive, it appears as if it were an endogastric disorder.

Gas in the large intestine overlapping with the stomach shadow can be differentiated as an exogastric factor. However, it is frequently said that the ligament of Treitz in the small intestine overlapping with the gastric angle may be misdiagnosed as an ulcer as a result of careless fluoroscopy and x-ray photography.

Figure 39 a was a radiograph of a barium filled stomach in the standing position displaying a tumor with a comparatively smooth surface. Clear margins could be noticed at the fornix of the stomach. The mucosal folds seemingly disappeared here, suggesting a similar observation to that with protuberances of type I. In a double-contrast study such as Figure 39 b, the folds did not disappear over the tumor surface and ran without a noticeable change in a lateral direction. Thus, it was difficult to diagnose instantly the presence of a tumor protruding into the stomach cavity.

In the right anterior oblique projection radiograph, as shown in Figure 39 c, this tumor projected outside the stomach wall, proving not to be an endogastric protuberant disorder. In the left projection photograph as well (Fig. 39 d), it appeared completely outside the stomach, indicating the importance of position conversion in observations and photography.

When a tumor is proved to be in the stomach, the measurement of its size can be carried out only by x-ray examination. It should be emphasized that a measurement of the size of the protuberant lesion and the degree of projection into the cavity can be performed only by stereoscopic observations through position conversions.

g. Suggestions for x-ray examination of protuberances

It is important in x-ray examinations to apply the above mentioned techniques as effectively as possible and to observe the affected part stereoscopically.

In the relief-pattern and double-contrast method, care should be taken on the following points during compression. A protuberance in the stomach can be observed in general as a defect in the barium thin layer, but when the barium lacks affinity for the mucous membrane, apparently a shadow defect can be observed even if no protuberance exists. Especially when intensified inflammatory edemata are found at the margins of ulcerous lesions, they appear to protrude into the stomach cavity because of the slight affinity of barium for the mucous membrane.

For example, in the activated ulcer of a Ul-IV on the anterior wall of the antrum which existed in combination with a pyloric ring ulcer shown in Figure 40 a, the ulcerous margins were surrounded by a border zone. On x-ray examination in the prone position of a barium filled stomach (Fig. 40 b), a broad border zone surrounding a round niche was noticed. Seemingly, it was a round-type shadow defect of the type observed in BORRMANN type II and flat-dish cancers. In the prone, double-contrast pattern (Fig. 40 c), it was observed as a broad shadow defect surrounding the barium deposits. When an increase in the depth of the niche was noticed through x-ray examination two weeks earlier, we felt it was imperative to make more comprehensive studies.

4. How to diagnose protuberant lesions

In this chapter, the concepts of differential diagnoses of polypoid lesions will be discussed.

a. Is there a protuberance in the stomach?

Firstly, x-ray and endoscopic examinations are carried out in the way described, and ruggedness is verified by insufflation of air and a comparison of the lesion with the surrounding mucous membrane.

Secondly, examinations are conducted to determine whether the protuberance is pedunculated or not. As shown in Figures 15 and 41, these examinations are very important for the identification of benign and malignant tumors. In order to perform the examinations, changes in position are important: for example, because in the supine position diagnosis is difficult when the tumor

39 a

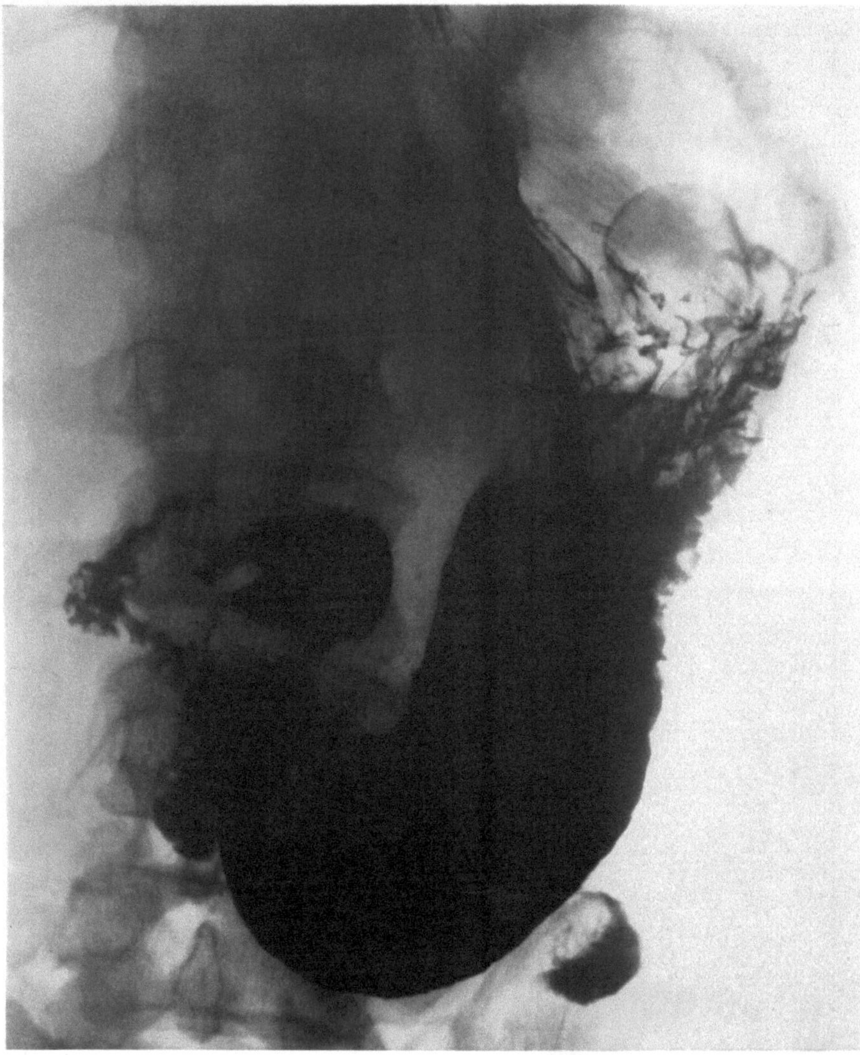

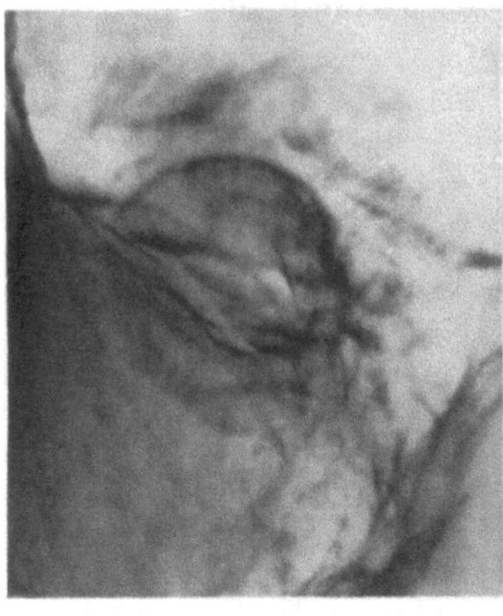

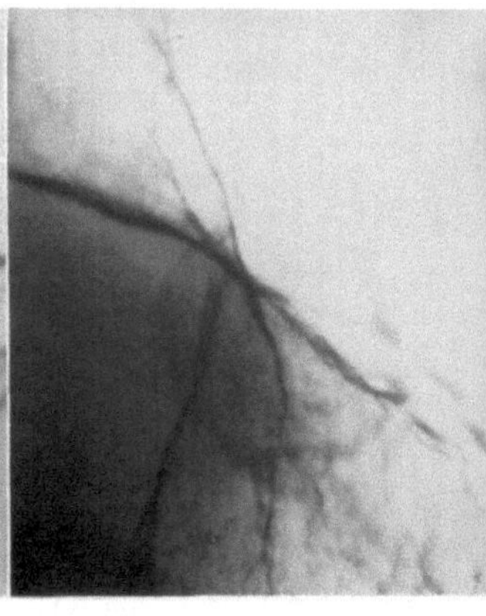

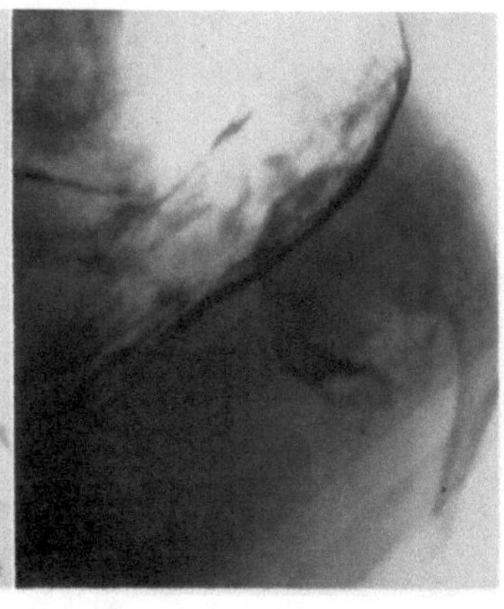

39 b 39 c 39 d

Fig. 39 a Standing position, filling study. A tumor-like shadow with smooth margins is noticed in the fornix of the stomach. The tumor had sharp outlines, suggesting the possibility of a protuberant type II lesion.

Figs. 39 b, c, d Double-contrast studies. When the mucosal folds surrounding the protuberance are photographed with sufficient air, they show a pattern displayed here. In the right projection (Fig. 39 c), half of the protuberance is observed to project from the stomach. When the position is altered to the left projection (Fig. 39 d), the protuberance is almost entirely found outside the gastric wall, proving it to be exogastric.

40a

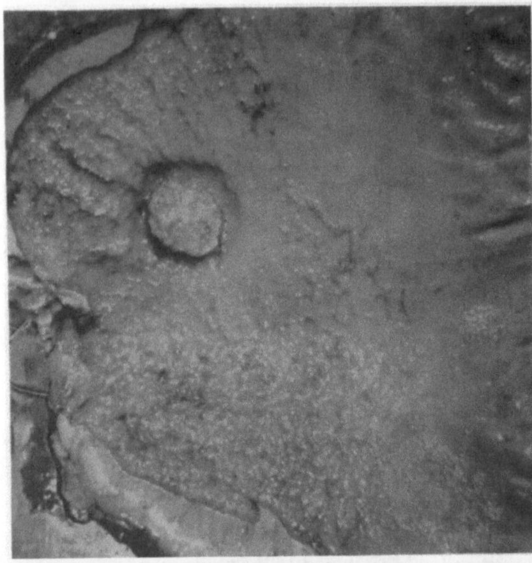

40b

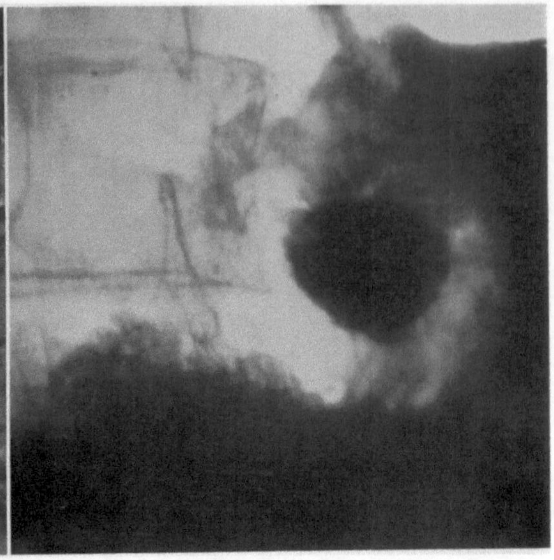

40c

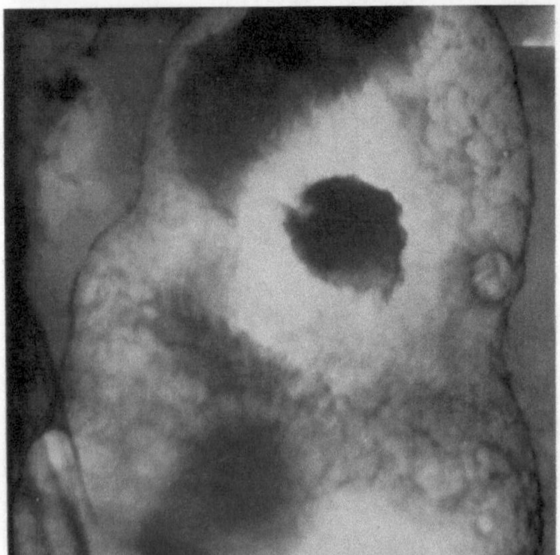

40d

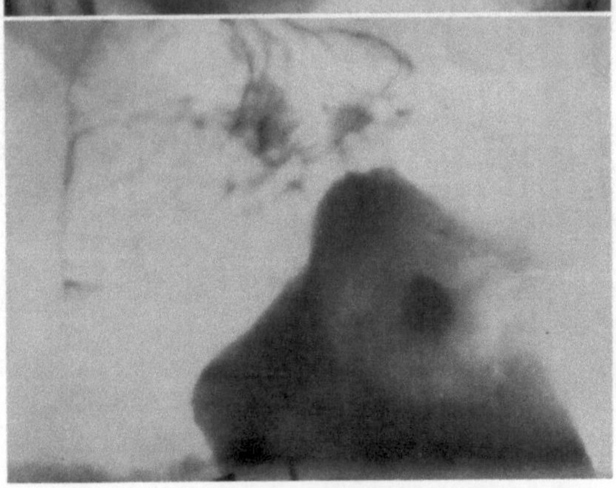

Fig. 40a Resected stomach. A round ulcer and an edematous protuberance around the ulcer are observed on the anterior wall of the antrum. A deep scar is also noticed on the pyloric ring.

Fig. 40b Prone position repletion. By means of a compressive factor, a broad border zone surrounding a circular niche is noticed in the antrum. It looks like the round-type shadow defect observed in BORRMANN type II, flat dish cancers.

Fig. 40c Prone, double-contrast study. The almost round niche and the surrounding broad border zone may be caused by deposits of barium, and the transparent pattern may be due to an edematous change.

Fig. 40d Prone, double-contrast study, two weeks earlier. The protuberance around the reactivity, together with the edema, is very akin to that of Fig. 40c.

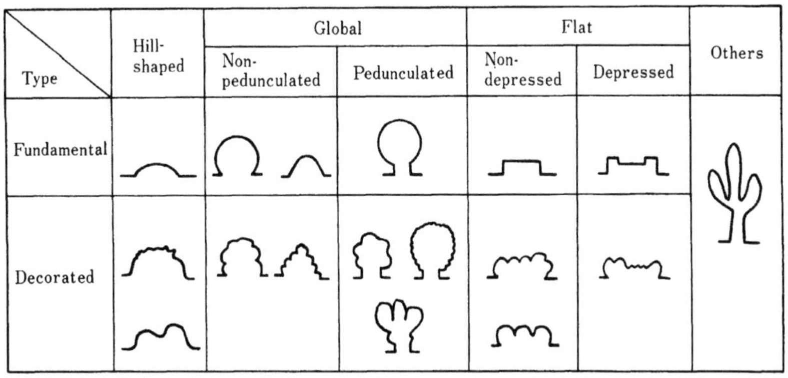

Fig. 41

Diameter \ Shape	Hill-shaped	Global: Non-pedunculated	Global: Pedunculated	Flat: Non-depressed	Flat: Depressed
– 1cm	○●●	●●●●●●●●●●●●●●●●●●	●●		○●●●
1 – 2cm	○○○○	●●●●●●●●●●●	●●●●●●●●	●	●●
2 – 3cm	○	●●●	○●●●	●	●●●●
3cm –	○○○○	●●	●●●●●●●	●●	●
Total	12	34	21	4	11

○ Nonepithelial ● Epithelial

Fig. 42 Is a phyma nonepithelial or epithelial?

and its stalk are located on the posterior wall, discrimination becomes easier when left in the recumbent to prone position, because the tumor is suspended in the gastric cavity due to its weight.

b. Is the gastric phyma nonepithelial or epithelial?

In nonepithelial lesions, no differences may be noticed other than a slight fading, if any, between the mucous membrane covering their surface and the surrounding mucous membrane. The fading is probably due to a slight shrinkage of the mucous membrane by compression. Thus, no distinct ruggedness can be observed. Since no difference in color is found endoscopically in comparison with the surrounding mucous membrane, the differentiation is very easy. In some cases when the protuberances are not very elevated, care should be taken because they can barely be recognized as protuberances in a stomach filled with air.

On the other hand, in epithelial protuberances (except accessory pancreas) with cases such as gastric hyperplastic polyps, no difference in color is found in comparison with the surrounding mucous membrane, but they are usually observed as reddish protuberances.

Protuberances are classified into the categories shown in Figure 42. Among 82 subjects, as seen in Figure 43, almost all cases with hill-shaped protuberances are nonepithelial submucosal tumors. It should be remembered, however, that with lesions less than 1 cm in diameter, mucosal protuberances occasionally exist instead of apparently hill-shaped lesions. In one case diagnosed as type IV appearing to be a global pedunculated protuberance (case 11), a submucosal tumor was detected. It must also be taken into consideration in that the data is one-sided coming from cases subjected to gastrectomy. These points for discrimination may be used as a standard, remembering that most hill-shaped tumors of about 1 cm in diameter are treated as noncancerous lesions.

c. If it is a tumor, is it benign or malignant?

A number of works dealing with this problem have been reported to date.

If the surface characteristics of a tumor protruding into the stomach are studied endoscopically in terms of changes in color, erosion, light reflection, etc., a tentative diagnostic hypothesis may be possible; but it is difficult to obtain the proper standard of differentiation in individual cases (Fig. 43).

Endoscopic findings	Benign polyp 26 cases 59 lesions		Cancer (advanced cancer + early cancer) 18 cases 59 lesions		Submucosal tumor 9 cases 10 lesions	
	Cases	%	Cases	%	Cases	%
Smooth surface	38	64	1	6	10	100
Granular surface	19	32	15	83		
Nodular surface	12	20	14	78		
Abnormal color tone to surrounding mucosa	21	36	9	50	4	40
Redness	21	36	8	44	4	40
Bleeding	6	10	7	39		
Erosion	7	12	5	28		
Light reflexion	55	93	6	33	※2	20

Fig. 43 Endoscopic findings of gastric protruded lesions.

YAMADA and FUKUTOMI noticed a close relationship between the type, size of tumor, and degree of malignancy on the basis of the characteristics of cross-sectional findings of gastric protuberances (Fig. 15). They reported that no cancer was detected in tumors of less than 2 cm dia. of type IV, of less than 1.0 cm dia. of type III and 0.5 cm dia. of type II (Fig. 44).

Size (mm) \ Type	I	II	III	IV	Total
− 4	○○	○○○○○○○○			10
5 − 9	○○	○○○○○○○○ ○○○○○ ◐◐	○○○○○○○○ ○○○○○○○○ ○○○○○○○○	○○○○○○○○ ○○○○	53
10 − 19	○○○○○○○	◐◐	○○○○○○○○ ◐◐◐◐	○○○○○○○○ ○○○○○○○○ ○○○○○○○○ ○○○○○○○	52
20 − 29	○	○○	◐ ●	○○○○ ◐◐	11
30 −	○	◐◐◐◐◐ ●	◐◐◐◐◐◐◐◐ ●●●●●●●● ●	○ ◐	26
Total	13	33	55	51	152

○ Benign ◐ Early cancer ● BORRMANN I

Fig. 44 Size and benignancy or malignancy in different types of protuberances (YAMADA and FUKUTOMI).

This indicates that only in pedunculated protuberances of greater than 2 cm dia. measured by x-ray examination should the possibility of cancerous polyps be considered. Subsequently, they added characteristics regarding protuberant surfaces to their classification. This work is very valuable because they established the proper standard through detailed histopathological examinations in contrast to the former classification, which had been conducted at random on the basis of personal experiences.

Figure 45 shows the standard for discriminating between benign and malignant tumors used in our department.

Diameter \ Shape	Hill-shaped	Global		Flat	
		Non-pedunculated	Pedunculated	Non-depressed	Depressed
− 1cm	○○○	○○○○○○ ○○○○○○ ○○○○○○	○○		●●●○
1 − 2cm	○○○○	●○○○○○ ○○○○○	○○○○○○ ○○	●	●●
2 − 3cm	○	●●●	●○○○	●	●●●●
3cm −	●●○○	●●	●●●●●○ ○	●●	●
Total	12	34	21	4	11

○ Benign ● Malignant

Fig. 45 Is a tumor benign or malignant?

Since most cases having a flat protuberance are malignant, hill-shaped or global protuberances will be considered directly. It is evident here that cases having protuberances of more than 3 cm dia. are for the most part malignant. Of cases showing hill-shaped protuberances more

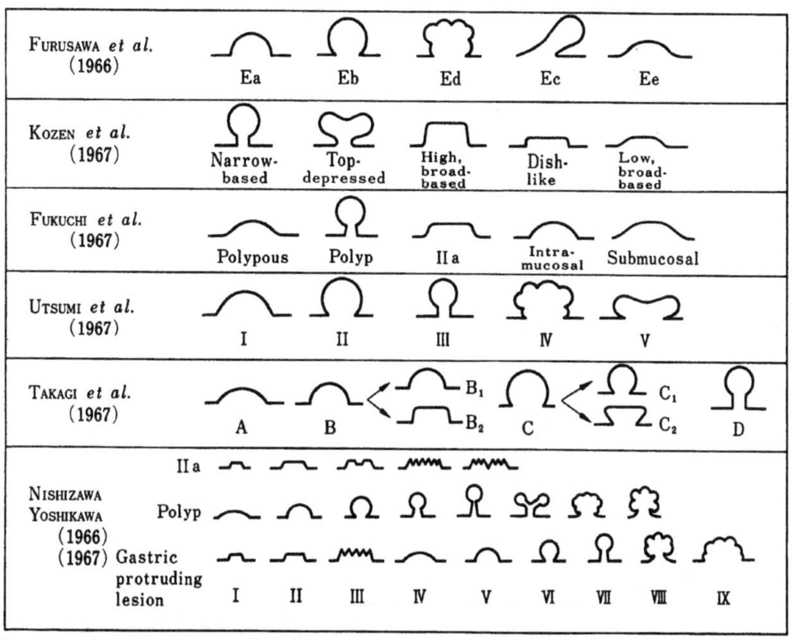

Fig. 46 Morphological classification of the protruding lesions of the stomach.

than 3 cm dia., two malignant cases were sarcoma. An additional important point is that there are malignant cases of global nonpedunculated tumors in lesions of 1 cm dia.. In global and pedunculated cases of more than 2 cm dia., cancer was found in one case out of four. Thus a close relationship exists between type and size.

There are still many reports of differential diagnosis of polypoid lesions, according to type and size (Fig. 46). Most reports agreed that there is a close relationship between type, size, and malignancy. However, classification must always be very simple. It is reasonable to think that these flat protuberances should be treated only on the basis of the shape of their protuberances entirely as flat ones without discriminating between type II and III of YAMADA's classification.

d. If it is an epithelial malignant phyma, is it an early cancer (type I or II) or an advanced case?

When a phyma is proved to be epithelial and malignant, in other words, the endoscopic examination before operation establishes it to be a cancer, the next problem is to determine the depth of the cancerous infiltration.

Generally, with global protuberances of less than 3 cm, the infiltration is found to reach only the lower regions of the mucous membrane. If more than 3cm, it sometimes reaches the muscular layer, especially in nonpedunculated protuberances. On the other hand, in pedunculated cases the infiltration rarely occurs at the basal portion of the protuberance. However, in flat protuberances it is difficult to show a definite relationship between the degree of infiltration and size.

The determination of whether a protuberant cancer in the stomach is advanced or early, depends solely on the histopathological observation of whether the cancerous infiltration remains within the mucous membrane and the muscular layer or not. In cases of adenomatous polyps, the mucous membrane and the muscle fiber branch encroach into the gastric polyps, so that histopathological diagnosis of the infiltration depth becomes difficult. Furthermore, in some cases the diagnosis is made as an advanced cancer of the BORRMANN type I.

When a tumor is more than 3 cm in diameter with an arid surface and hemorrhage, together with a rugged appearance, it is commonly judged as an advanced cancer of the BORRMANN type I. In this case, the hardening pattern of the margin on x-ray filling studies can be used as a standard for the diagnosis of infiltration, and the marginal irregularity is not noticeable because the proliferation of the connective tissue is seldom seen in an early cancer of the type I.

An early cancer of the type IIa is observed as a flower bed-like protuberance of the gastric mucous membrane. This type is rarely judged as benign histologically. In some cases, however,

Shape / Diameter	Global		Flat	
	Non-pedunculated	Pedunculated	Non-depressed	Depressed
− 1cm				○○◑
1 − 2cm	○		◑	◑◑
2 − 3cm	○○◑	○	◑	○○◑◑
3cm −	●●	○◑◑◑●	○◑	○
Total	6	6	4	10

○ m ◑ sm ● pm~

Fig. 47 How deep is the infiltration in an epithelial malignant tumor?

the judgment between benign and malignant tumors is difficult as they are sometimes diagnosed as any of the following: hyperplasia, regenerated mucous membrane of an erosive gastritis, "a borderline lesion or atypical epithelium". As far as a resected stomach is concerned, however, it may be concluded that the discrimination between a benign or malignant, flower bed-like protuberance is comparatively easy.

e. Malignancy judged by surface characteristics

The correlation of surface properties of protuberances, *i.e.*, small-granular-patterned areas on the surface, with the degree of infiltration by cancer was examined. Most of the hill-shaped phymata were smooth in accordance with the following classification: Grade 1 (smooth), Grade 2 (granulated), Grade 3 (small knotted), and Grade 4 (large knotted) (Fig. 48). Considering that most of them are submucosal tumors, it is natural that the presence of a small knotted lesion in the submucosal region suggests the necessity of a comprehensive examination.

In cases of nonpedunculated tumors, early cancers of the protruding type were found in 1 out of 3 granulated cases and 3 out of 4 small knotted cases. All the large knotted cases were found to be advanced cancers.

Of cases having pedunculated tumors, however, early cancer was found in 2 out of 6 small knotted cases and in 3 out of 4 large knotted cases. This suggested a one-step divergence in comparison with nonpedunculated lesions in the relationship between surface property and infiltration.

Shape / Grade	Hill-shaped	Globular		Flat	
		Non-pedunculated	Pedunculated	Non-depressed	Depressed
Smooth 1	○ ○ ○ ○ ○ ○ ○ ◎ ◎	◎ ◎	◎ ◎		○
Granulated 2	○ ○	◎ ◎ ◑	○ ◎ ◎ ◎ ◎ ◎ ◎ ◎ ◎		◑ ◑ ◑ ◑ ◑
Small knotted 3	○	◎ ◑ ◑ ◑	◎ ◎ ◎ ◎ ◑ ◑	◑ ◑	◑ ◑ ◑ ◑ ◑
Large knotted 4		● ●	◑ ◑ ◑ ●	◑ ◑	
Total	12	34	21	4	11

○ Submucosal tumor ◎ Gastric polyp ◑ Early cancer ● Advanced cancer

Fig. 48 Malignancy judged by surface characteristics.

C. The fundamentals of endoscopic diagnosis

In the gastrofiberscopic diagnosis, it is very important to know the macroscopic characteristics of gastric diseases.

The diagnostic process of endoscopy is almost the same as that of radiologic diagnosis. It is not too much to say that since the development of the gastrofiberscope, all portions of the stomach are now observable. There is no special method of endoscopic procedure for protruding or excavated gastric lesions. Needless to say, it is necessary to scrutinize lesions according to the fundamentals of endoscopy. The first step in skillful endoscopy is to observe the entire mucosa of the stomach and, simultaneously, to observe and photograph lesions dynamically and stereoscopically in "sharp focus". In practice, the choice of an instrument and the method of observation and photography is highly important. There is one more problem, the choice of patients.

The final diagnosis of gastric lesions should not simply rely on x-ray or endoscopic findings, but should include cytological or biopsy examination under direct vision.

1. Basic problems of endoscopic examination

a. Subjects for endoscopy

As a rule, x-ray examination is the first choice for gastric disorders and the second is endoscopic examination. The role of endoscopy in diagnosing gastric diseases is ultimately to find lesions which are missed or to diagnose doubtful lesions observed by fluoroscopy. Lesions missed fluoroscopically may be diagnosed with endoscopy, which indicates the possibility of diagnosing lesions in which a color change is the only macroscopic finding. This is the particular advantage of endoscopic over radiologic examinations.

There are two problems of clinical limitations. One is whether lesions exist that have no radiological abnormality but only a change in color. The other is whether all patients without x-ray findings should be examined endoscopically. These are by far the most difficult problems and will be discussed further.

Usually lesions which are not discovered due to insufficient x-ray studies or whose radiological findings are too slight to consider abnormal can easily be practically diagnosed with an endoscopic examination. From this point of view, it is practical to decide the indications for endoscopic examination with reference to the x-ray findings and preciseness of the radiological examination. If endoscopic examination is limited to patients who have some pathological findings radiologically, the x-ray diagnosis must be of high quality. So if x-ray examination is precise enough, endoscopic examinations may be limited to patients who are radiologically abnormal. On the other hand, if the radiological examination is not reliable, endoscopic examination should be extended to radiologically normal persons. When the judgment of "no findings" is made from rough x-ray diagnosis, lesions which have slight or no fibrosis may be overlooked.

b. Instruments for gastric endoscopy

Although there are many kinds of instruments for gastric endoscopy, the gastrocamera and various types of gastrofiberscopes are chiefly used now. The advantages and disadvantages of each instrument must be understood. Commonly used instruments are briefly explained as follows.

1) Gastrocamera (Olympus, GT type V, type Va, type Pa)

The gastrocamera (Fig. 49) has no finder but its tip can be made to flex 100 degrees upward and downward and can be equipped with a short-focus lens. The photographic field is 108° wide so that a wide area of the gastric mucosa can be photographed. The film placed at the tip of the camera is 4 or 5 mm wide and has 30 frames.

Advantages

1. Photographic pictures are quite clear and fine.
2. A wide area of the gastric mucosa can be covered by a skilled technician.
3. Manipulation of the gastrocamera is simple, and the time required for examination is relatively short.

Disadvantages

1. The gastrocamera has no finder, so a naked observation is not possible.
2. It is difficult to take photographs of the intended site of the stomach.

2) Gastrofiberscope (FGS-Machida)

The gastrofiberscope has been widely used and the gastric mucosa has become easy to observe with the naked-eye. However, photography is more difficult, and photographs are rather coarse compared to those taken with the gastrocamera.

3) Gastrocamera with a Fiberscope (Olympus GTF, GTFa, GTF-S)

This instrument (Fig. 50) is a combination of the gastrocamera and the gastrofiberscope. The gastrofiberscope is used as the finder for the gastrocamera.

Advantage

The photographic picture is clear and fine, and at the same time, dynamic observation is possible.

Disadvantages

1. Focus of the view-lens is fixed, and dynamic observation is not sufficient.
2. When one lesion is found, the examiner is apt to observe only that portion and to neglect the other areas.

4) Gastrofiberscope for Biopsy and Cytology (Olympus, GF type B and type C; Machida FGS type B and type C)

A special gastrofiberscope has been developed with which a gastric biopsy and/or cytology is made possible during direct vision (Figs. 51 and 52).

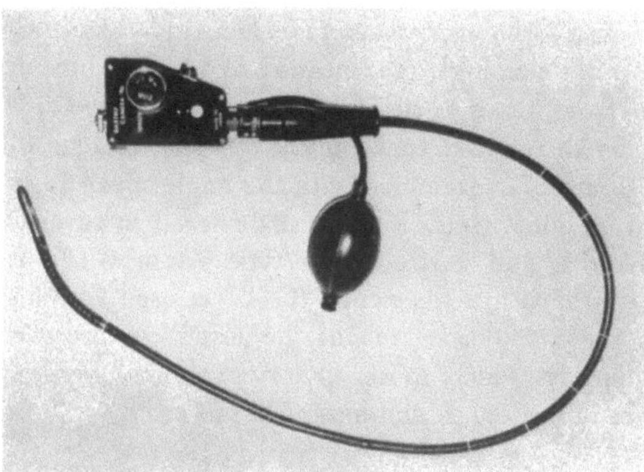

Fig. 49 Gastrocamera (Olympus, type Va)

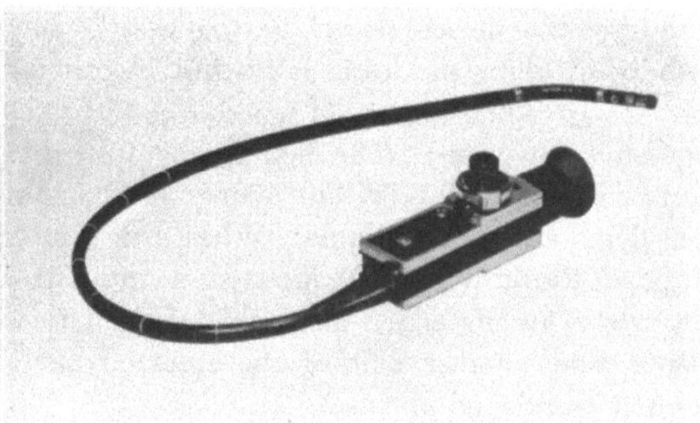

Fig. 50 Gastrocamera with Fiberscope (Olympus, type GTF-S)

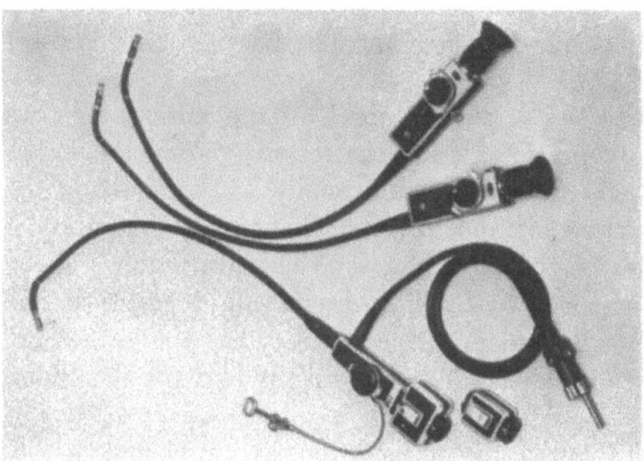

Fig. 51 Gastrofiberscope for Biopsy and Cytology (Olympus, GF-B and GF-C)

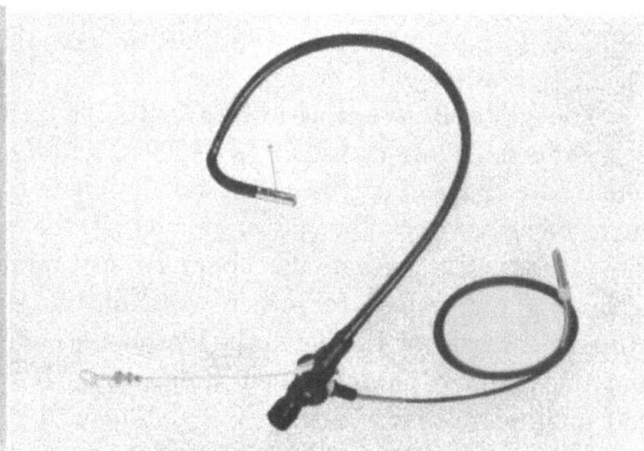

Fig. 52 Gastrofiberscope for Biopsy (Machida, FGS-BL)

2. Clinical application of endoscopy

The authors present two indications for endoscopy. One is to observe x-ray examination positive abnormalities, and the other is to find lesions in patients who have slight or no abnormalities radiologically, but have long histories of gastroenterological disorders.

a. Routine examination (Endoscopic examination for the radiological "no findings" group)

This is an examination to seek pathological alterations in the stomach or to confirm that there are no lesions. It is obvious that blind photography with the gastrocamera is not sufficient for this purpose and that scopic photography, which permits a choice of sites in the stomach and distance from the lens to the mucosa, is a more desirable method. However, it is not difficult for those who are skillful with the gastrocamera to take pictures of almost any part of the stomach. Currently, very fine pictures can be obtained with the gastrocamera, and handling of the camera has been simplified. Being reliable and durable, the gastrocamera type Va or Gastrocamera with a fiberscope has been used for this purpose.

It is desirable to use the gastrocamera in a relatively dark room so that the flash can be seen through the abdominal wall to locate the tip of the camera. The authors use a GTFa, FGS and a secondary gastrofiberscope for biopsy or cytology.

There are some differences in the methods of observation, especially the order of photography with a gastrocamera and a gastrocamera with a fiberscope (GTF). The patient is laid on his left side and the camera or GTF is inserted. It is important for the examination that the patient is relaxed and that the entire procedure be carried out gently without any force.

As shown in Figure 53, the authors usually insert the gastrocamera sufficiently deep into the antral sinus and then take the pictures; then using the angle mechanisms of the instrument, withdraw the device slowly to the gastric angle from the pyloric antrum. As the camera is withdrawn along the lesser curvature, air should be introduced to keep the proper distance of the lens from the object. Then the body of the stomach is examined with the angle mechanism regulated downward. The final photography is carried out with the camera shaft flexed in reverse. Gastrocameras and GTF are mainly used in this order, and gastrocamera type Va or GTFa is considered the most suitable. When the gastrocamera with a fiberscope (GTF) is used for this purpose, the instrument is inserted to the gastric angle, and the arch of the lesser curvature is observed. Finally excess air is voided, and the scope is guided to the pyloric antrum. Figures 54 a–e show another part of the stomach being examined and photographed according to the method mentioned above.

b. Accurate examination (Gastrofiberscopic examination for the radiological abnormal group)

In this group, the site of the lesion radiologically revealed should be carefully observed and photographed. Then the rest of the stomach should be examined according to the method mentioned above. Initially, the GTF or gastrofiberscope is recommended, because direct observation is possible.

The gastrofiberscope is inserted into the gastric angle, and the arch of the lesser curvature is examined. Then excess air is expelled and the scope is guided to the lesion. When the lesion comes into the field of the scope, the lesion is observed frontally and anally while adjusting the angle mechanism of the scope, regulating the volume of the air, and changing the posture of the patient. The authors use about twenty frames of the GTF film for the main lesion and the remaining ten frames for other parts of the stomach. With the ordinary blind gastrocamera, utilizing the halo of the flash, the lens of the camera is guided to the lesion by the above method, and the lesion is photographed intensively. It is advisable to use one roll of film for the lesion and another roll for the rest of the stomach.

Generally speaking, the left-side position is adopted for observation by most gastroendoscopists, but the supine position or the right-side position is selected for best visualization of the pyloric antrum and the upper portions of the gastric body.

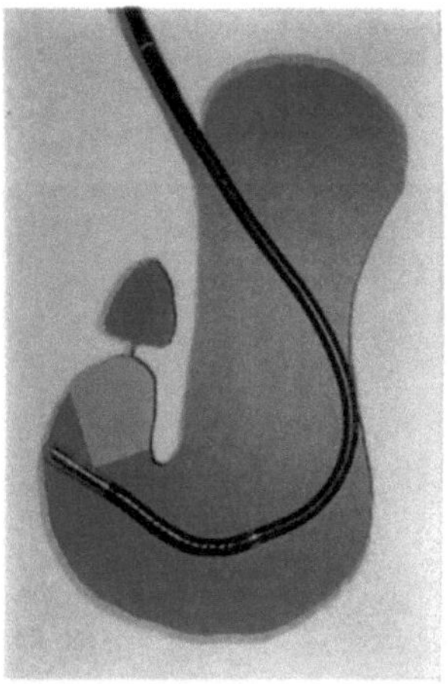
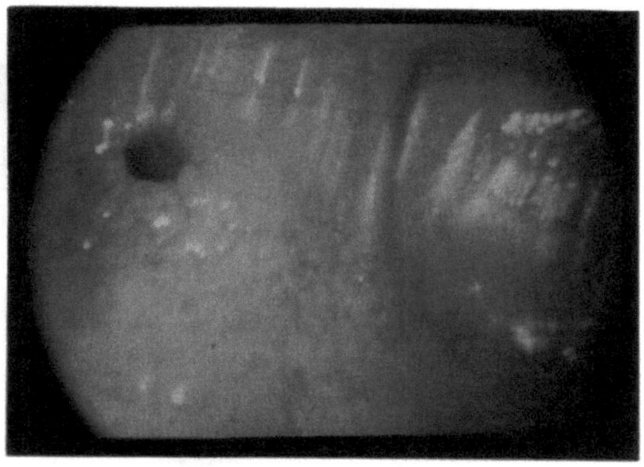

a a′

The gastrocamera should be sufficiently inserted into the antral sinus (a), then the pyloric ring is seen on the left side (a′).

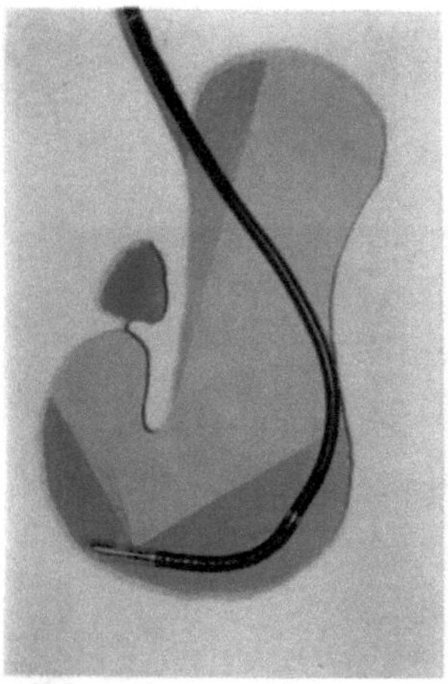
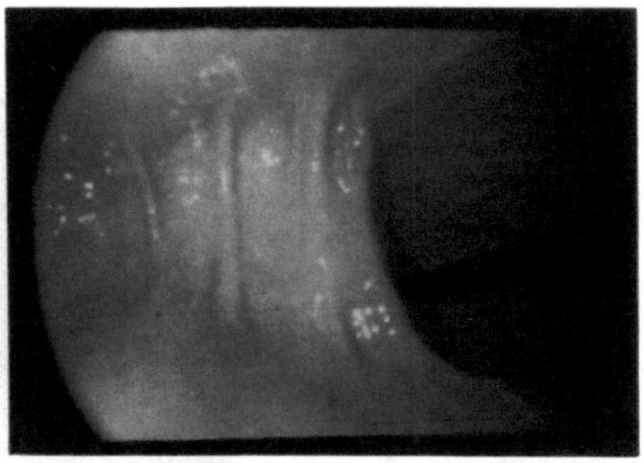

b b′

Withdrawing the gastrocamera slowly, photograph the pyloric sinus and antrum (b). Most of the left side in this picture (b′) is the lesser curvature of antrum. The angular arch is photographed from the antrum side.

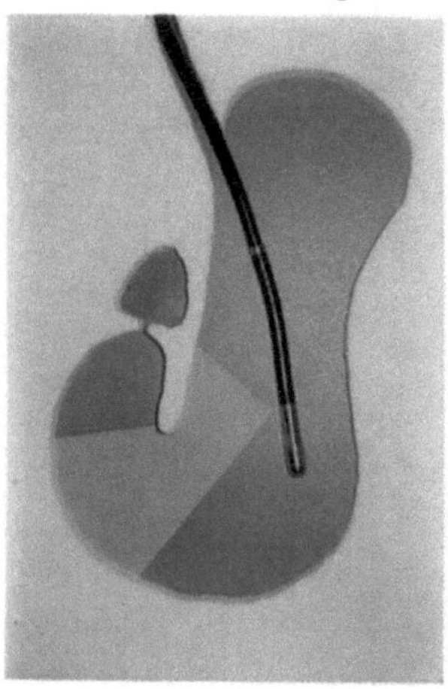
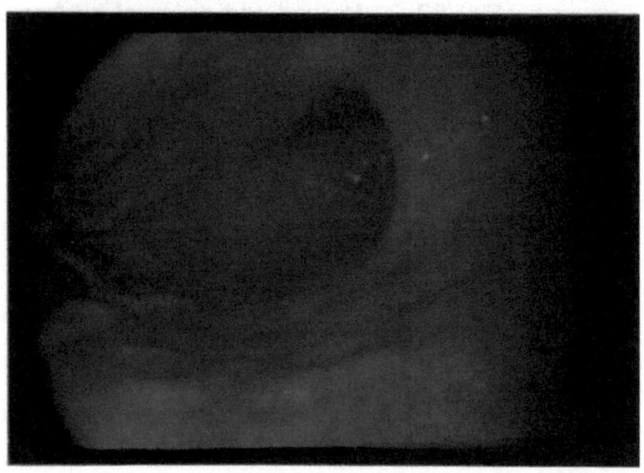

c c′

With further withdrawal of the gastrocamera to the gastric angle (c), the gastric angle is seen as the arch (c′).

Fig. 53-1 Method and order of routine endoscopic examination

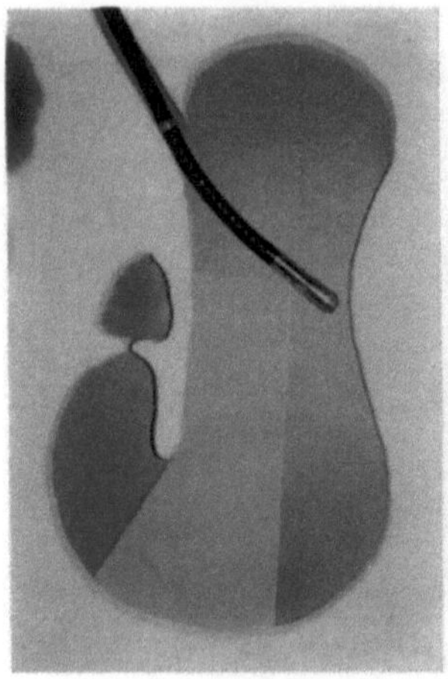
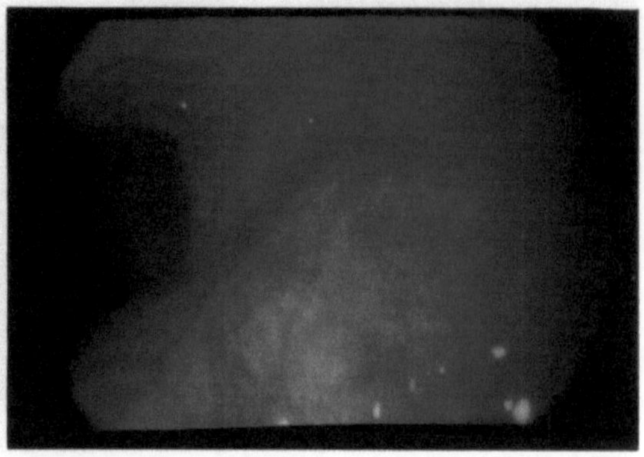

d d′

The gastric corpus is photographed at this camera position (d and d′).

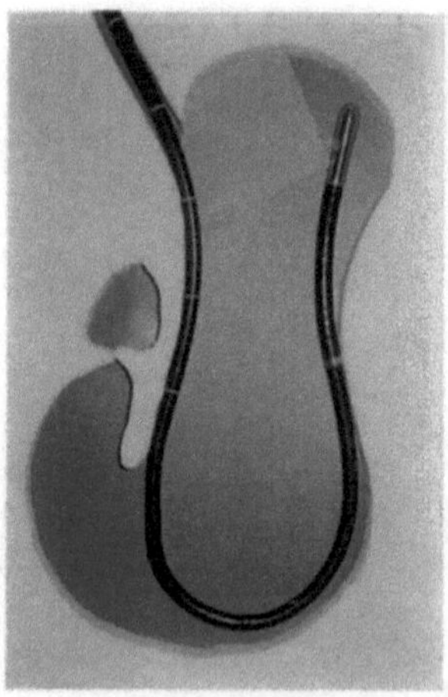
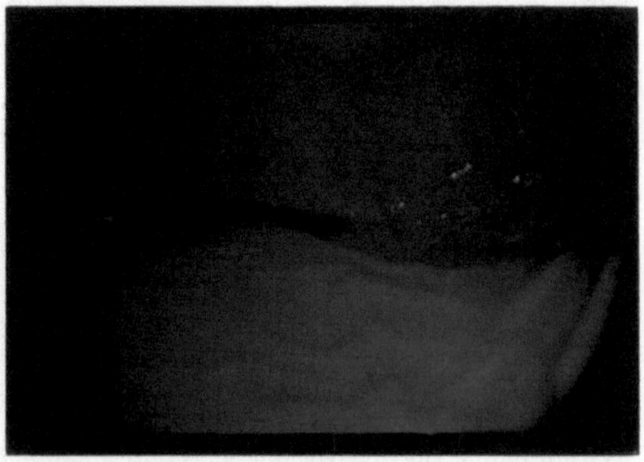

e e′

When the gastrocamera shaft is reversed by the "U-turn" method (e), the cardiac and fornix area can be photographed (e′).

Fig. 53-2 Method and order of routine endoscopic examination.

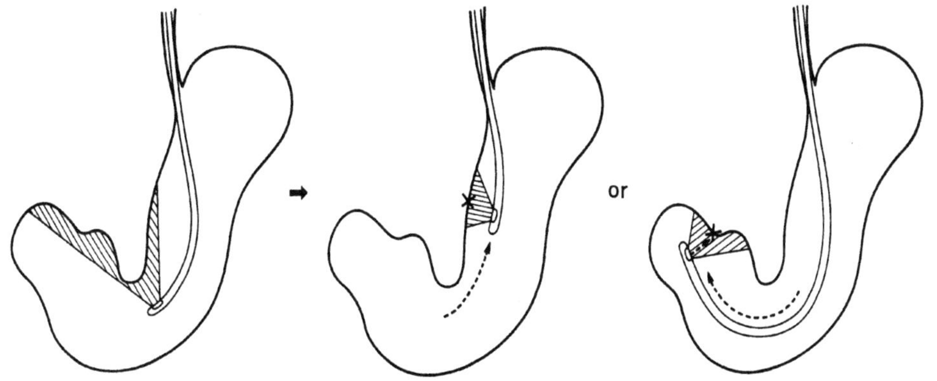

a. Radiological "abnormal findings" group.

1. Carefully observe the gastric angle.
2. Make the tip of the scope face the lesion or intended position of the stomach.
3. Observe the lesion from all directions and photograph it.
4. Observe and photograph the other parts of the lesion, according to the method of (a), from antrum to cardia.

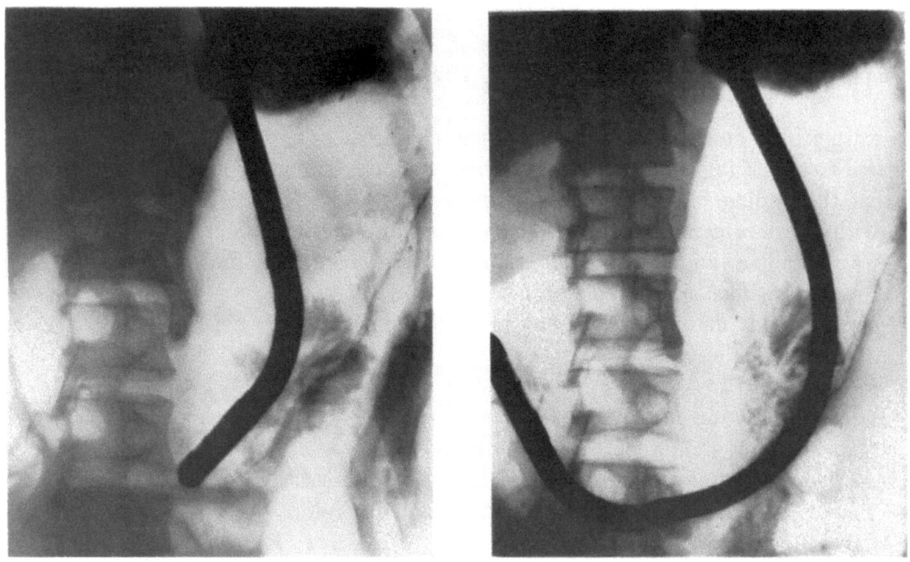

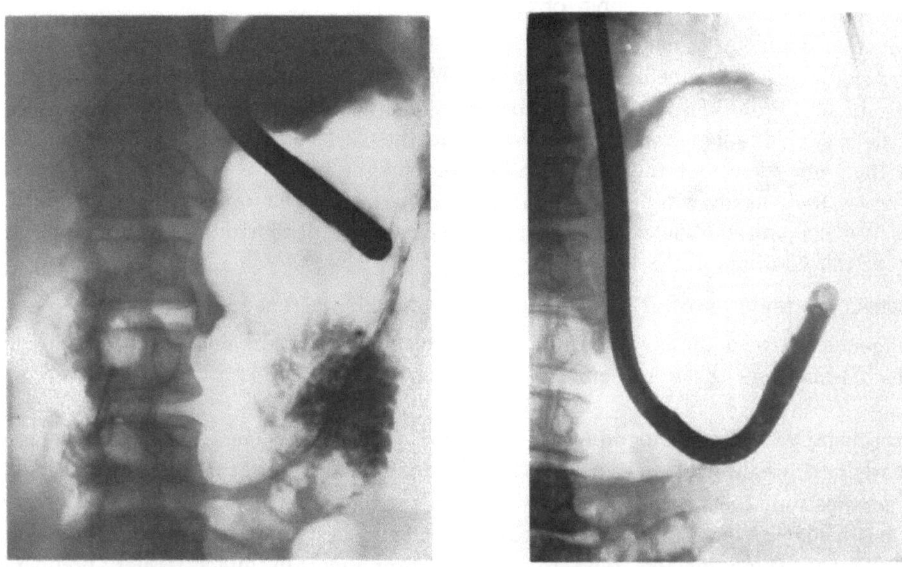

d. Gastric corpus e. Cardia and fornix

Fig. 54 Method and order of accurate endoscopic examination.

3. Technical details of endoscopy

In this chapter, the value of endoscopic examination especially with regard to excavated lesions will be discussed.

a. Endoscopic fundamentals for excavated lesions

The diagnostic basis for endoscopy of excavated lesions of the stomach is a knowledge of the macroscopic features of lesions as well as the radiological viewpoint. For this purpose, the macroscopic findings of resected stomachs are carefully observed, and the macroscopic and pathological features of various gastric diseases must be studied in great detail.

1) Excavation: deep or shallow

The depth of the defect in reference to the surrounding mucosa, the color of the lesion, and the exposed base are of help in the diagnosis.

2) The nature of the base of the lesion

There may be bases covered with thick fur, or exposed the part for being very thin, or only disclosed without fur. It is helpful for diagnosis of the base of lesion to observe the nodular and granulated pictures.

3) Sharpness of the border of the defect

Whether the margin of the defect is clear-cut or obscure in relation to the surrounding mucosa is important for differential diagnosis. The defect should be observed frontally and obliquely.

4) The existence of converging folds and their character

A lesion with converging folds is fibrotic to some extent. In endoscopy the stomach expands with air so that the findings are sometimes diminished.

In cases with rugal convergence, the following findings should be carefully observed:

1. Are the rugae interrupted or continuous to the center of the crater?
2. Are they swollen at the end or not?
3. Are the rugae flattened or narrowed at the end?
4. Are they discolored or bleeding?
5. Are they hard or soft in appearance?

5) The nature of the surrounding mucosa

Likewise the following should be carefully observed:

1. Are there elevations or protrusions around the defect?
2. What is the consistency of the elevation and its color?
3. Is there evidence of hemorrhage?
4. Is the defect surrounded with a shallow defect or a discolored zone?

b. Practical suggestions in endoscopic observation

An excavation 4 mm in diameter and 1.5 mm in width prepared on a model stomach was photographed with a gastrocamera (Figs. 55 a and b). The picture taken from a distance of 4 cm was the best. Figure 55 a was taken almost straight upward, and Figure 55 b was an oblique view. The details of the base of the excavation or the surface of the protuberance are well observed in the front view, but the depth and/or the height are not. On the other hand, in the oblique view, the shadow and excavation are emphasized. The oblique view is useful, for discovery of defects and the determination of their margins. The front view is essential for discernment of the contour of the lesions.

c. The endoscopic features of the excavation in vivo and the resected stomach

The difference between these two is due to the blood circulation and tonus of the living stomach which sometimes make the endoscopic findings more obvious than those of a resected stomach.

When preoperative gastrophotography is compared with gastrocamera findings of a resected stomach in early gastric cancer of the type III+IIc, the contour of the excavation is almost identical in the two pictures, but the margin of the excavation appears sharper in the preoperative gastrocamera findings. The spasms of intact gastric muscles emphasize the shallow depression of the gastric wall. Since shallow defects tend to be more prominent in intact tissues, preoperative diagnoses should be made with these points in mind (Figs. 56 a and b).

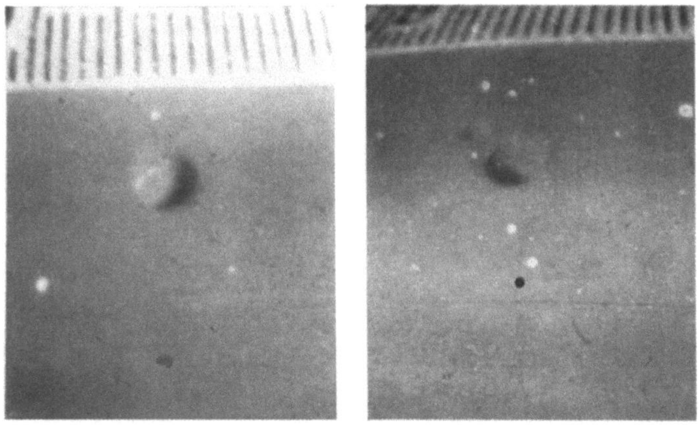

a b

Fig. 55 Experimental gastrophotography with an excavation on a model stomach.
a. Almost straight upward view at a distance of 4cm.
b. An oblique view at a distance of 4cm.

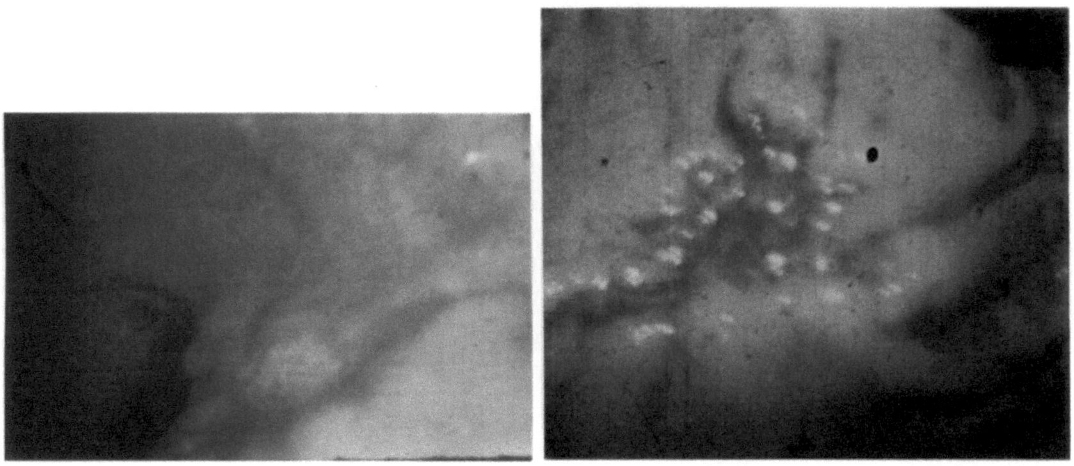

a b

Fig. 56 Comparison between preoperative and postoperative gastrophotography.
a. Preoperative picture taken with the gastrocamera.
b. Postoperative picture taken with the gastrocamera.

One more difference is the fur at the base of the defect. The fur is chiefly composed of exudates from the tissue defect. It is thick and clearly observed in the preoperative picture, thin and slimy in the postoperative picture. The differentiation and elimination of mucus must be kept in mind during endoscopy.

d. Protruding+excavated type lesions in endoscopy

As stated previously, in x-ray examinations excavated lesions in elevated mucosal areas or excavations surrounded by mucosal protrusions are better demonstrated by compression studies than by the double-contrast method.

Diagnosis of this type of lesion is similar to that of protruding lesions. Endoscopic examination is very efficient for diagnosing excavated lesions with protruding mucosal areas. On the other hand, care must be taken not to overdiagnose these lesions in endoscopy, because the endoscopic findings of protrusions are sometimes more prominent than in resected specimens.

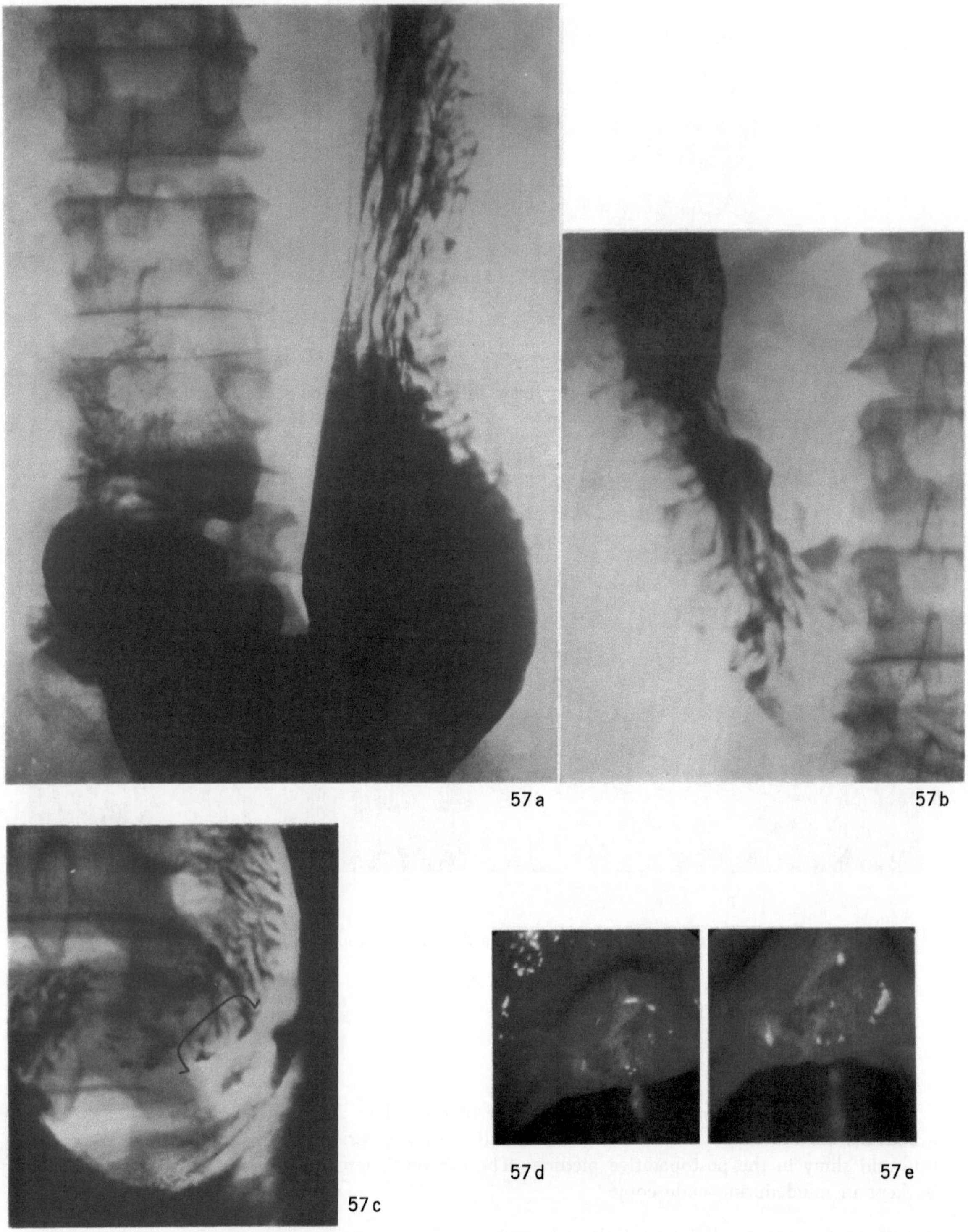

Fig. 57 Endoscopic examination is valuable in finding "Protruding type+Excavated type" lesions, however, it is necessary to be careful of overdiagnosis.

a. Radiograph of a barium filled stomach in the upright position.
b. Mucosal picture in the prone position.
c. Compression picture in the upright position. Compression observation under fluoroscopy is the best way to find small lesions.
d. Observation of the entire lesion (FGS picture).
e. Close-up frontal observation (FGS picture).

A case of an advanced gastric cancer is shown in Figure 57. The appearance of this lesion resembled that of an early cancer of the type II a+II c. This was a small "protrusion+excavation" type lesion, 20 mm × 20 mm, and cancer cells had partially reached the muscle layer proper. On x-ray examination, it was apparent that the lesion must have been in the angular region, because of the angular deformity and mural rigidity. The lesion was also demonstrated in a mucosal study done in the prone position (Fig. 57 b) and in a compression radiograph (Fig. 57 c). The indication of malignancy was a small irregular niche surrounded by a mucosal embankment. Endoscopically, when the fiberscope was inserted to the gastric angle, the lesion was easily visualized (Figs. 57 d, e). The mucosal embankment was prominent. It seemed to be an early cancer of the type II a+II c by endoscopy, because the protrusion had a soft mucosal appearance. An oblique observation of the entire lesion (Fig. 57 d) and a proximal frontal observation (Fig. 57 e) allowed a vivid macroscopic visualization. Endoscopically, it is rather easy to diagnose this type of lesion morphologically, but differential diagnosis of whether it is advanced or early is much more difficult.

Let us consider the gastrocamera picture of another case (Fig. 58). An excavation of the mucosa with a surrounding mucosal embankment was seen on the lesser curvature of the angulus. It could be diagnosed as benign with the findings of a clean white fur with a lack of rigidity and a discoloration of the surrounding mucosa. However, it was not easy to confirm precisely whether this lesion was not a III type early cancer, a IIa+IIc type early cancer, or a Borrmann II type advanced cancer.

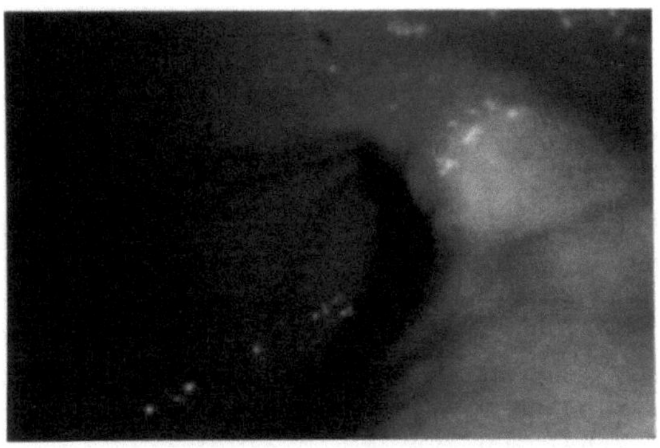

58 a

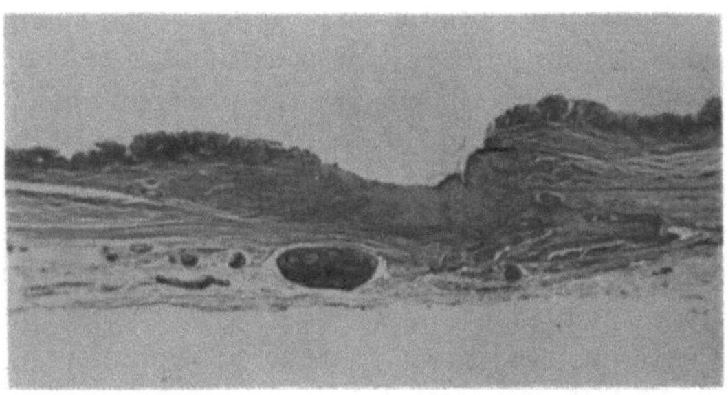

58 b

Fig. 58 Close-up endoscopic picture and differential diagnosis of an excavated lesion.
a. Acute ulcer. It is not easy to confirm malignancy or benignancy because of an exaggeration of the surrounding mucosal embankment. Endoscopic diagnosis of a "Protruding type+Excavated type" is liable to be an overdiagnosis.
b. Histopathological findings. This lesion was revealed as an acute ulcer (two weeks after the endoscopic examination).

As shown in the histology of the lesion (Fig. 58 b), this was a case of an acute gastric ulcer. The confusion came from the endoscopic appearance of the swelling due to an exaggeration of the edema in the mucosa adjacent to the ulcer. The swollen zone surrounding the ulcer left no room for doubt radiologically. Endoscopic examination is efficient, but there are dangers with the diagnosis.

4. Special remarks on endoscopic examination

The procedure for endoscopic examination is discussed above. Additional practical problems will be discussed in this chapter.

a. Lesions on the anterior wall and multiple lesions

The combined usage of endoscopy with radiology is convenient. In diagnoses of the gastric anterior wall, abnormalities and lesions must be discovered in the first x-ray examination. For this purpose, mucosal and compression studies and the double-contrast method in the prone position are essential. If abnormalities are discovered on x-ray examination, it is apparent that endoscopy has an advantage over radiology. For diagnosis of duplicated lesions, it is important to observe the entire mucosa of the stomach to avoid overlooking coexistent lesions.

b. Difficulties in observing lesions from the frontal view

Blind areas in endoscopy of the stomach have almost vanished with the development and dispersion of the gastrocamera, type Va, and the development of the gastrofiberscope. The first goal for endoscopists is to observe without any blind areas. Endoscopic observations should meet certain conditions in order for the physician to grasp the macroscopic features of gastric lesions. A precise observation of macroscopic findings is the basis for differential diagnosis of excavated or protruding lesions. Accordingly, when qualitative diagnoses are attempted with endoscopy, it is essential to obtain accurate frontal views under good conditions. Otherwise, endoscopy is merely complementary to frontal view x-ray photographs.

In endoscopy, it is chiefly due to technical difficulties that adequate frontal views of the lesions cannot be obtained. In general, the posterior wall of the body and the neighborhood of the pylorus are parts of the stomach that are difficult to observe.

With radiology, it is difficult to show frontal views of lesions in the marginal portions of the lesser or greater curvature, but rather easy with endoscopy. An example of an excavated lesion is shown in Figure 59. This lesion, demonstrated in a double-contrast study in the upright position (Fig. 59 a), appears on the posterior wall of the upper body like a II c type of early cancer. It is possible to determine the contours of the excavation, its uneven base, and the surroundings of the defect. Figure 59 b is the GTF picture of this lesion.

Regulation of the air volume introduced into the stomach and changes of the patient's position make it possible to observe lesions of this height without reversing the scope. The straight frontal view, however, is difficult to obtain, making the picture somewhat of a "bird's-eye view". This case was an advanced cancer with the appearance of a II c+III type early cancer.

The next is a prepyloric lesion (Fig. 60). As shown in the picture of the resected specimen (Fig. 60 a), this is a small II c type early cancer adjacent to the pyloric ring. A close observation by GTF was impossible, and the frontal view was also unsatisfactory. From the findings of the resected stomach, a diagnosis could not be accurately predicted (Fig. 60 b). Radiological compression study was performed based on these endoscopic findings (Figs. 60 c, d). In this radiograph, the frontal view of the mucosal depression was portrayed accurately.

One must be careful to diagnose qualitatively when working with long-distance endoscopic observations or without adequate frontal view. Especially when the lesion is on the upper body or pyloric region, the diagnostic value of endoscopy is limited.

On the contrary, when the lesion is on either of the curvatures, endoscopy is of great value. For example, Figure 61 is an advanced cancer of the Borrmann II type. A niche is seen on the lesser curvature of the antrum in the barium-filled study (Fig. 61 a). A diagnosis of cancer may be made with only this picture, but the double-contrast and compression method failed to show the frontal view of the defective surface. It is not difficult to diagnose this lesion qualitatively with these findings, but they are not sufficient for portraying the gross findings of the resected specimen (Figs. 61 b, c).

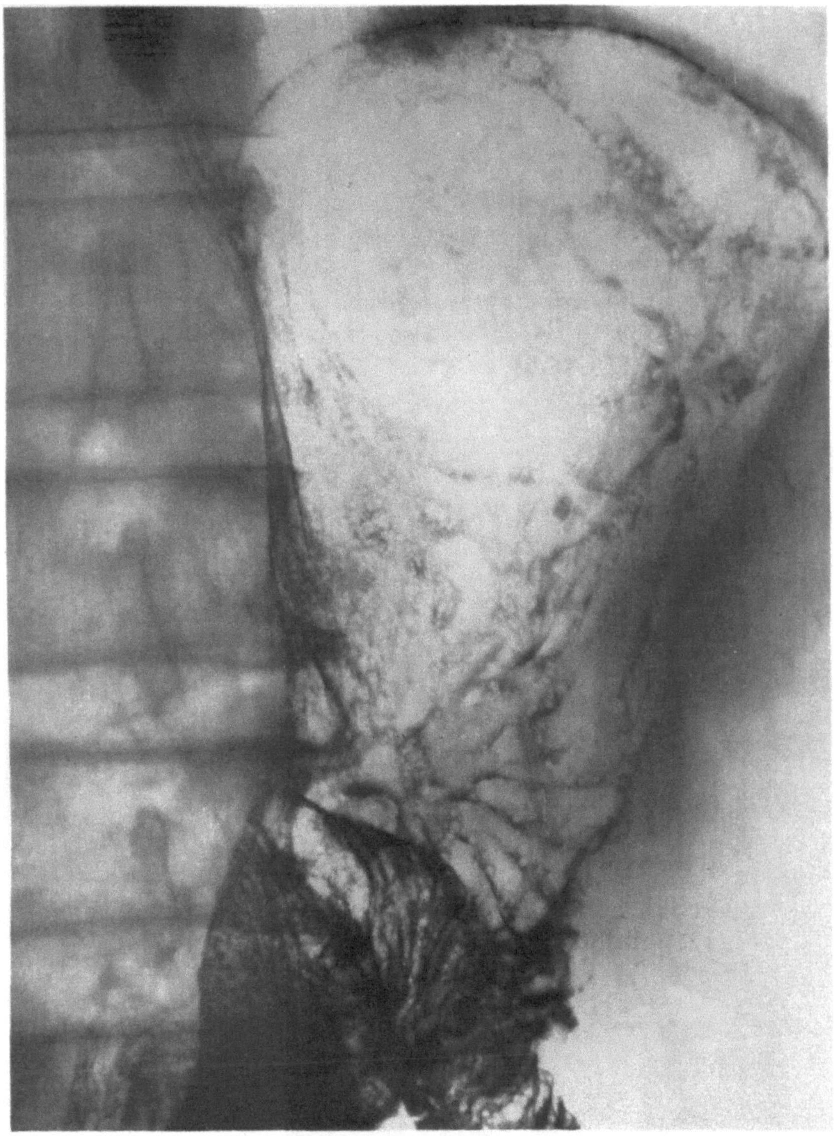

59 a

59 b

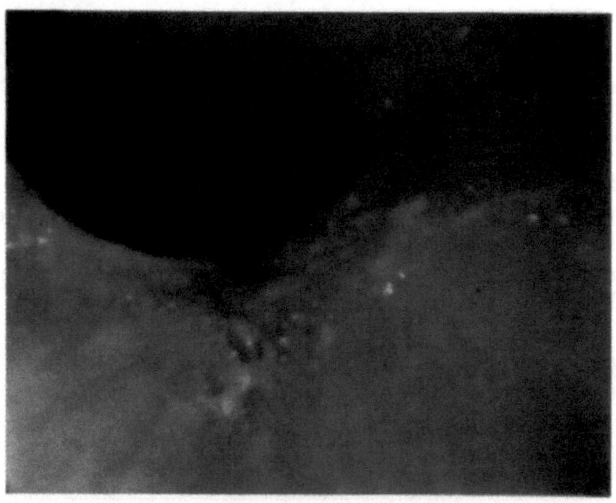

Fig. 59 Lesion of the upper portion and the endoscopic picture.
a. Double-contrast study in the upper position. Frontal view is observed.
b. GTF picture. It is possible to observe the lesion in position without inversion, but it is not easy to observe it frontally.

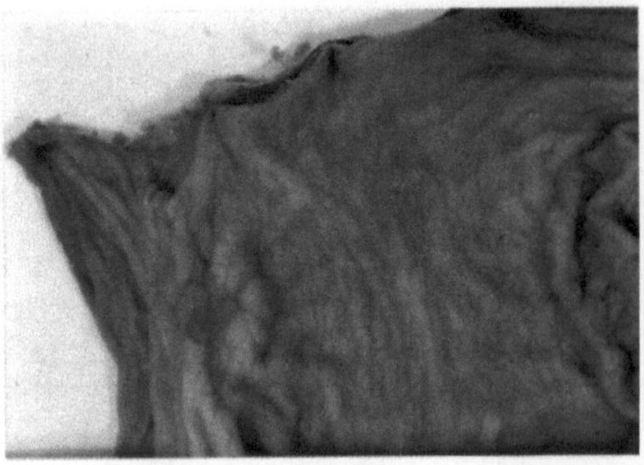

60 a

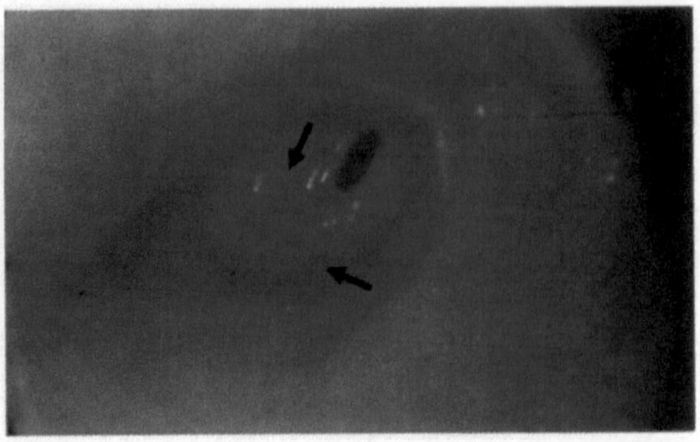

60 b

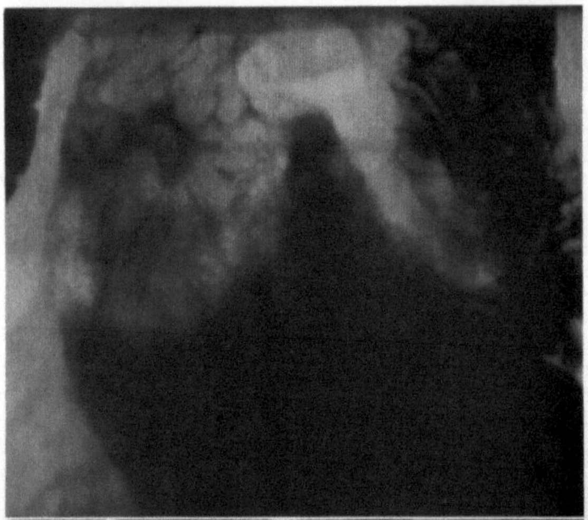

60c

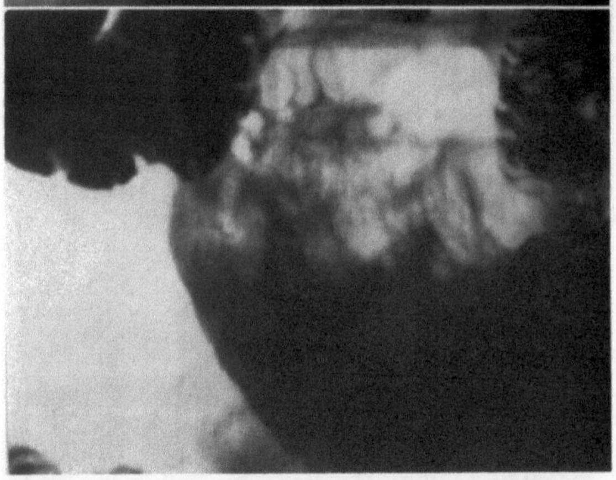

60d

Fig. 60 Endoscopic diagnosis of a prepyloric lesion. Many cases are apt to be observed from a long distance using fixed-focus endoscopy. In addition, it is comparatively difficult to observe the frontal view.

a. A IIc type early gastric cancer adjacent to the pyloric ring.
b. GTF picture. The lesion can be seen, but it is impossible to read it in detail because of the great distance.
c. Compression study in the upright position.
d. Compression study in the upright position.

61a

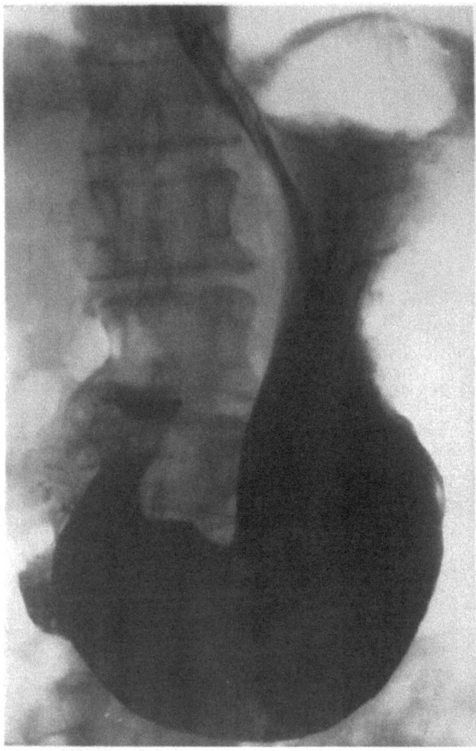

61b

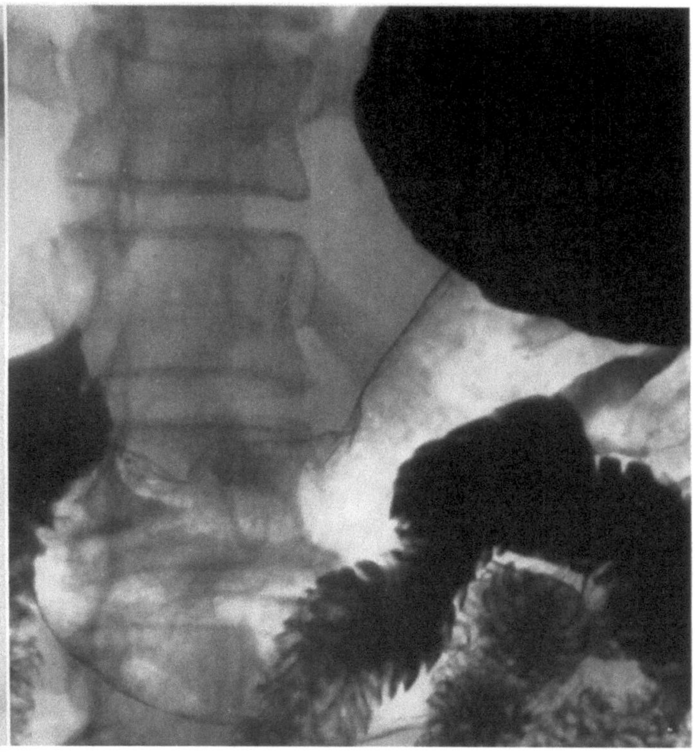

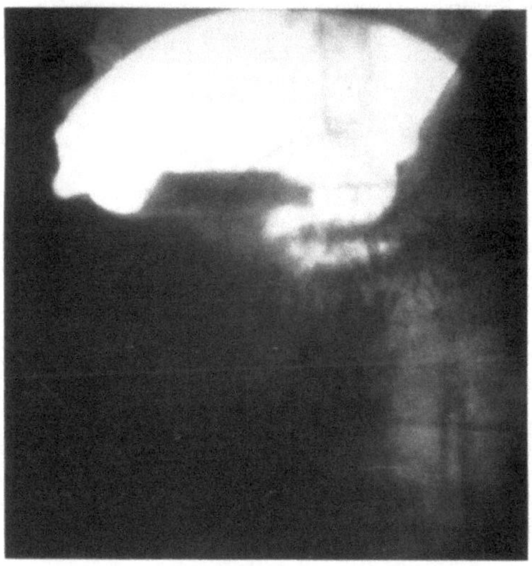

61c

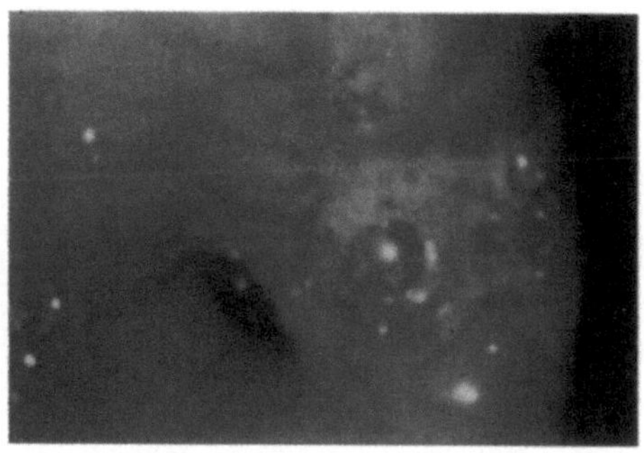

61d

Fig. 61 Lesions on the lesser curvature and the greater curvature are easily observed by endoscopy.
a. Barium filled stomach in the upright position.
b. Double-contrast study.
c. Compression study in the upright position. Excavation with a semi-circular wall is seen.
d. GTF picture. It is not difficult to observe the frontal view endoscopically.

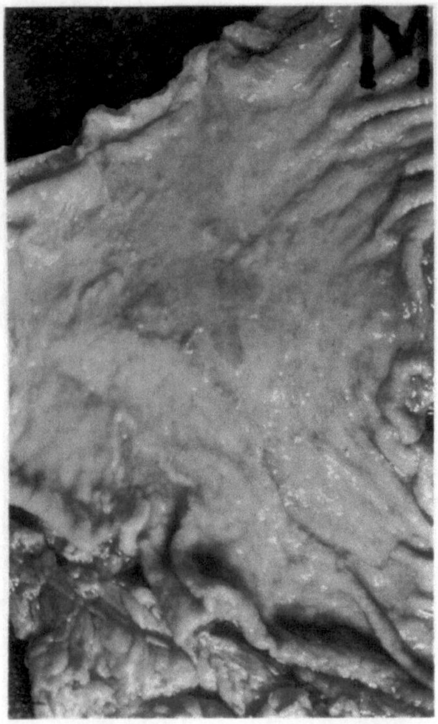

62a

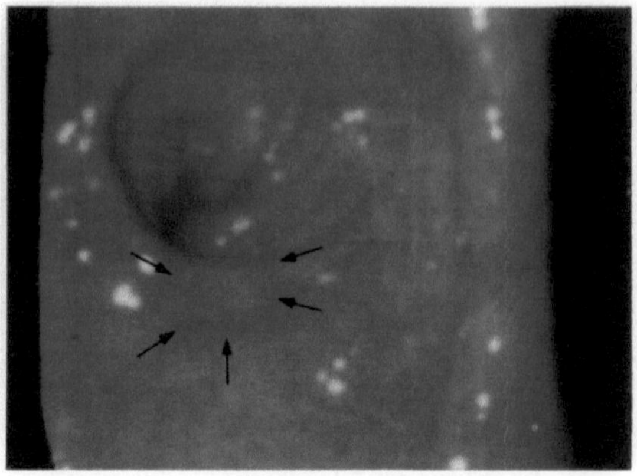

62b

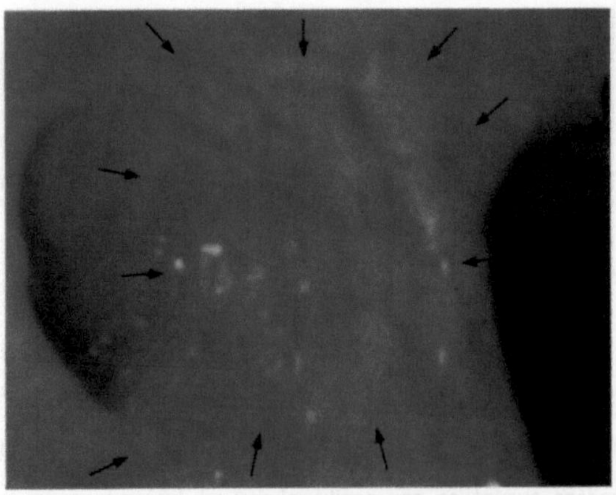

62c

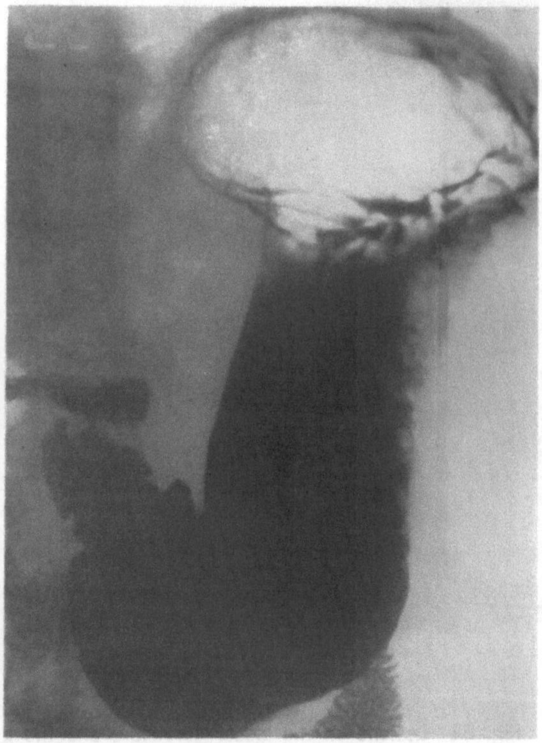

62d

Fig. 62 Endoscopic diagnosis of a shallow excavated lesion and its limits.
a. Resected specimen of a duplicated IIc-type early cancer (Cancerous invasions were limited to only the mucosal layer).
b. GTF picture. A IIc type can be observed on the greater curvature.
c. GTF picture. Peculiar reddening and patchy discoloration can be observed, but an accurate diagnosis is not easy.
d. Radiograph of the barium filled stomach in the upright position.

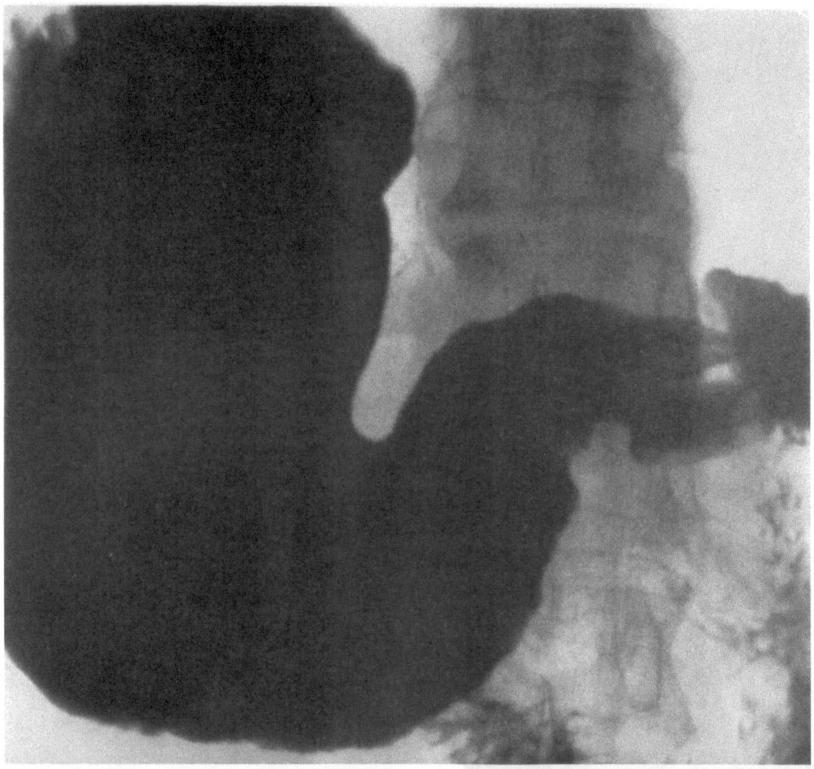

62e

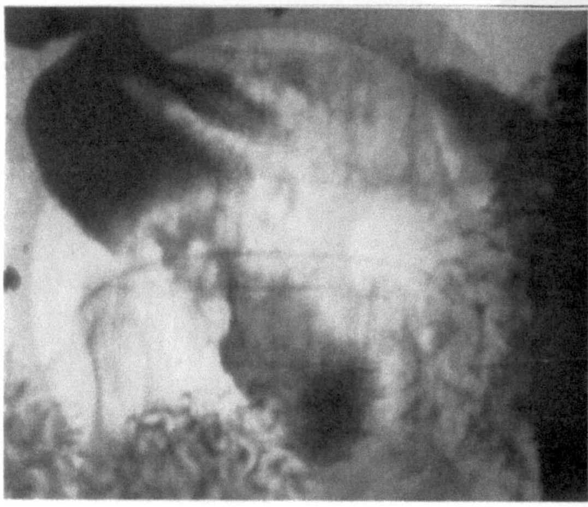

62f

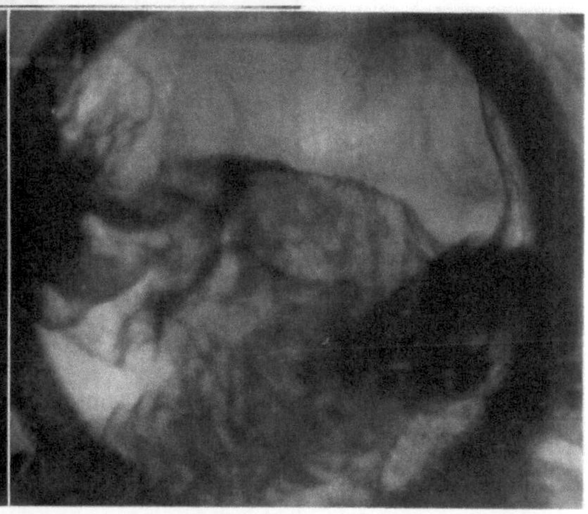

62g

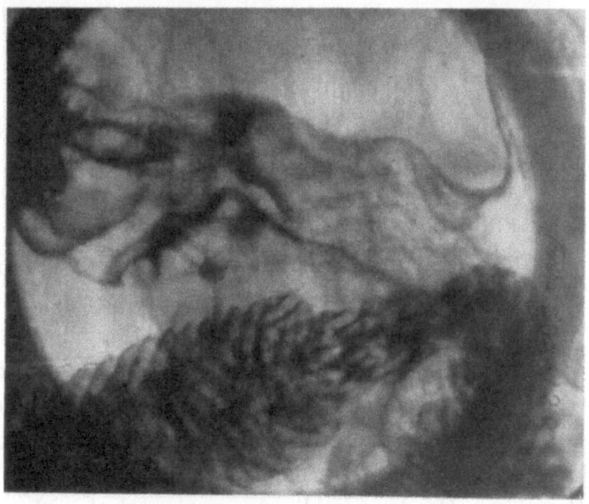

62h

Fig. 62 Endoscopic diagnosis of a shallow excavated lesion and its limits.

e. Radiograph of the barium filled stomach in the prone position.
f. Compression study in the upright position. The finding of a IIc type on the greater curvature is portrayed well.
g. Double-contrast study with compression.
h. Double-contrast study with compression. Irregular granules and a reticular surfaced, shallow depression are seen.

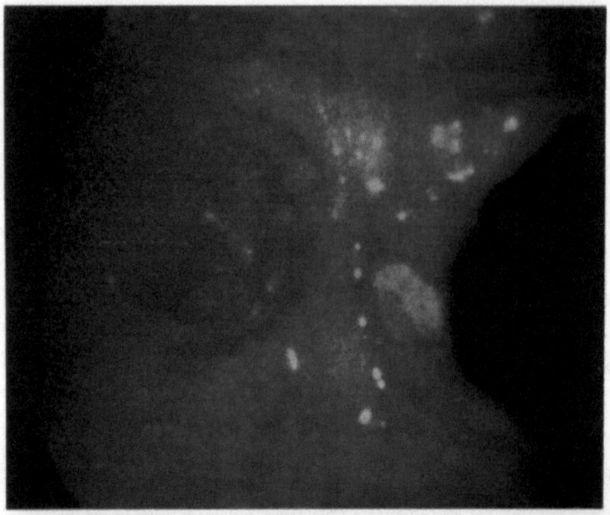
63a

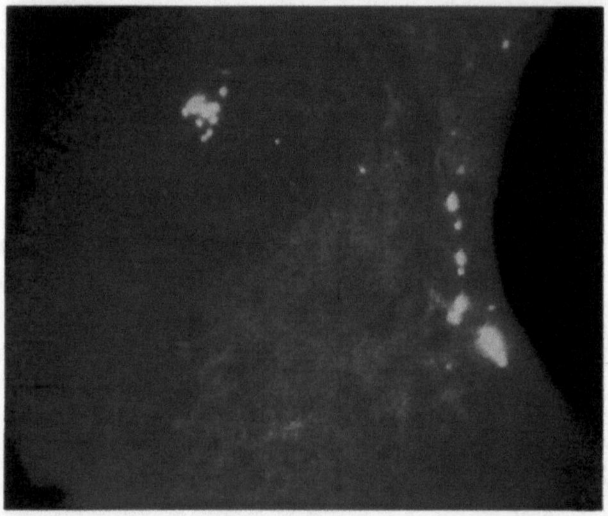
63b

Fig. 63 Malignant cycle.
a. Gastocamera finding on the first examination.
b. Gastrocamera finding one month after hospitalization. After the ulcer healed, it was too difficult to point out the superficial depressed carcinoma in the antrum. However, endoscopic biopsy at this scarred phase is inevitably necessary.

It is not difficult to obtain frontal views of lesions in given areas of the stomach with endoscopy (Fig. 61 d). Endoscopy should not be overrated for the observation of lesions even in the curvatures, pyloric region, or upper body.

c. Limitations in observing the existence and quality of lesions

It is sometimes difficult to diagnose whether shallow defects without rugal convergence or mucosal elevation are malignant or merely discolored. When there is a rugal convergence or mucosal elevation, the contour and the margins of the defects are clearly observed, and there are fewer difficulties in diagnosing shallow defects.

Peptic ulcers can develop in cancerous mucosa as well as normal mucosa. If they are encountered with benign gastric ulcers, the neighboring mucosa should be observed to detect cancer tissue. When benign ulcers are observed endoscopically, attention should be paid to whether there is a II c type malignancy around the ulcer. Furthermore, slight discoloration and minute mucosal roughness should be carefully observed. These may be within the limits of endoscopy.

With duplicated early cancers (Fig. 62), a triangular irregular defect is seen on the greater curvature of the antrum of the resected specimen as shown in Figure 62 a. There was a slight mucosal elevation, and the surface of the defect was rough and granulated. On the anterior wall, another II c type was seen which had no rugal convergence and a shallower almost flat surface as compared with the prepyloric lesion. The appearance of the defect and the peculiar finding of a II c type on the greater curvature, seen in the GTF picture (Figs. 62 b, c), were confirmed by gross findings of the resected specimen.

An abnormally discolored and reddened area could be observed in the picture of the anterior lesion, but it was difficult to differentiate whether the change was due to gastritis or a cancerous erosion. Diagnosis was difficult because the lesion, being so large, was only partially seen. The depression was very slight with no rugal convergence and a slight mucosal elevation. The existence of lesions was easily pointed out in the stomach barium filled (Figs. 62 d, e). The finding of a II c type on the greater curvature was well portrayed in the compression study (Fig. 62 f), as well as by endoscopy. The lesion on the anterior wall was shown in a radiograph taken with the double-contrast compression method (Figs. 62 g, h). Thin, irregular barium flecks with a granular appearance were the findings, suspicious of a II c type even though the findings were overlapped by a bone shadow.

As in this case, it is essential that when endoscopic examination is insufficient, radiological examination should supply the needed information, and vice versa. But as far as excavated lesions are concerned, the contours of the excavations should be accurately shown radiologically with reference to the endoscopic findings. In such cases, the value of biopsy becomes apparent. The lesions that are easy to find but difficult to diagnose are minimal polypoid lesions, ulcers in the malignant cycle, or III type early cancers. For instance (Fig. 63), a round ulcer was seen by the gastrocamera on the lesser curvature of the angulus. When examined by the gastrocamera after four weeks of treatment, the ulcer had diminished. It was diagnosed as a II c type early cancer. This case was operated on shortly after the second gastrocamera examination. It was a case of a malignant cycle (see Fig. 24), and a retrospectively eroded mucosa could be seen around the ulcer in the gastrocamera picture.

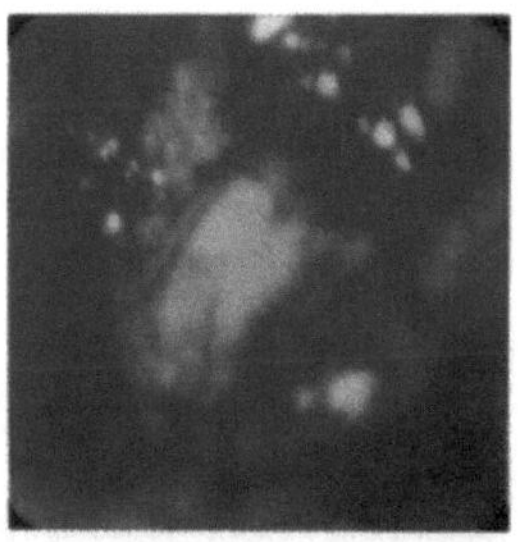

64 a

64 b

Fig. 64 a Cytological examination of an excavated lesion under direct vision.
Fig. 64 b Biopsy of a small excavated lesion under direct vision.

Perhaps initially (Fig. 63 a) acute inflammatory findings were added to the surrounding cancerous mucosa making the diagnosis difficult. It is not rare to see such findings in benign gastric ulcers. As stated previously, thinking that "these findings may be seen in benign ulcers" may lead to misdiagnoses.

d. Cytology and biopsy in diagnosing gastric lesions

When performing a biopsy on an excavated, protruding or flat lesion, the forceps must be controlled at the center of vision and must extend perpendicularly. The longer the forceps in the gastric cavity, the more difficult it is to get a mucosal particle from the target lesion.

1) Biopsy techniques for excavated lesions

Cytology and biopsy are chiefly for differential diagnosis of malignancy. For this purpose, cells and biopsy materials should be obtained from (1) the base, (2) the marginal areas of the defect, (3) the mucosa adjacent to the defect, and (4) the surrounding normal areas of the excavated lesion. Routinely, as shown in Figures 64 a, b, when the defect is rather deep and covered with thick fur, the specimens are taken from the marginal portion of the defect and from the mucosa adjacent to the defect and not from the base. On the other hand, when the defect is shallow and the base of the defect is prominent, it is necessary to take the specimen from the base.

In a small excavation, the specimen is taken directly from the base, and then from the marginal region to continue the biopsy. Cytology and the biopsies should be aimed at the discolored areas, the mat or rough surfaces and granulated portions in the area surrounding the defect.

2) Biopsy techniques for protruding lesions

For protruding lesions, the biopsy specimen must be obtained not only from the top of the protuberance but also from the stalk and the base of the lesion (Fig. 65).

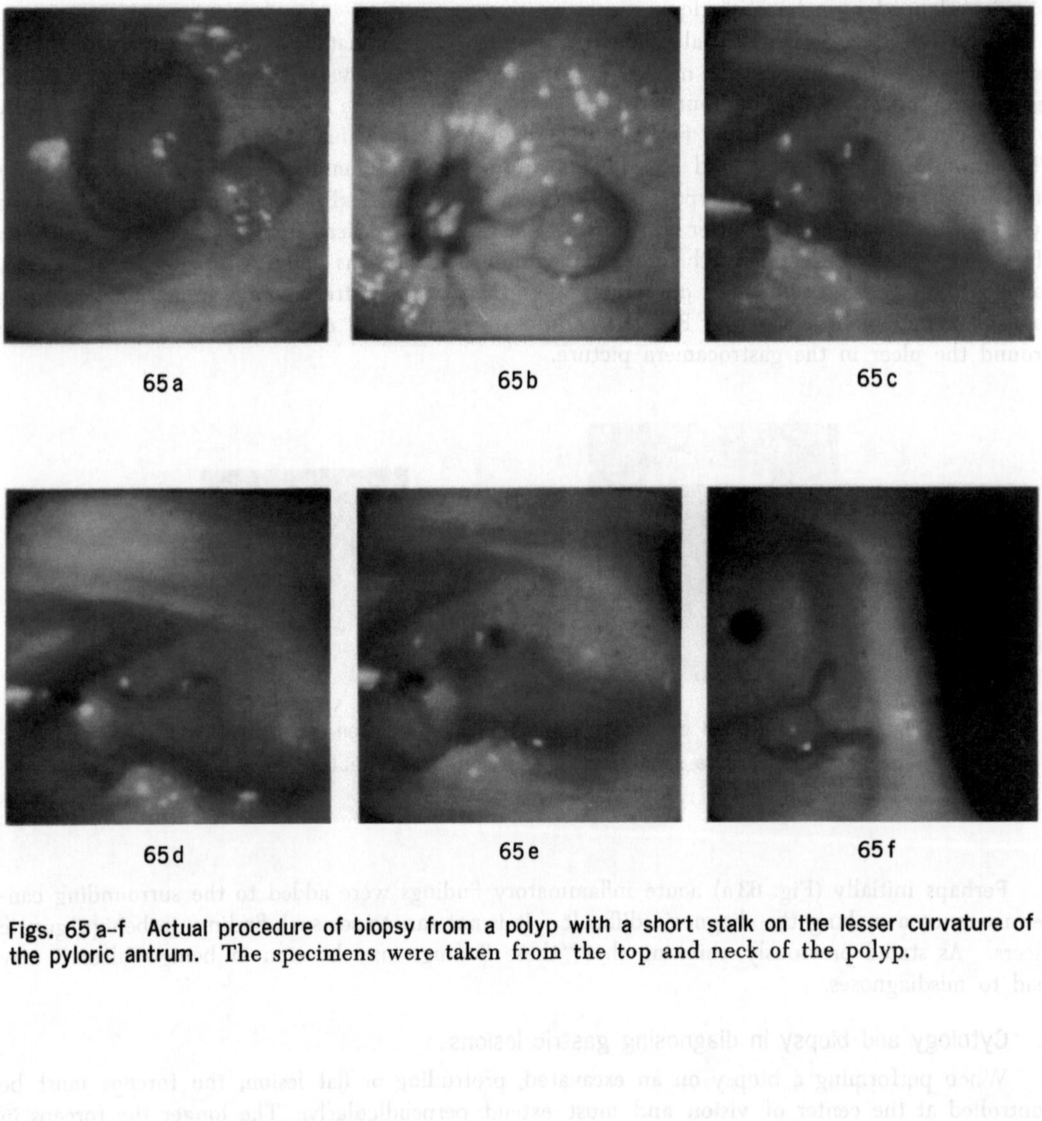

Figs. 65 a–f Actual procedure of biopsy from a polyp with a short stalk on the lesser curvature of the pyloric antrum. The specimens were taken from the top and neck of the polyp.

II. Case Presentations

Protruding type

A. Typical cases of gastric polypous lesions

1. Protruding types of advanced cancer of the stomach

a. BORRMANN I type (Fungating type)

The frequency of this type occurs in about 3 to 17 per cent of all advanced gastric cancers. Radiologically the lesion can be demonstrated as a filling defect or an intragastric tumor, which is generally huge with marked lobulated surfaces, making its diagnosis relatively easy.

Case 1

c.c.: Epigastric distress for one month.

62 year-old female.

In the radiograph of the barium filled stomach in the upright position (Fig. 66 a), a rigidity of the lesser curvature and a filling defect extended from the lower part of the corpus to the antrum. In the mucosal picture in the prone position (Fig. 66 b), a filling defect with rigidity of the gastric wall was noted on the lesser curvature. In the double-contrast study in the supine position (Figs. 66 c, d), a huge tumor shadow was found superimposed upon a few of the parallel mucosal folds of the posterior wall.

Thus, it could be reasonably concluded that the lesion was a localized tumor, circumscribed sharply from the surrounding normal mucosa and lying mainly on the anterior wall. Usually we regard a nonpedunculated tumor over 3 cm as a fungating cancer (BORRMANN I type). Further, the noticeable irregularities of the surface described as barium flecks in the radiographs made this tumor look like the fungating type of an advanced cancer.

Endoscopically (Fig. 66 e), it was a tumor protruding abruptly from the mucosa, the surface of which was nodular and covered with a pale coat. Generally the surface of this type of cancer is dirty because of a dark brown coat on the eroding, bleeding, or necrotic tissue. Macroscopically (Fig. 66 f), it was a fungating cancer, 6.5×6.0 cm in diameter, with irregularly shaped ulcers on its surface.

Histologically the cancerous tissue had invaded the muscular layer proper.

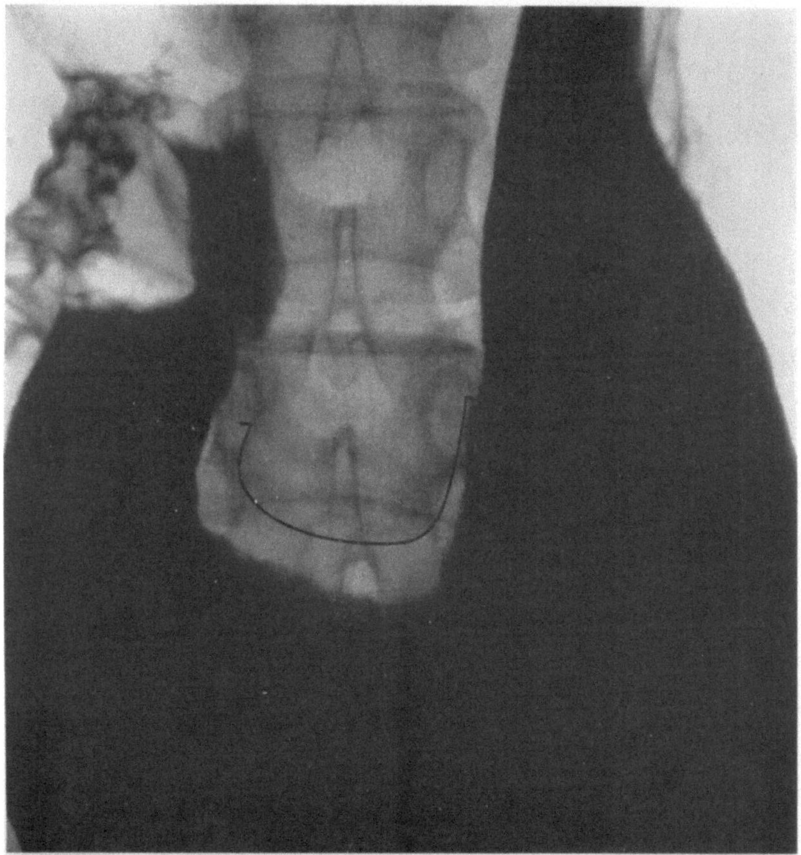

66a

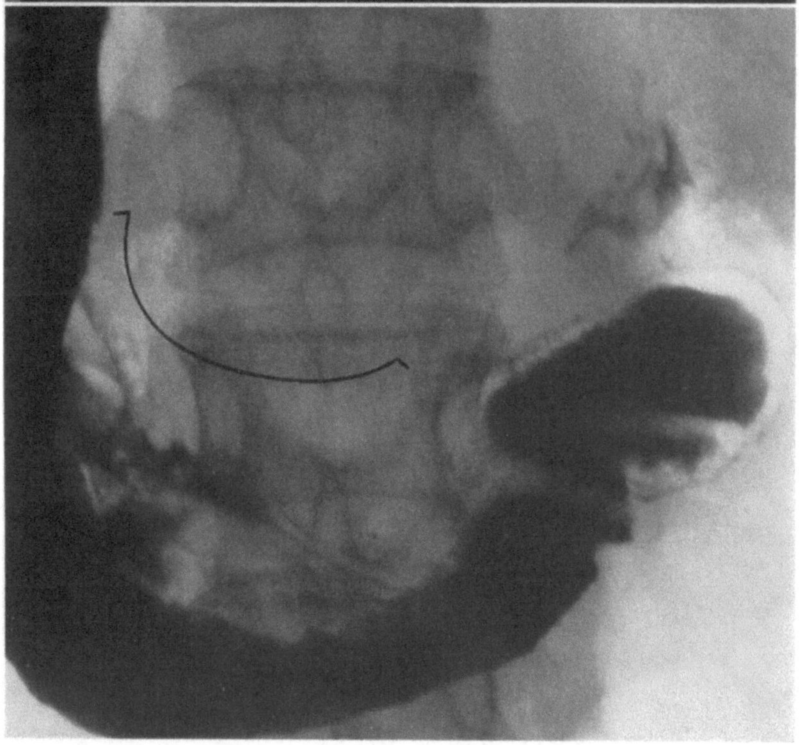

66b

Fig. 66a. Radiograph of the barium filled stomach in the upright position. The rigidity of the lesser curvature, showing a local filling defect, extends widely from the lower part of the corpus to the antrum. Also on the greater curvature of the prepyloric region filling-defect-like findings are seen, but it is impossible to distinguish whether these are really filling defects or not.

Fig. 66b. Mucosal picture in the prone position. The rigidity of the wall described in Figure 66a is seen as a huge filling defect. This filling defect may occupy the lesser curvature and the anterior wall from the lower part of the body to the antrum. The prepyloric region is well distended in this figure.

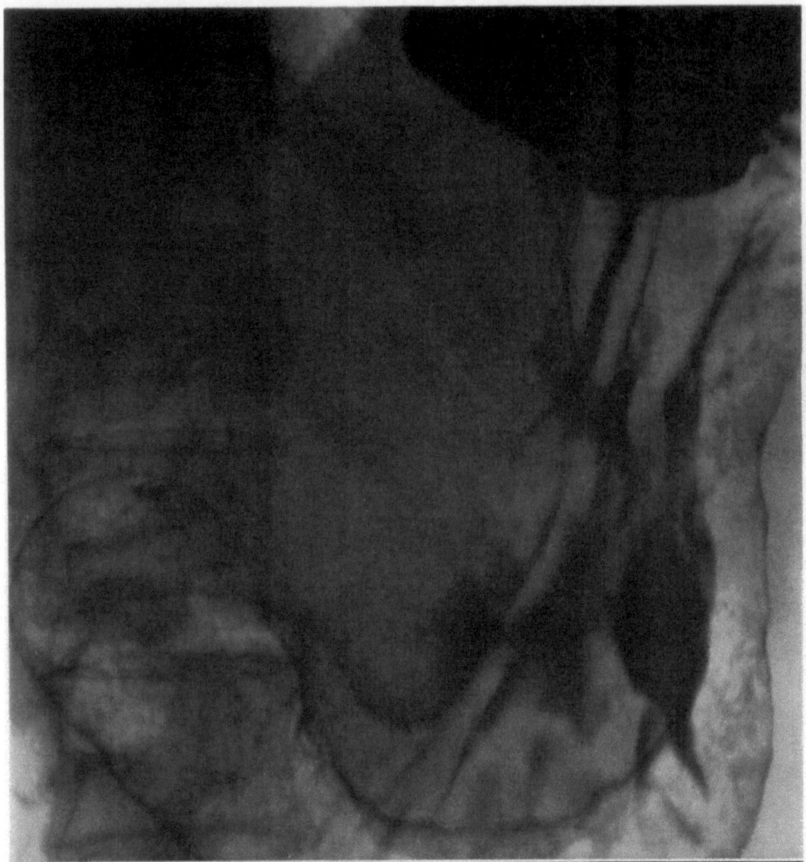

66c

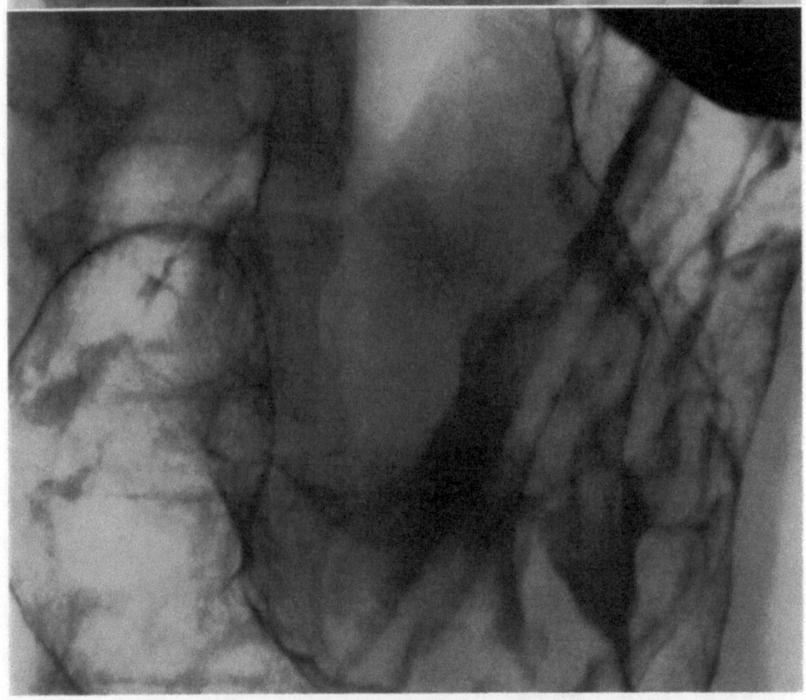

66d

Fig. 66c. Double-contrast study in the supine position. A huge filling defect, superimposed on a few of the regularly arranged mucosal folds of the posterior wall, is seen from the lower part of the body to the antrum. The lesion appears to be a localized tumor, which is mainly developing on the anterior wall and is relatively sharply circumscribed by the surrounding mucosa.

Fig. 66d. Double-contrast study in the supine position (first oblique position). The surface of the tumor shows a remarkable irregularity, so it is readily diagnosed as epithelial. Moreover, it is considered to be a fungating type of advanced cancer.

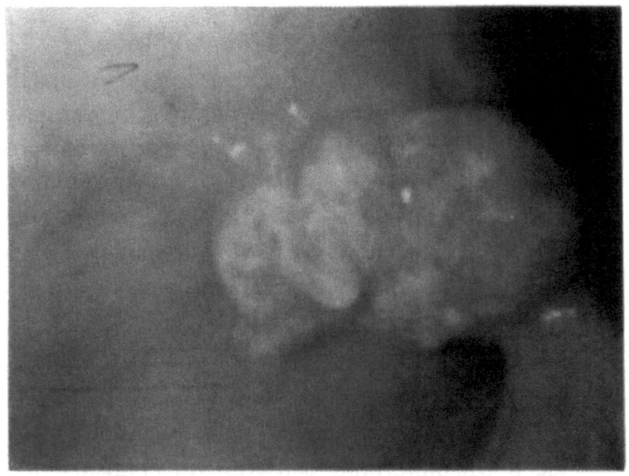

66e

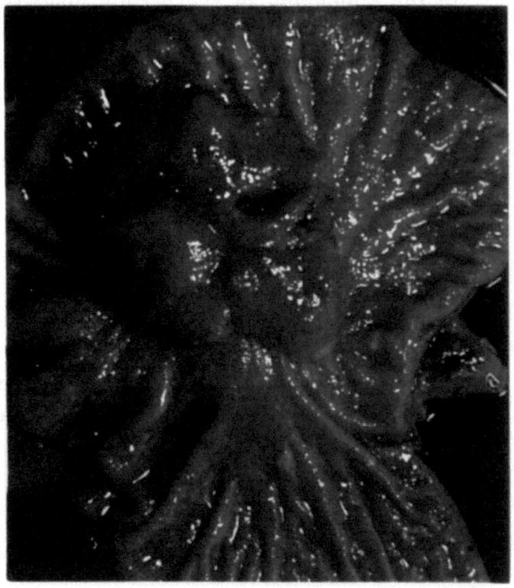

66f

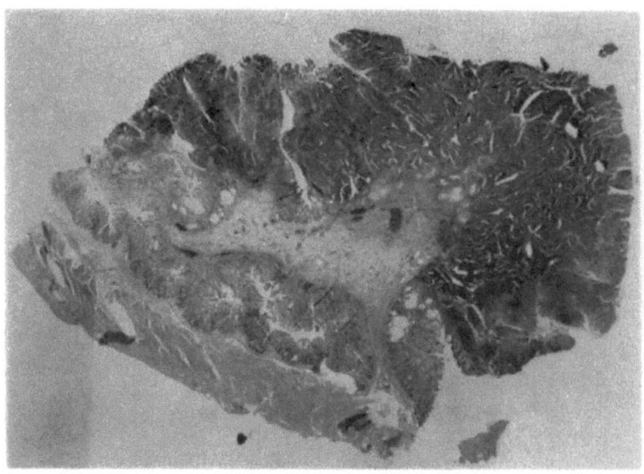

66g

Fig. 66e. Endoscopic picture. A tumor steeply protruding from the surroundings is seen on the anterior wall of the angular region. The markedly uneven surface is covered with a whitish coat in map-like patches. These findings represent a malignancy.

Fig. 66f. Resected stomach. The tumor, 6.5 × 6.0 cm in size, is seen on the anterior wall of the angular region. Its surface shows irregular ulcerations.

Fig. 66g. Histopathological findings. Histologically, cancer cells had spread all over the tumor and had infiltrated to the muscular layer proper.

b. BORRMANN II type (Ulcerating type)

Among the protruding cancers in the stomach is the Borrmann II type cancer, an irregularly shaped ulcer with marginal swellings. In our investigation, 33% of the advanced cancers belong to this type. Macroscopically the lesion is elevated like a flower bed with a large ulceration in the center, that is, a dish-like cancer. Marginal swelling is distinctly demarcated from the surrounding normal mucosa. Radiological appearance has the feature of a doughnut-shaped filling defect from the frontal view. From the profile view, however, a crescent, or so-called meniscus sign, can be observed. Carcinomatous cells are usually restricted to the bottom of the ulceration.

Case 2

c.c.: Uncomfortable sensation in epigastrium.

56 year-old male.

In the radiograph of the barium filled stomach in the upright position (Fig. 67 a) no particular change was noted except a slight rigidity in the angular region. However, in the double-contrast study, in the supine position (Fig. 67 b) and the right oblique position (Fig. 67 c), an irregularly shaped ulcer surrounded by a marginal swelling was detected on the posterior wall of the lower part of the body. The lesser curvature side of this protrusion had been slightly destroyed. On the other hand, in the compression studies (Figs. 67 d, e), the doughnut-shaped marginal swelling did not disappear even under a fairly strong compression, so the protrusion was believed to be high and rigid.

Endoscopically (Fig. 67 f), an irregularly shaped ulcer with an uneven bottom could be seen within the low marginal swelling. Histopathological examination of the resected specimen (Fig. 67 g), revealed the cancerous infiltration extending to the subserosal layer.

Since the narrow marginal swellings surrounding the large ulceration are pathognomonic for cancers of the BORRMANN II type, its diagnosis is relatively easy. The marginal swelling in a cancer of the BORRMANN III type also protrudes. but is at least partially broken away.

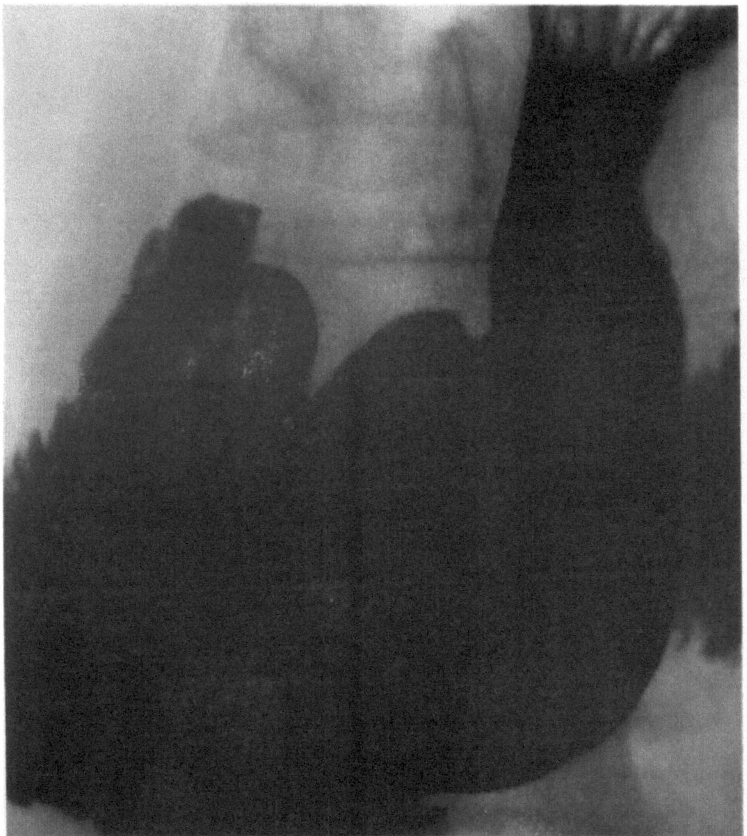

67 a

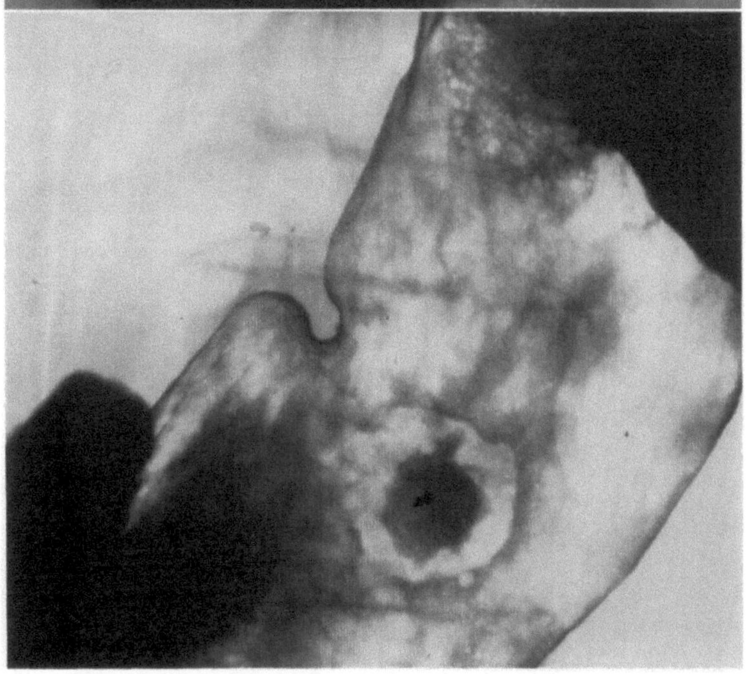

67 b

Fig. 67 a. Radiograph of the barium filled stomach in the upright position. There is no remarkable change except a slight deformity of the angular region.

Fig. 67 b. Double-contrast study in the supine position. An irregularly shaped, considerably deep niche is detected on the posterior wall of the angular region. The niche is clearly circumscribed by a rigid marginal swelling, but it is difficult to estimate the height of the swelling by this figure alone.

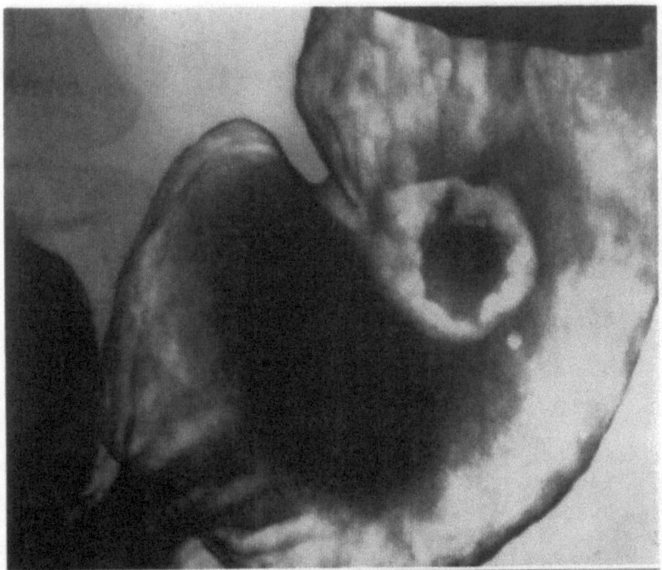

67c

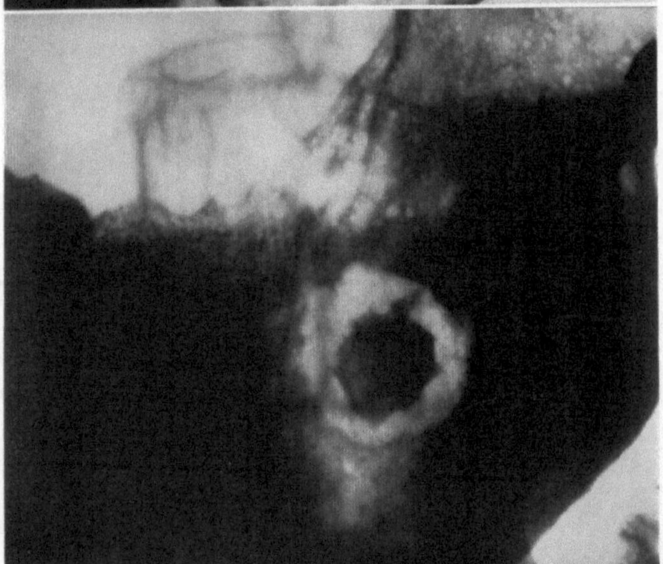

67d

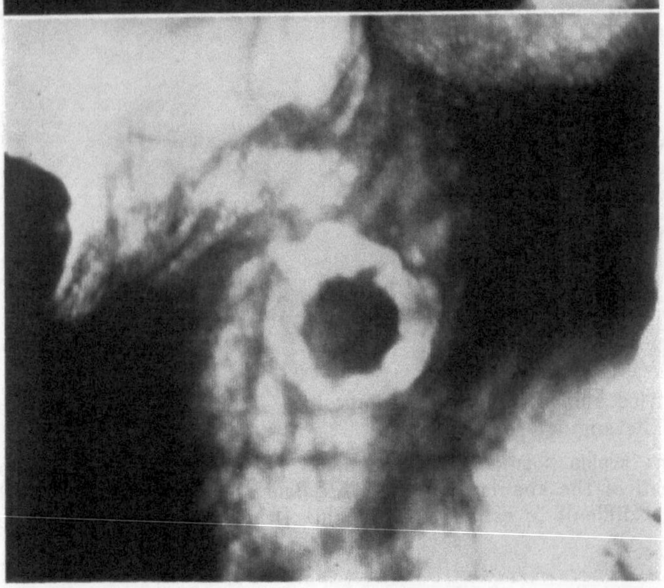

67e

Fig. 67c. Double-contrast study in the supine position. By making use of the effect of thin layers of a barium meal, the lesion on the posterior wall of the angular region is observed. As seen in this figure and Figs. 67d, e, the marginal swelling surrounding the crater pushes away barium, which shows the extensive height of the swelling.

Fig. 67d. Compression study.

Fig. 67e. Compression study. On strong compression, the marginal swelling did not disappear.

67 f

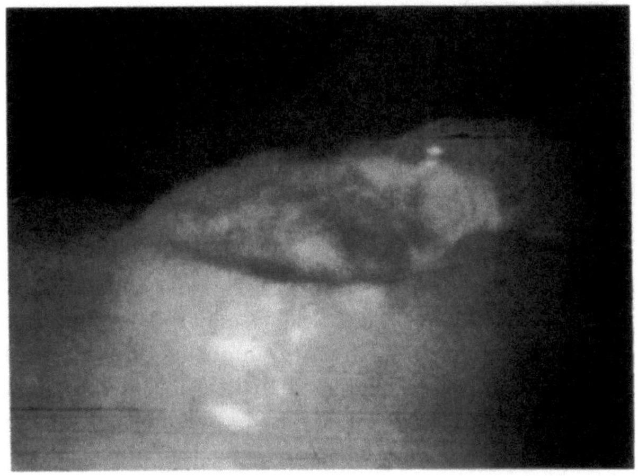

67 g

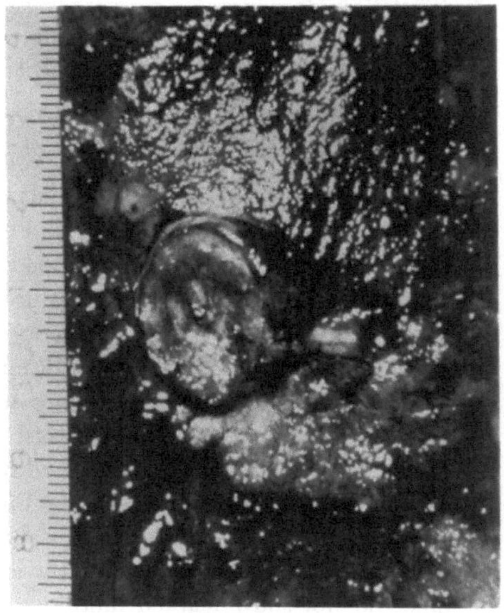

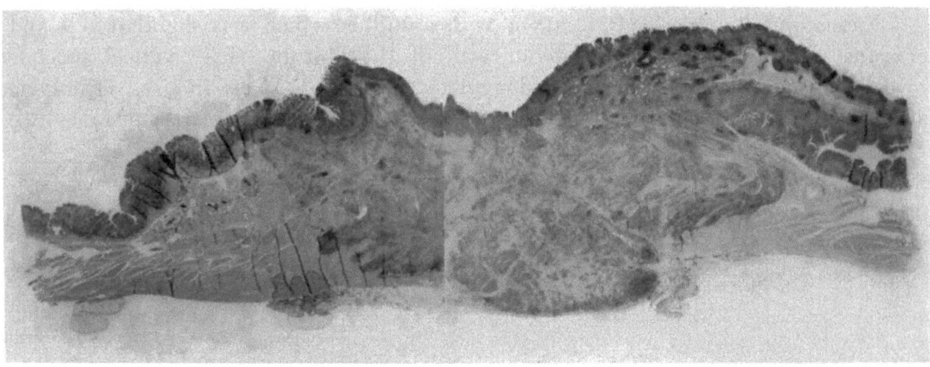

67 h

Fig. 67 f Endoscopic picture. An irregularly shaped, white-coated ulcer of which the bottom is markedly uneven is surrounded by a marginal swelling independent of the mucosal fold.

Fig. 67 g Resected stomach.

Fig. 67 h Histopathological findings. Histologically the cancer infiltrates expansively to the subserosal layer in the region showing the mucosal depression. The horizontal invasion of cancer cells, however, is relatively circumscribed.

2. Protruding types of early gastric cancer

a. Type I (Protruding type) early gastric cancer

As stated before, the type I early gastric cancer has been defined as one in which the cancerous tissue is localized only in the protrusion itself, without infiltration to the muscular layer proper. Even when radiographs give good descriptions of the outline of the lesion, it is very difficult to differentiate this type from an advanced cancer.

Thus far, there have been many reports concerning differential diagnoses of gastric polypous lesions. As mentioned above, YAMADA stated that cancer was not encountered in the following cases: type IV polypoid lesions under 2 cm in diameter, type III lesions under 1.0 cm, or type II lesions under 0.5 cm. Also in our investigation, cancer was found neither in pedunculated polypoid lesions under 2 cm in diameter nor nonpedunculated lesions under 1 cm. HAY and CARLSON have reported that broad-based, polypoid lesions over 2 cm in diameter with uneven, dark-red surfaces can be suspected of being cancerous.

Malignant changes of benign polyps of the stomach are discussed here from the standpoint of the pathologist and of the endoscopist observing the processes of polypoid lesions.

Case 3

c.c.: Epigastric discomfort for half a year.

62 year-old female.

The radiograph of the barium filled stomach in the upright position (Fig. 68 a) exhibited a slight irregularity on the lesser curvature of the antrum.

In the mucosal picture in the prone position (Fig. 68 b), however, a walnut-sized, irregular tumor was noted on the antrum. It must be emphasized that a mucosal picture was essential for the diagnosis of protruding lesions of the stomach.

Furthermore, in the double-contrast study in the supine position (Fig. 68 c), this tumor was described as a definite filling defect with a clover-shaped barium fleck on the surface which corresponded to the irregular shadow in Figure 68 b.

Thus, this tumor with a short stalk protruded like an unfolded umbrella. As seen in the double-contrast studies in the slightly left lateral position (Fig. 68 d), the tumor, though having a stalk, did not show marked motility.

In the compression study (Fig. 68 e), a shallow barium fleck was noted on top of the tumor. This probably represented an ulceration of the surface of the tumor.

Endoscopically (Fig. 68 f), a tumor with a surface which was slightly rough and spotted with erosions was observed on the anterior wall of the antrum. The surgical specimen (Fig. 68 g) revealed a tumor of the spherical, pedunculated type, 3.5×3.5 cm in size. Histologically, this was a well-differentiated adenocarcinoma partially invading the muscularis mucosae (Fig. 68 h).

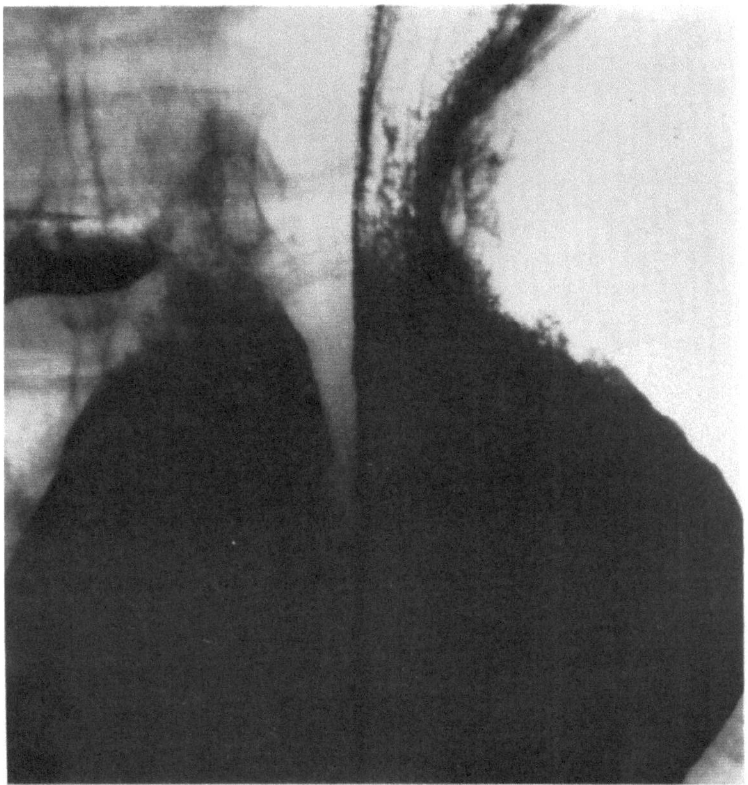

68 a

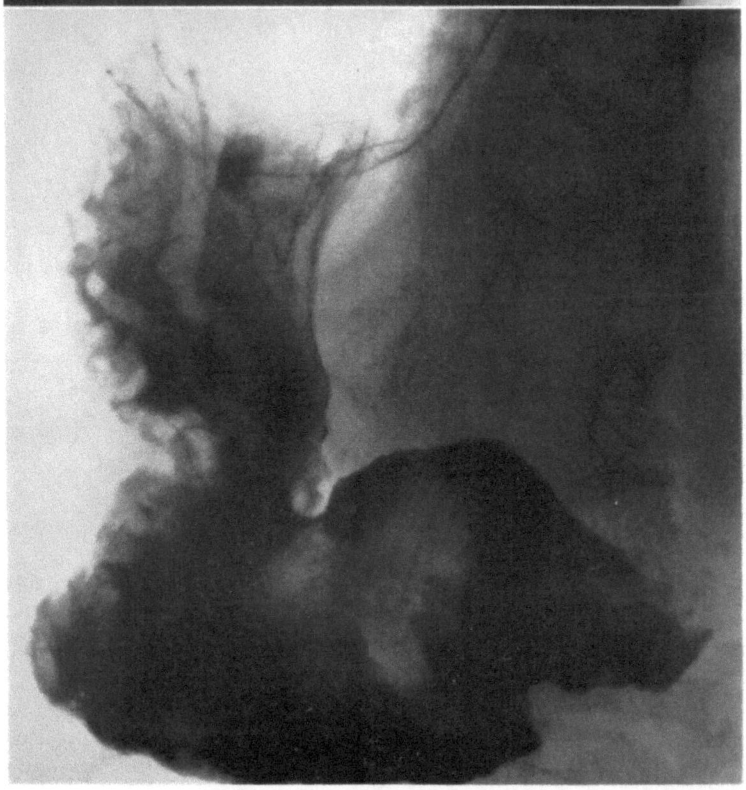

68 b

Fig. 68 a Radiograph of the barium filled stomach in the upright position. There is no particular change except a slight irregularity on the lesser curvature of the antrum.

Fig. 68 b Mucosal study in the prone position. A walnut-sized filling defect is detected on the antrum. Mucosal pictures with a small amount of barium meal are often effective for the diagnosis of protruding lesions of the stomach.

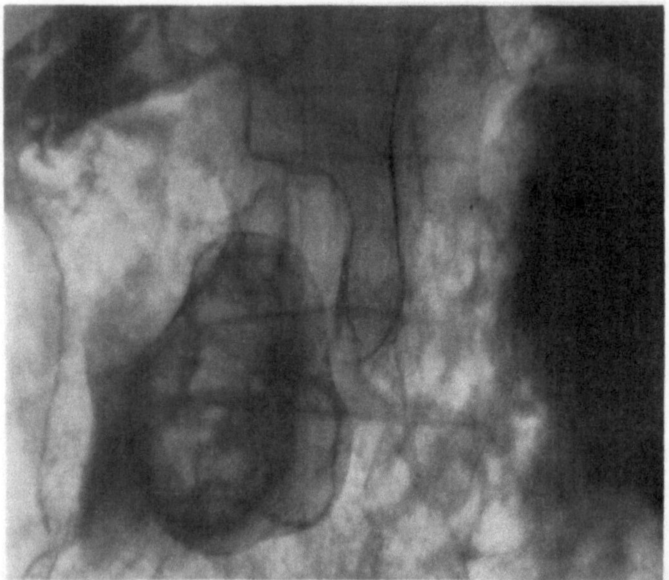

68 c

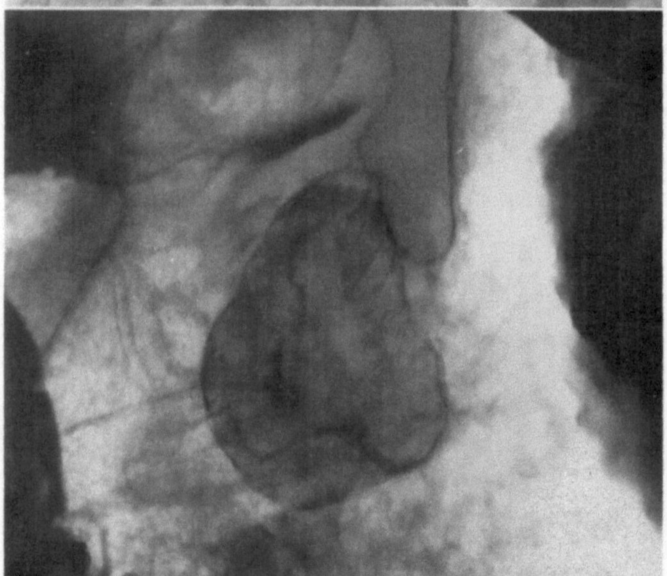

68 d

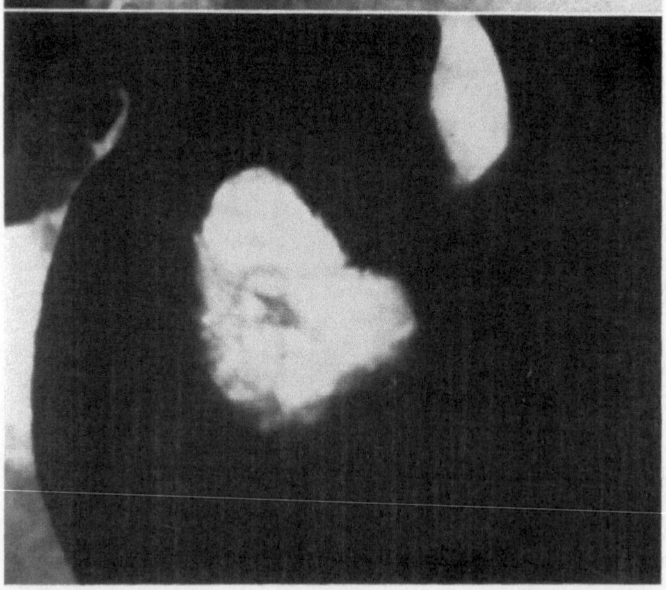

68 e

Fig. 68 c Double-contrast study in the supine position. A walnut-sized tumor is noted on the antrum. The double-contrast method makes minute markings on the surface of the tumor clear. A tortous shadow overlapping the tumor shadow represents the stalk of the protrusion.

Fig. 68 d Double-contrast study in the supine position (right oblique position). The stalk is more pronounced.

Fig. 68 e Compression study. The irregular mucosal surface of the tumor is more distinct.

68 f

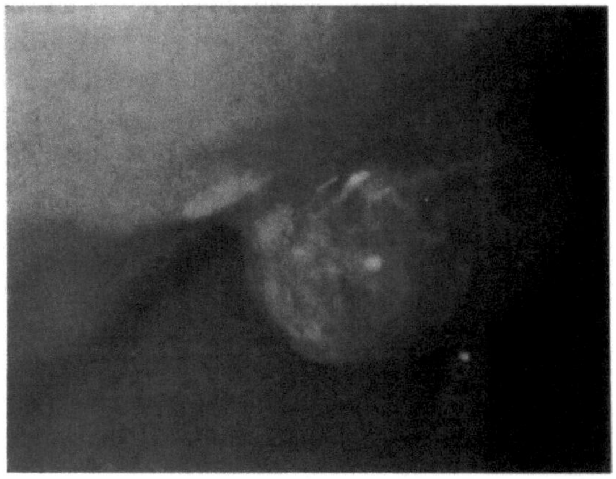

68 g

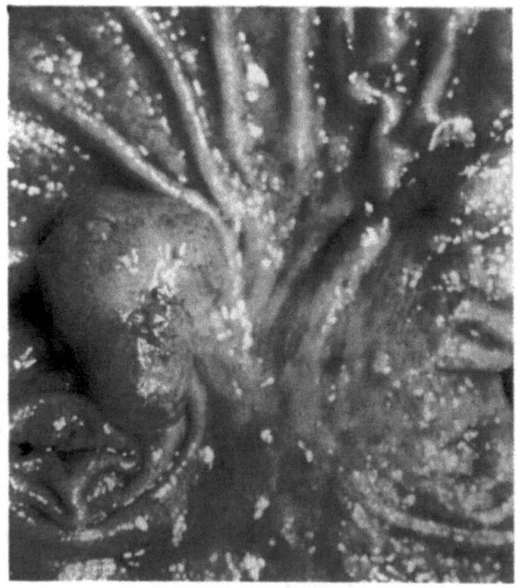

68 h

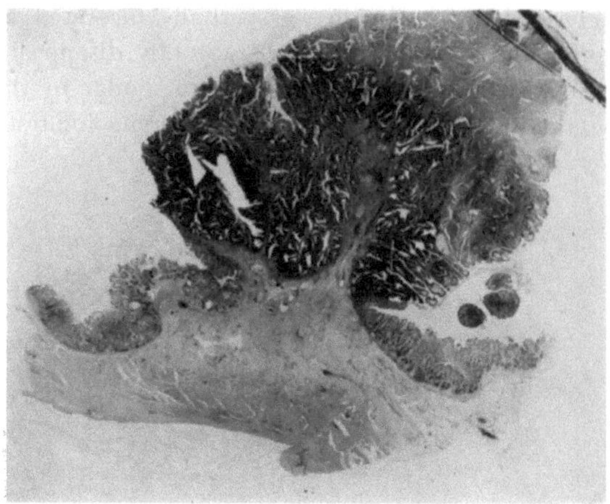

Fig. 68 f Endoscopic picture. A tumor with slight bleeding and adherent mucus protrudes abruptly from its surroundings on the anterior wall of the antrum. From these findings, this tumor is suspected of being cancerous.

Fig. 68 g Resected stomach. A protruding lesion, 3.5×3.5 cm in size, of the spherical, pedunculated type is observed. Its surface is rough and shows a slight erosion on the top.

Fig. 68 h Histopathological findings. An adenocarcinoma is revealed which partially infiltrates the muscularis mucosae.

b. Type IIa (Superficial elevated) early gastric cancer

This type of early gastric cancer is macroscopically unsuitable for inclusion in YAMADA's classification of protruding lesions. We have added another category for protruding lesions with mucosal irregularities, the so-called "disk" or "parterre" type. The disk type of tumor shows as its profile a "sake-cup" figure protruding from the surrounding mucosal surface at an acute or right angle, and the frontal view shows an oval or chrysanthemum form.

Recently many cases of early gastric cancer have been discovered in aged people showing nonacidity or hypoacidity in their gastric juice. Our attention has been attracted to their relationship to atypical epithelia. Having investigated 78 cases of operated stomachs with protruding lesions, we discovered that the disk type tends to be malignant, with or without a central depression. It is a fact, however, that few of the benign mucosal hyperplasias are included in this type. Therefore, histological examinations using biopsy methods are necessary for the differentiation of malignant lesions from benign ones.

Case 4

c. c.: Dullness in her epigastric region.

66 year-old female.

Both radiographs of the barium filled stomach exhibited nothing in particular from the cardiac to the pyloric region (Figs. 69 a and b), but in the supine, double-contrast study (Fig. 69 c), a thumb-head-sized mucosal irregularity was seen on the posterior wall of the antrum.

Without adequate care, this irregularity would be overlooked in a general radiographic examination. In the supine, double-contrast study of the first projection (Fig. 69 d), a slightly elevated lesion with a rough mucosal surface was markedly demonstrated. If barium sufficiently adhered to the mucosal surface as in Figure 69 e, a "parterre" type of elevated lesion, *i. e.*, a group of polypoid prominences, might be suspected. With different degrees of pressure (Fig. 69 f), the irregular shape of the elevated lesion with rough surfaces could be sharply demarcated from the surrounding mucosa. When the lesion was firmed pressed, its border disappeared (Fig. 69 g). This lesion was shown to be a "parterre" type or a slightly elevated protrusion.

Endoscopically, there was observed on the posterior wall of the antrum an elevated lesion with a rough and irregular surface, *i. e.*, a group of small polypoid prominences without stalks (Fig. 69 h). The lesion was partially ulcerated and dirty. Mucosal folds coming from the posterior and the pyloric regions abruptly disappeared at the borders of the lesion. In the operated stomach, macroscopic findings were similar to those of endoscopy (Fig. 69 i). Histologically, it was a well-differentiated adenocarcinoma infiltrating into the submucosal layer.

69a

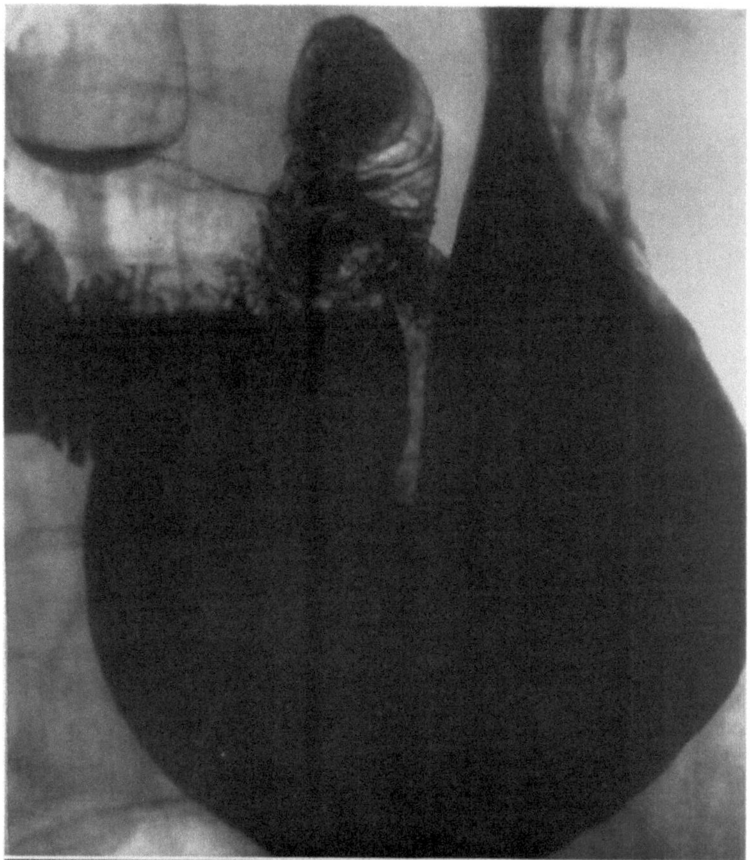

69b

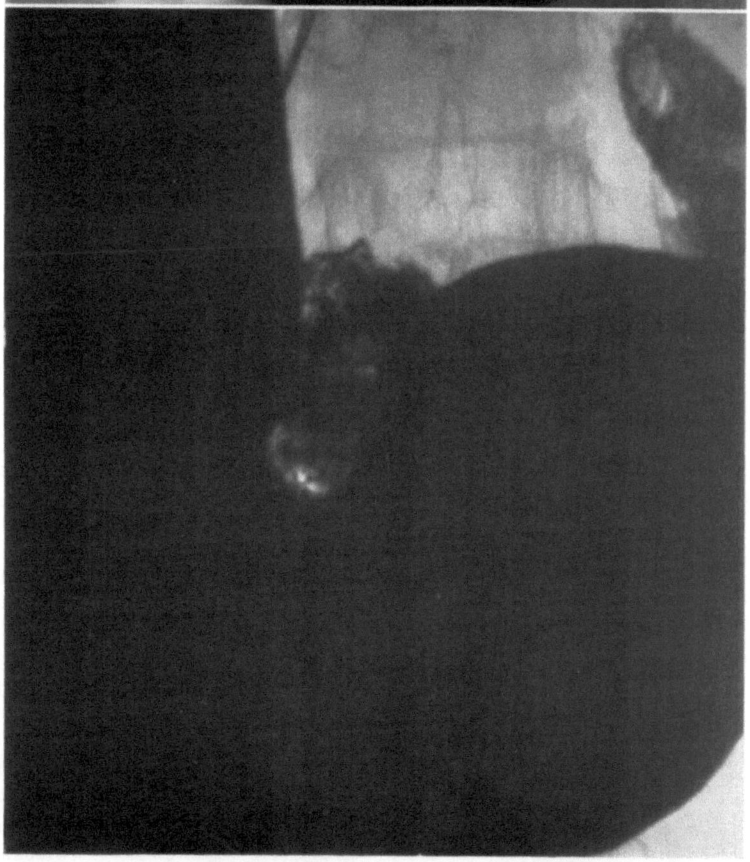

Fig. 69a Upright, filled study.

Fig. 69b Prone, filled study. In both filled pictures, nothing unusual can be seen.

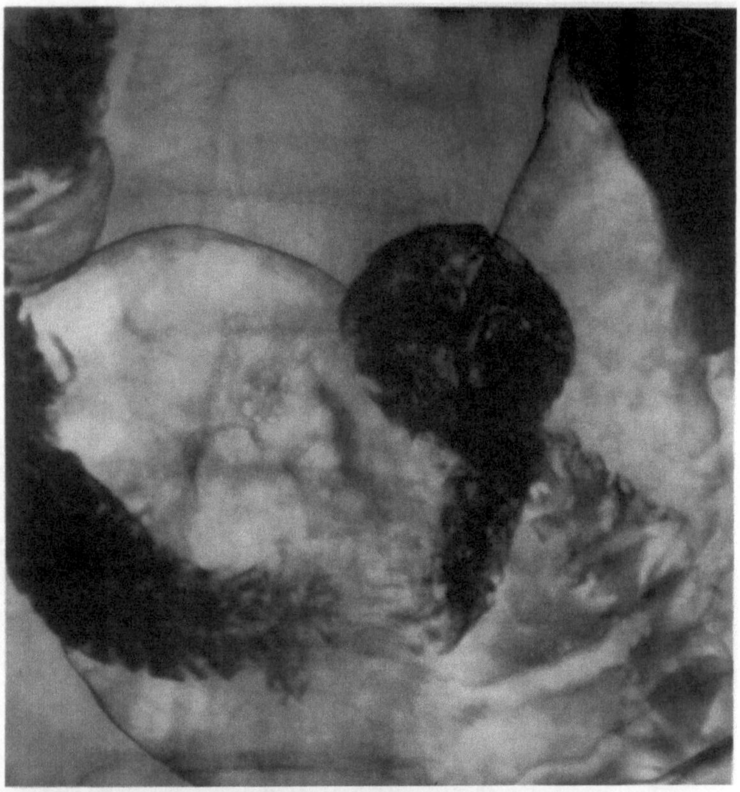

69c

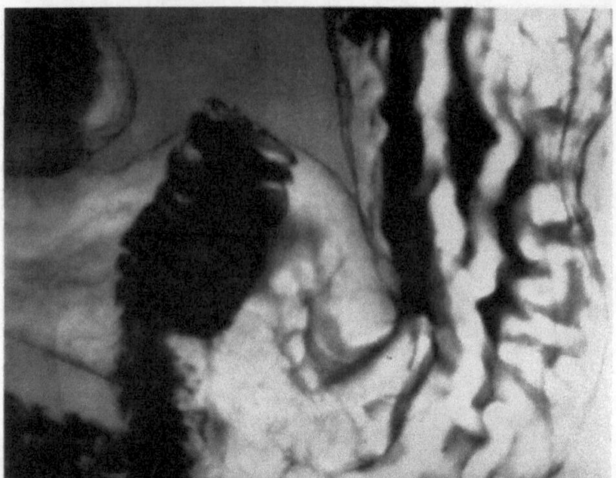

69d

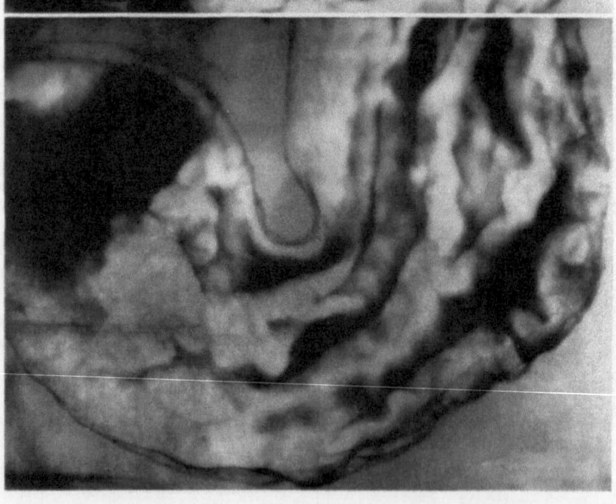

69e

Fig. 69c Supine, double-contrast study. A prominence consisting of several knotted granules is demonstrated at the posterior wall of the antrum. In this picture, the fine structure of the surface is not clearly shown because of insufficient adherence of the barium to the mucosal surfaces.

Fig. 69d Supine, double-contrast study in the right oblique projection. If the volume of air is decreased so that the mucosal folds may be demonstrated, the tubercle can be seen on the posterior wall of the antrum.

Fig. 69e Supine, double-contrast study in the right oblique projection. On the posterior wall of the antrum, a tubercle with a rough surface is markedly demonstrated.

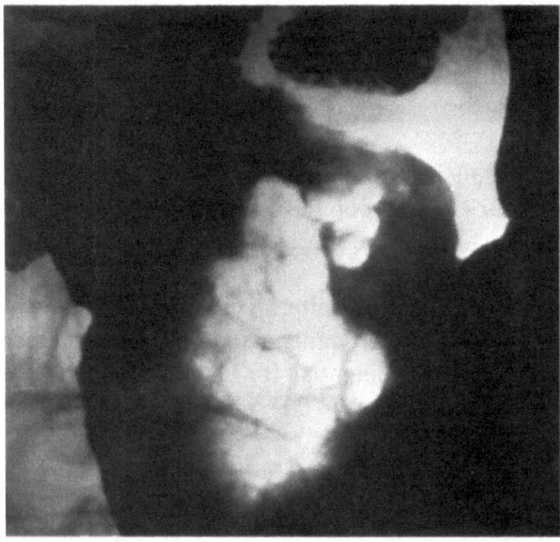

69f

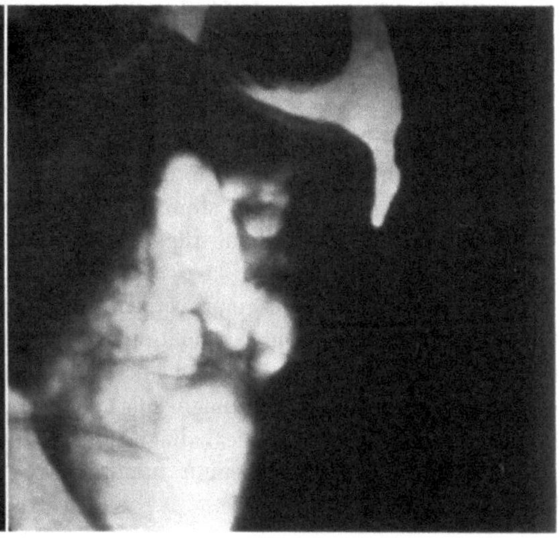

69g

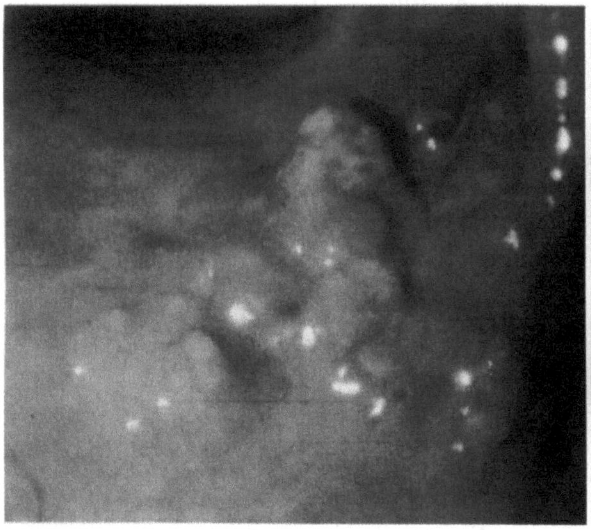

69h

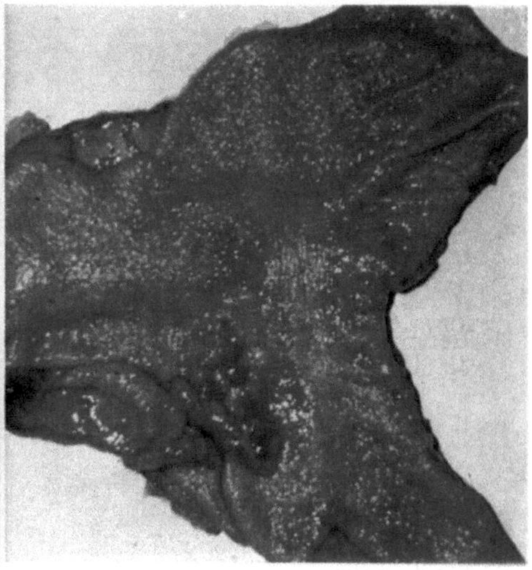

69i

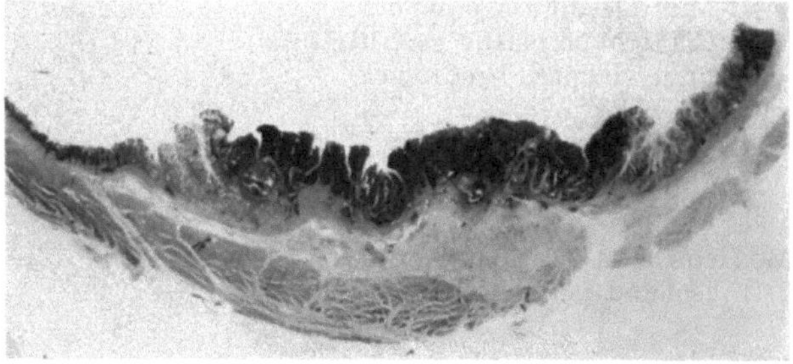

69j

Fig. 69f Compression study. The prominence, with its rough and knotted surface is markedly separated from the surrounding hyperplastic mucosal changes, is observed with a change of pressure.

Fig. 69h Endoscopic picture. On the posterior wall of the antrum, there is a tuberculous prominence with mucus. From the shape and the color of its surface, it is diagnosed as a type IIa early gastric cancer.

Fig. 69i Resected stomach. Macroscopic findings are similar to the endoscopic findings.

Fig. 69j Histopathological findings. Histologically the lesion is a well-differentiated adenocarcinoma, partly infiltrating the submucosal layer.

3. Gastric epithelial, benign tumor (Gastric polyp)

The frequency of gastric tumors has been reported to be 22.9% (STEWART) and 25.8% (RIGLER) in autopsy cases, 1.3% (EUSTERMAN) and 2% (KIRKLIN) in resected stomachs, and 0.07% (MASON) in roentgenographic observations.

In our country, it has been reported that the frequency of nonneoplastic tumors is about 3.7% of all cases of resected stomach, according to OI's report obtained from operated cases in 93 main hospitals throughout the country. Sixty-three and two-tenths per cent of them are gastric polyps.

However, with recent improvements in the x-ray apparatus as well as technical advances with the progress of endoscopic examinations, the frequency of gastric prominences has greatly increased. Furthermore, with the marked advances of clinical diagnostic potential for small gastric lesions, we cannot be content with diagnosing them as gastric polyps. We are obliged to get further information for a basic clinical diagnostic technique.

Gastric epithelial and benign tumors have been classified differently by many authors, as follows:

KATSCH's Classification
1) Adenoma
2) Tumor villosus
3) Adenopapilloma

PALMER's Classification
1) Simple adenomas
   a. Isolated adenomas
   b. Part of generalized gastrointestinal adenomatosis
2) Hyperplastic adenoma of atrophic gastritis
   a. Circumscribed adenomas
   b. Diffuse polypoid
3) Heterotopic adenomas
   a. Aberrant pancreatic tumors
   b. Brunneriomas
4) Benign argentaffinomas
5) Compound forms
   a. Undifferentiated adenomyomas
   b. Inflammatory fibroid polyps

CARLSON's Classification
1) Single polyp
2) Multiple isolated polyps
3) Multiple diffuse polypoid
4) Giant hyperplastic gastritis
5) PEUTZ-JEGHERS syndrome

EKLÖF's Classification
1) Single
2) Multiple
3) Polyposis

MONACO's Classification
1) Isolated polyps (number 1–10)
2) Localized polyps (number 50–100)
3) Diffuse polyposis

EVANS & MING's Classification
1) Adenomatous polyp
2) Regenerative polyp

MATSUMOTO & OOTA's Classification
1) Hamartomatous polyp
2) Hyperplascogenic polyp
3) Solid inflammatory polyp

NAKAYAMA's Classification
1) Fibro-adenoma
2) Hyperplastic mucosa (adenomatous, inflammatory)
3) Transitional type

SANKI's Classification
1) Fibro-adenoma
2) Adenomatous hyperplasia
3) Inflammatory hyperplasia
4) Transitional type

NAKAMURA's Classification
1) Adenomatous epithelial type
2) Regenerative epithelial type
3) Intestinal metaplasial type

SCHINDO's Classification
1) Gastric epithelial type
2) Colonic epithelial type
3) Small intestinal epithelial type
4) Adenomatous type
5) Atypical epithelial type
6) Carcinomatous polyp

Either macroscopically or microscopically, gastric benign tumors have been classifed in many ways. A clinically convenient classification is desired.

a. Hyperplastic polyps

The term hyperplastic polyp is used in the case of a macroscopic, low protruding lesion when there is a localized proliferation of the surface epithelium and a prolongation of the gastric foveolae, but no evidence of an adenomatous structure microscopically. Berg has reported that adenomatous structures are connected to gastric glands in gastric hyperplasia, but are not so in adenomatous polyps.

According to Muto's report, adenomatous polyps have been characterized by the following factors: 1) prolongation, kinking, and cystic dilatation of gastric pits; 2) hyperplasia and cystic formation of gastric glands (fundic or pyloric glands); 3) proliferation of gland structures caused by an increasing production of gastric pit-like gland structures and pink ducts; 4) branch or loop formation of productive gland structures; 5) an interstitial edema, production of new capillary blood vessels, and round cell infiltration.

The prominence caused mainly by prolongation or kinking of gastric glands is also encountered in focal hyperplasias. This is a histological characteristic of hyperplastic polyps. Although a focal hyperplasia can be differentiated from an adenomatous polyp because of the absence of a production of gland structures, the former can clinically be considered as a precursor to adenomatous polyps.

Questions still remain as to whether a hyperplastic polyp is caused by an inflammatory gland proliferation or a tumorous proliferation, and what percentage of focal hyperplasia develops into an adenomatous polyp.

Evans and Ming have called this hyperplastic polyp a regenerative polyp.

Case 5

c. c.: Epigastric pain and stiffness.
39 year-old female.

In the upright (Fig. 70 a) and prone (Fig. 70 b) filled studies, nothing in particular could be seen. As seen in this upright filled study, however, the remaining air in the antral portion was suspicious. In this case, after getting the patient to assume a prone position and having let the remaining air go to the fornix or the duodenum, we made her stand up. By this technique, we could easily take excellent upright, filled photographs.

In the supine, double-contrast study (Fig. 70 c), a spherical protruding lesion without a stalk, measuring 0.8×0.7 cm in size, was demonstrated on the greater curvature of the antrum. On radiographs after applying the proper compression (Figs. 70 d and e), the protruding lesion did not seem to be so elevated. Because of its sharply demarcated border, it was radiographically diagnosed as an epithelial tumor. An epithelial tumor can easily be differentiated from a non-epithelial one by observing the shape roentgenographically. Almost all of the flat type of protruding lesions are submucosal tumors.

Endoscopically (Fig. 70 f), a reddish prominence on the greater curvature of the antrum could be seen. According to the relation between the size of the protruding lesion and the cancer as stated before, this lesion could be diagnosed as benign.

In the resected stomach (Fig. 70 g), we found a flat, disk type of protruding lesion sharply demarcated from the surrounding mucosal surface. Histologically (Fig. 70 h), this tumor was shown to be a hyperplasia of the gastric pits.

70a

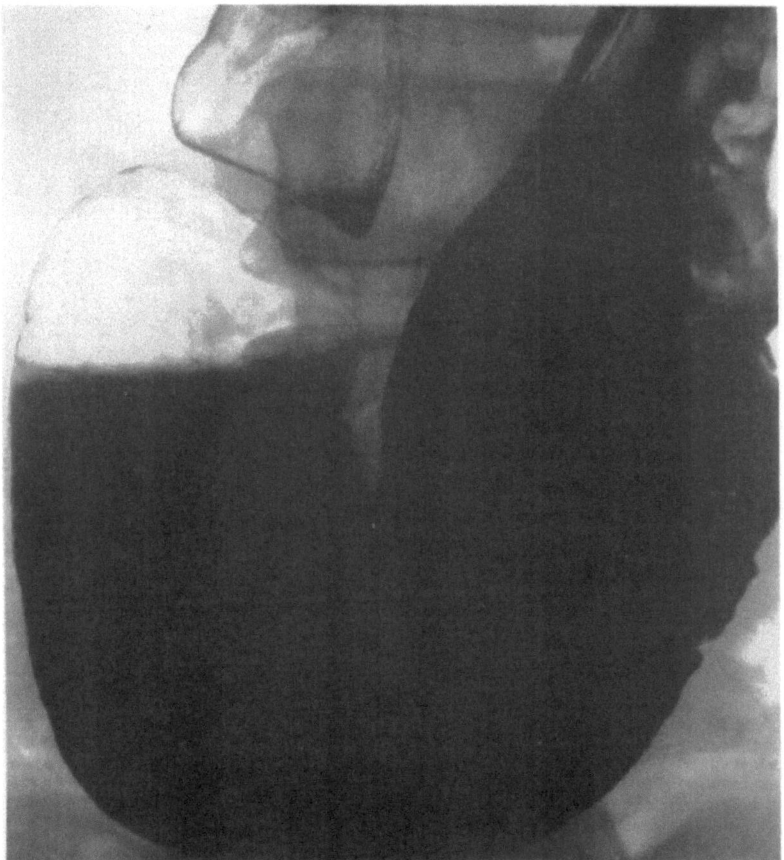

70b

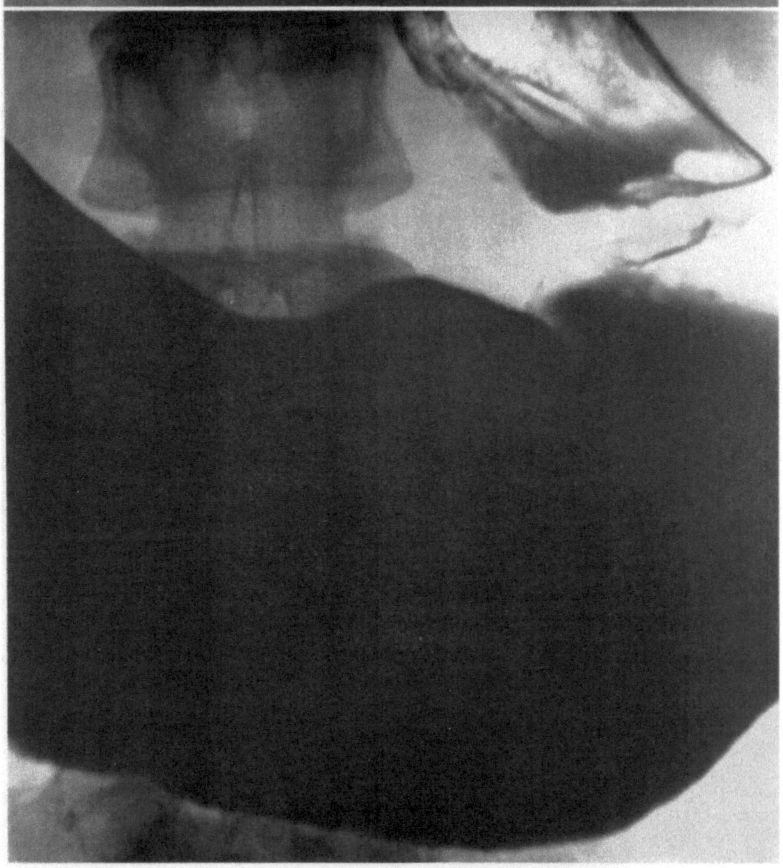

Fig. 70a Upright, radiographs of the barium filled stomach. In the prepyloric portion, the remaining air must be removed.

Fig. 70b Prone, radiographs of the barium filled stomach. Nothing unusual can be seen.

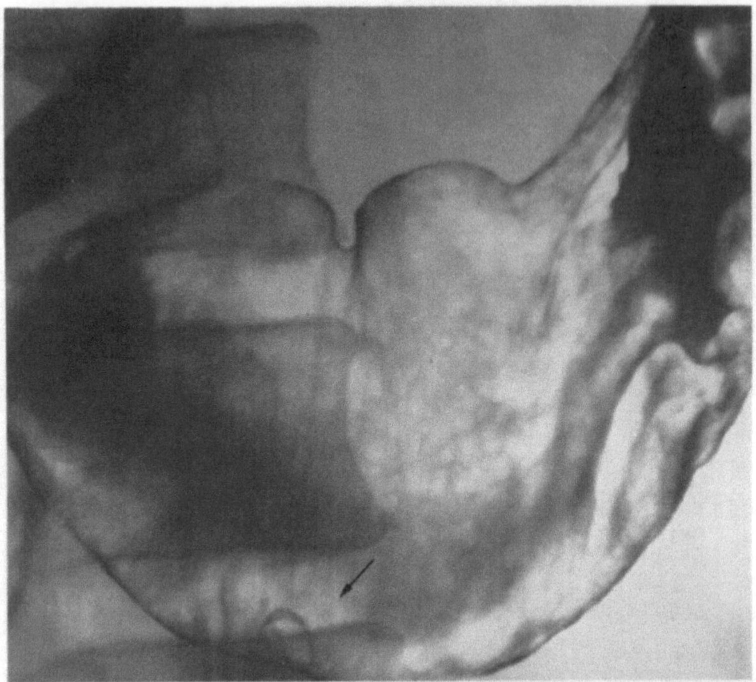

70c

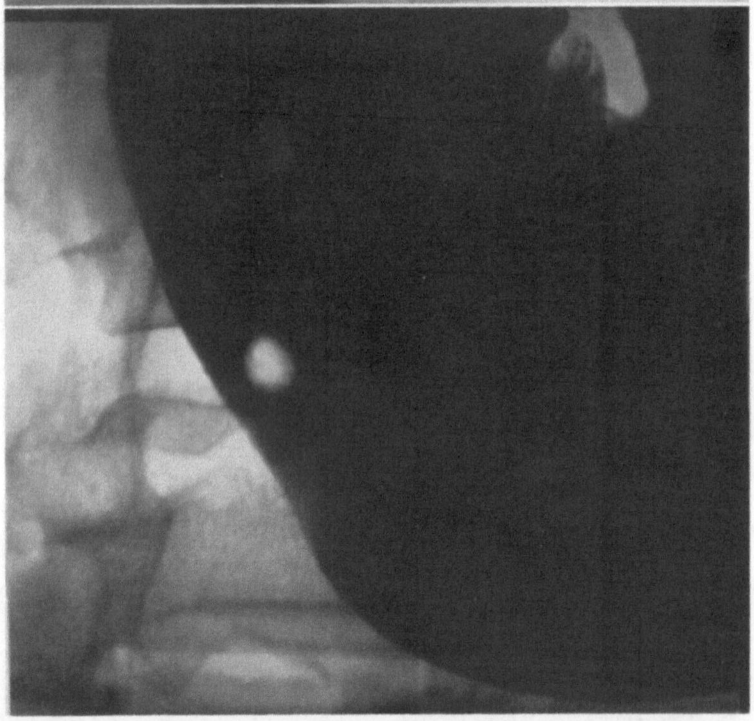

70d

Fig. 70c Supine, double-contrast study. On the greater curvature of the antrum, a small round protruding lesion with a smooth surface, measuring 0.8×0.7 cm in size, is demonstrated.

Fig. 70d Radiograph taken with sufficient compression. The fine structures of the lesion become clear with a compression study.

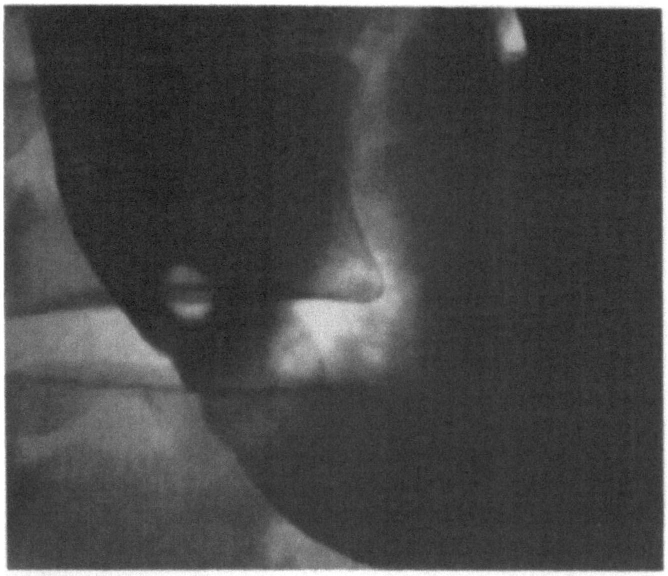

70e

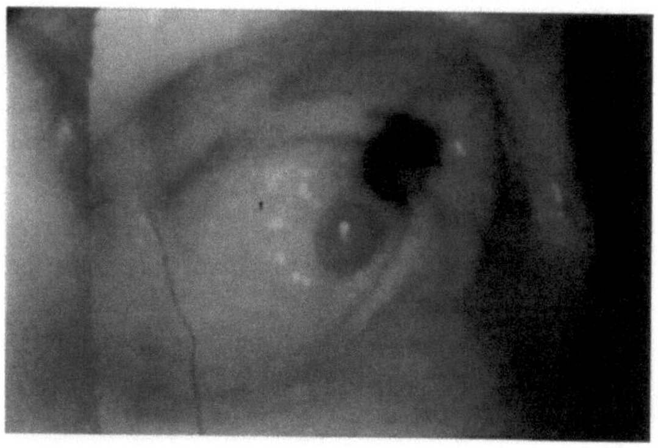

70f

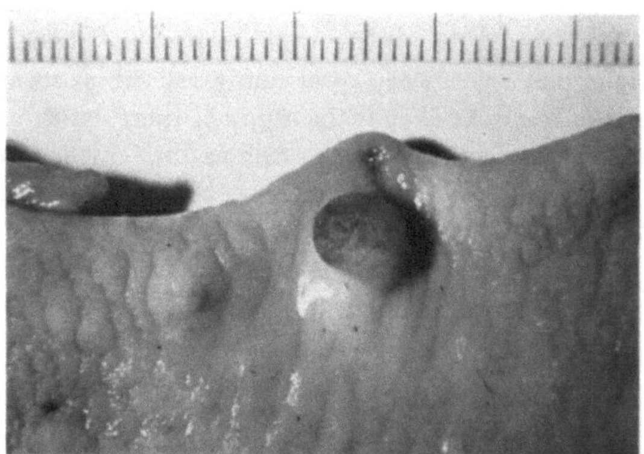

70g

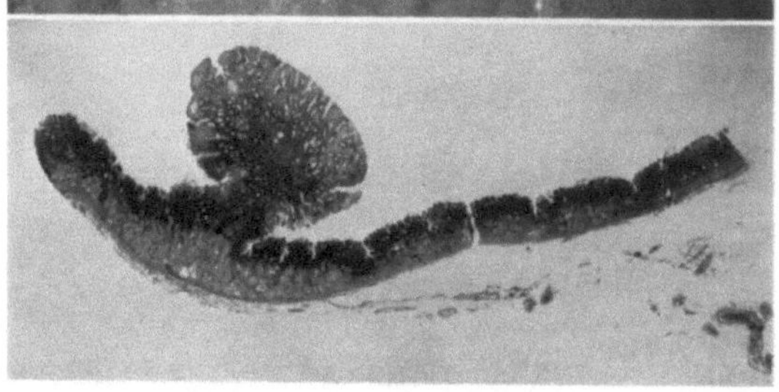

70h

Fig. 70e Radiograph taken with proper compression. The proper compression method should be used to take sufficient pictures to demonstrate the surrounding mucosal surface as well as the lesion.

Fig. 70f Endoscopic picture. On the greater curvature of the antrum, a round, reddish polypoid prominence with smooth surfaces is demonstrated. It was diagnosed as a benign epithelial tumor from its shape, size, and color.

Fig. 70g Resected stomach. A disk type of a spherical protruding lesion which is sharply demarcated from the surrounding surface and shows fine granules on the greater curvature of the antrum.

Fig. 70h Histopathological findings. Histologically, a hyperplastic change in some gastric pits and the proliferation of the pyloric glands could be seen, but changes of the muscularis mucosae or cyst formation could not be observed.

b. Adenomatous polyps

Case 6

c. c.: No subjective symptoms.
52 year-old female.

A thumb-head-sized protruding lesion with rough surfaces was demonstrated in the prepyloric region in a radiograph of the barium filled stomach in the upright position (Fig. 71 a). In the radiograph of the barium filled stomach in the prone position, the lesion was not very clearly observed (Fig. 71 b), because it was covered by the ascending part of duodenum. In the radiograph of the barium filled stomach in the prone position taken with the double-contrast method, several small indistinct prominences with smooth surfaces were demonstrated in the antrum (Fig. 71 c). The base of these lesions seemed to be hyperplastic mucosal folds, and these fold-like structures signified the existence of a stalk. In the radiograph of the barium filled stomach in the supine position taken with the double-contrast method (Fig. 71 d), several rough areas could be observed on the surface of this lesion. It could be diagnosed as a spherical type of epithelial tumor with a stalk, measuring 2.0×2.0 cm in size. In the radiograph of the barium filled stomach in the other supine position taken with the double-contrast method (Fig. 71 e), we could not detect the existence of a stalk, although the separated features of the surface was observed. The longer the stalk of a polyp, the more difficult the roentgenographic description becomes.

Profile views of the polyp allow easy differentiation of the stalk, but frontal views make a demonstration of the existence of a stalk difficult. In the radiograph of the barium filled stomach in the upright position taken with the compression method (Fig. 71 f), the whole stature of the polyp with its stalk was clearly demonstrated. In the radiograph of the barium filled stomach in the upright position taken with the compression method (Fig. 71 g), another polyp was shown on the lesser curvature of the antrum.

Endoscopically (Fig. 71 h), besides the roentgenographic polyp with its stalk, two other polyps were encountered on the greater and lesser curvatures of the antrum. These findings indicated that endoscopic examinations were most useful for the discovery of related lesions.

Macroscopically (Fig. 71 i), the mucosal surface from the polyp to the pyloric ring was rough and uneven. The changeable distance from the polyp to the pyloric ring and the radiographic changes of the surface might be the result of gastric peristalsis.

Rigidity of the gastric wall, as seen in ulcerated lesions, can not be demonstrated in filled radiographs, even when protruding lesions exist along the greater or the lesser curvatures of the stomach. As already mentioned, there is little difficulty in showing small polyps roentgenographically, even those measuring as little as 0.5 cm in diameter. Roentgenographic efforts must be made to discover small polyps, because these efforts provide a chance to discover early gastric cancers of the protruding type.

71a

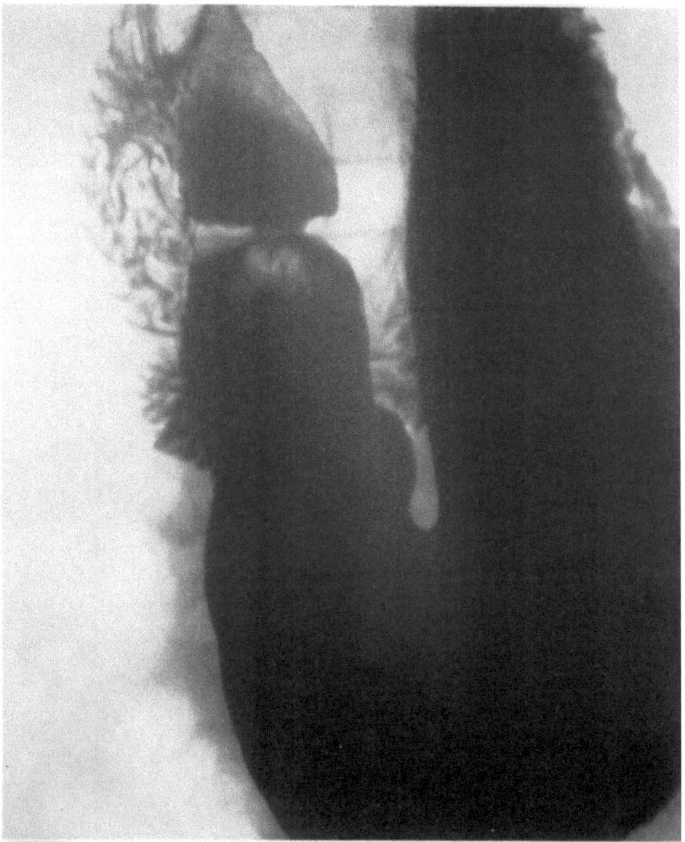

71b

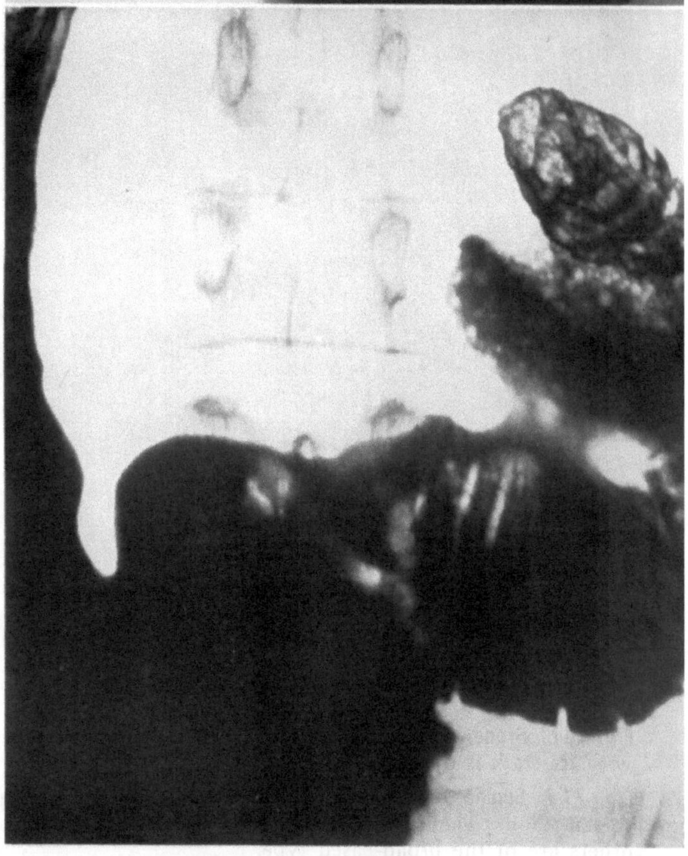

Fig. 71a Upright, barium filled study. A thumb-head-sized protruding lesion in the prepyloric region is shown, but rigidity of the wall could not be demonstrated.

Fig. 71b Prone, barium filled study. Small indistinct prominences are demonstrated on the antrum.

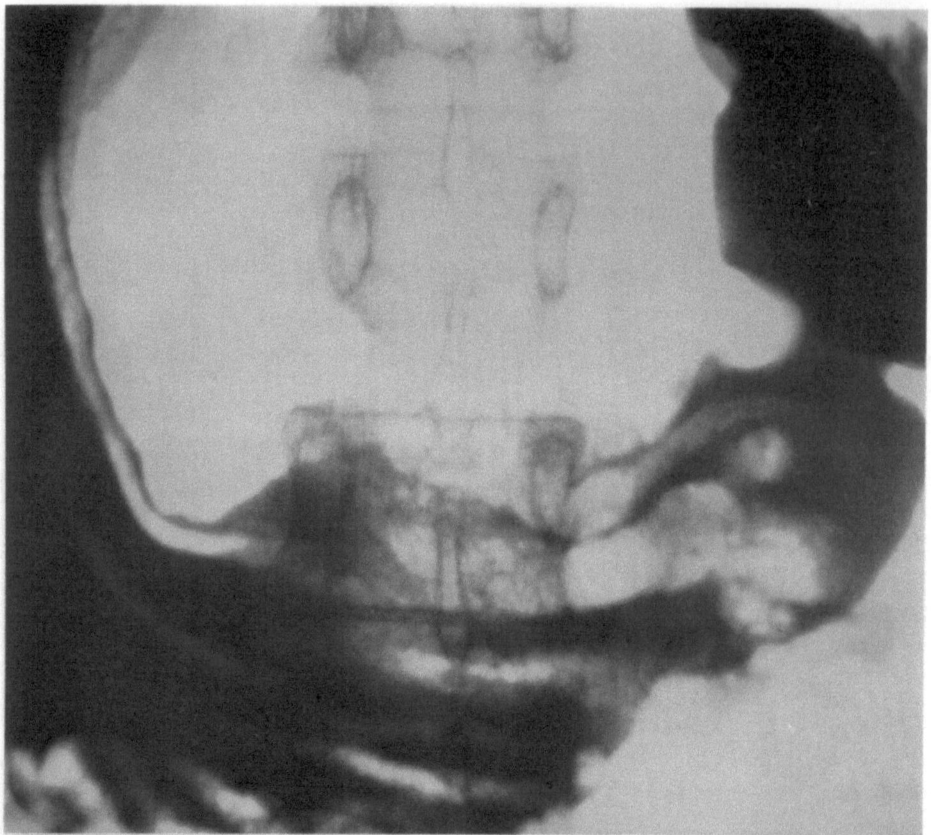

71c

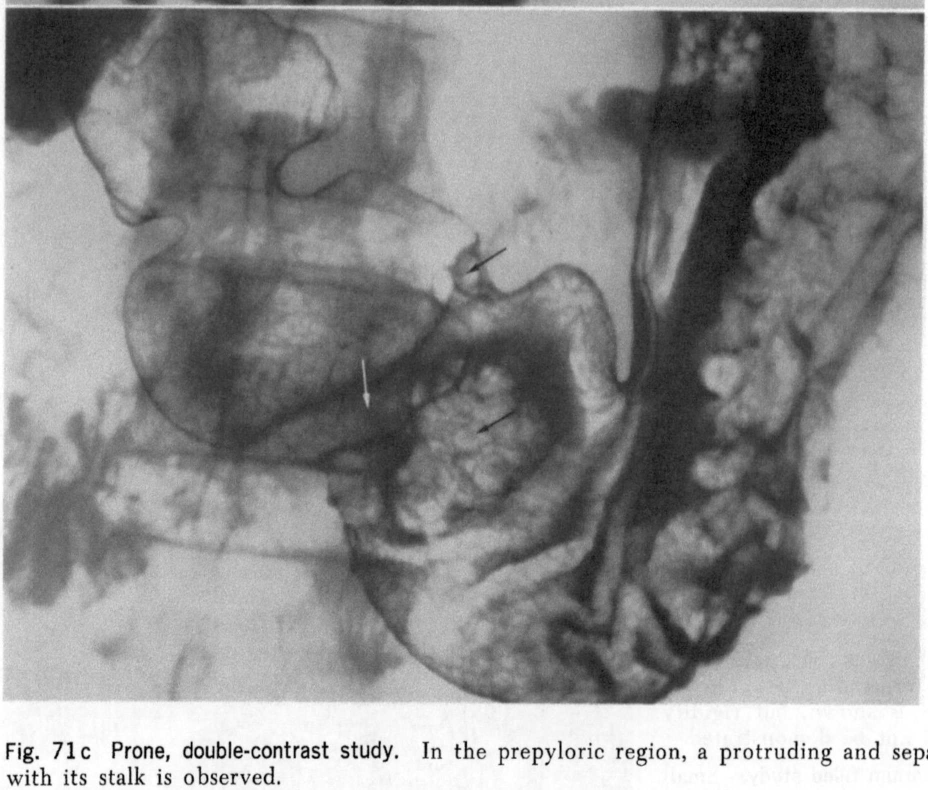

71d

Fig. 71c Prone, double-contrast study. In the prepyloric region, a protruding and separated lesion with its stalk is observed.

Fig. 71d Supine, double-contrast study. Multiple protruding lesions can be seen on the antrum by this method. The lesion consists of the three prominences, the largest one has a stalk and the others are of the broad-based type.

71e

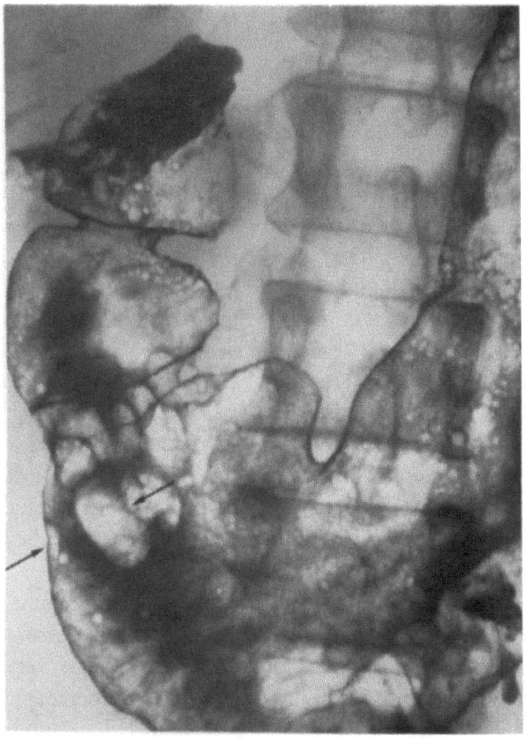

71f

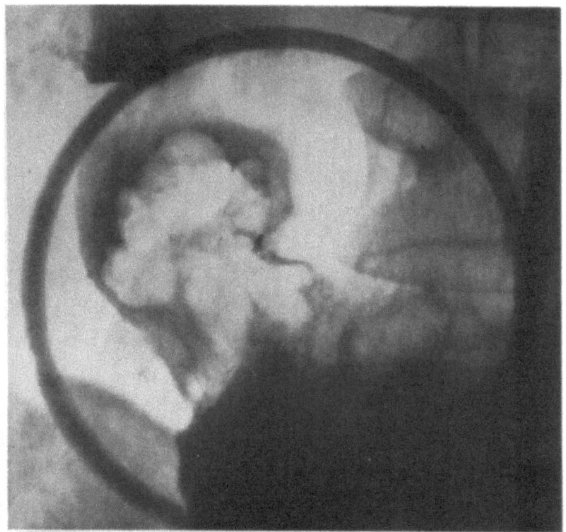

71g

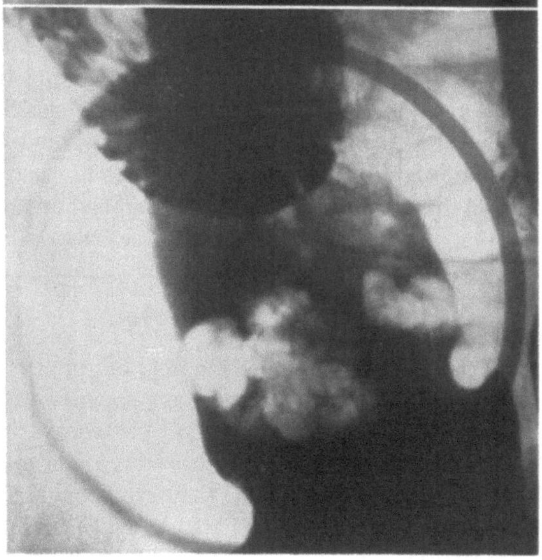

71h

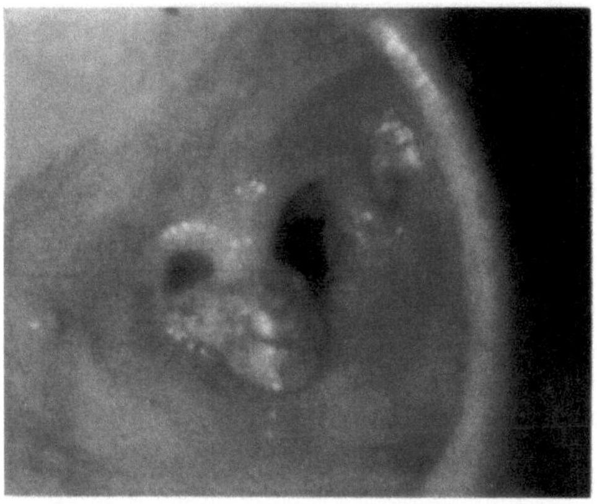

71i

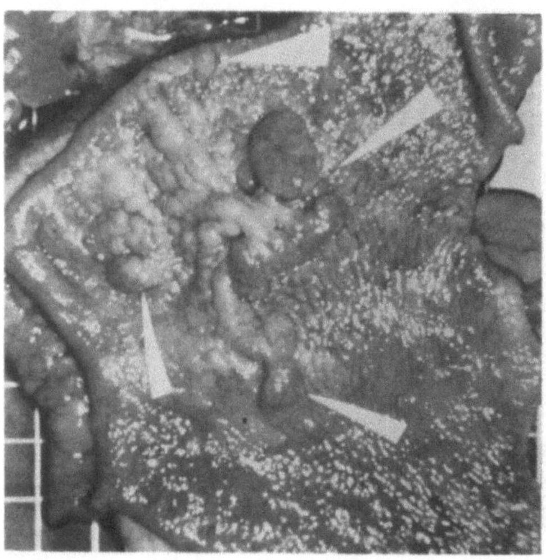

Fig. 71e Supine, double-contrast study. Description of the findings is difficult because of gastric peristalsis.

Figs. 71f, g Compression study. By changing the pressed center, the head of the polyp with its stalk can be moved and its surface is clearly demonstrated.

Fig. 71h Endoscopic picture. A large polyp with its stalk and two other small and broad-based ones are shown in the antrum.

Fig. 71i Resected stomach. In the antrum, three polyps are encountered, one of which is similar to the surrounding hyperplastic mucosa.

4. Nonepithelial tumor (Submucosal tumor)

Strictly speaking, a "nonepithelial tumor" is not synonymous with a "submucosal tumor", because the accessory pancreas is histologically classified as an epithelial tumor, but would be considered as a submucosal tumor according to its type of growth.

The incidence of nonepithelial tumors depends on the physician's judgment and its surgical treatment. Of 1,368 cases of noncancerous tumors in 93 large institutions in Japan, 17.3% were malignant and nonepithelial, 15.2%, benign and nonepithelial, 63.2%, benign and epithelial, and accessory pancreas accounted for 4.3 percent (reported by Oi).

Radiologically, nonepithelial tumors tend to form protrusions with smooth borders, covered with intact mucosa. Majority of these belong to the type I polypoid lesions. Usually the contours of barium filled stomachs show neither irregularities nor abnormal peristalsis. Compression studies reveal round- or oval-shaped filling defects with smooth borders that slope gently toward their bases. Gastroscopically, the surfaces of the protrusions are covered with intact mucosa.

In some cases, ulcer craters are found on the domes of the protrusions; in others, several mucosal folds disappear, smoothly bridging the surfaces of the protrusions. Benign epithelial gastric tumors, which are generally called adenomatous polyps, clearly indicate the circumscribed filling defects without bridging or interrupting the folds.

Nonepithelial tumors are histologically classified as follows (according to Palmer): leiomyoma, fibroma, neurinoma, lipoma, hemangioma, and lipo-muco-fibroma; in addition, cysts, accessory pancreas, and eosinophilic granulomas, etc., may be included. From our experience, it is very difficult to diagnose nonepithelial tumors preoperatively even with the aid of gastrofiberscopic biopsies, because they grow under the submucosal layer of the stomach. A nonepithelial tumor can be found in any segment of the stomach.

a. Leiomyoma

This tumor is of smooth muscle origin. Its size mainly ranges from 2 to 6 cm in diameter. Among benign gastric tumors, the frequency of leiomyomas is next in numbers to adenomatous polyps. According to Palmer, 58 per cent of 273 cases of benign nonepithelial tumors were leiomyomas. Usually leiomyomas are single and located in any segment of the stomach. As for the direction of growth, they grow mainly toward the lumen of the stomach but rarely to the serosa. Fifty per cent have shown ulcer formation on their convexities.

Yamagata classifies submucosal tumors into 4 types: endogastric, exogastric, intramural, and mixed types. Skandalakis classifies them into 6 types: endogastric, endogastric ulcerated, intramural endogastric and exogastric, exogastric ulcerated, and exogastric.

Case 7

c. c.: Upper abdominal pain.

27 year-old male.

Radiologically, picture of the barium filled stomach (Fig. 72 a) showed a slight irregularity at the lesser curvature of the antrum. Another radiograph (Fig. 72 b) revealed a filling defect with smooth borders in the prepyloric region. The defects with smooth surface looked like flat, spherical, sessile protrusion, and their sizes are up to 2–3 cm in diameter. As seen in compression studies (Figs. 72 c, d), a few folds went around the protrusion with relatively sharp borders. Another study made under appropriate compression (Fig. 72 e) revealed a shallow depression in the center of the dome, a so-called central ulceration. Double-contrast studies in the supine position taken with a small amount of air showed no particular sign except a smooth filling defect at the antrum. In conclusion, the tumor was radiologically diagnosed as a submucosal tumor. Endoscopically (Fig. 72 g), the color of the flat protrusion was similar to that of the surrounding intact mucosa. The gross specimen as well as the cut section (Figs. 72 h, i) revealed a leiomyoma, measuring 3.0×2.8 cm, with a shallow, central ulceration in the prepyloric region.

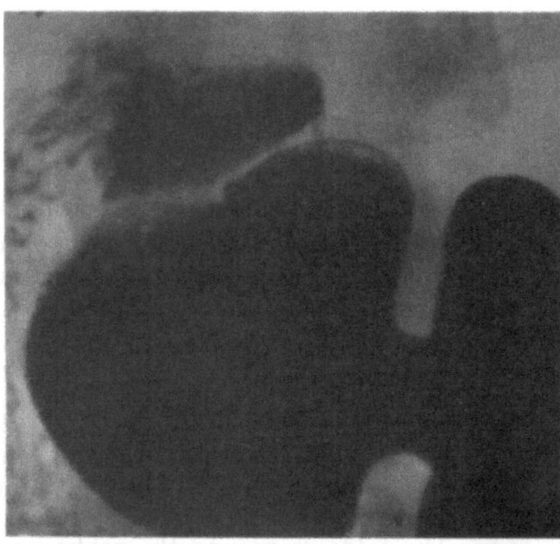

72 a

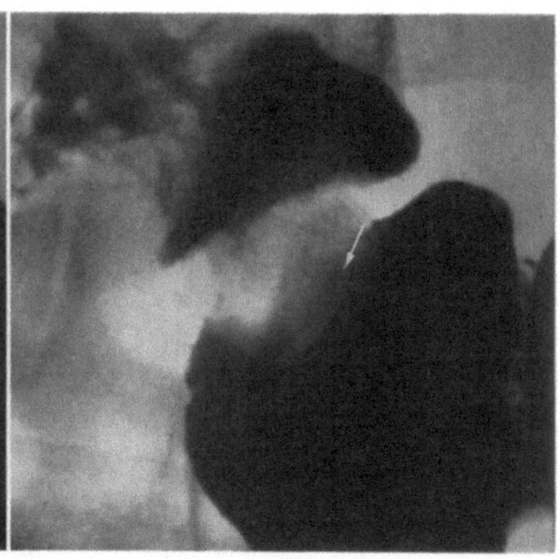

72 b

Fig. 72 a Upright, barium filled study (prepyloric region). Note no abnormality at the lesser curvature of the antrum.

Fig. 72 b Upright, barium filled study. Note the filling defect with a smooth border in the prepyloric region (arrow) under conditions of peristalsis.

72c

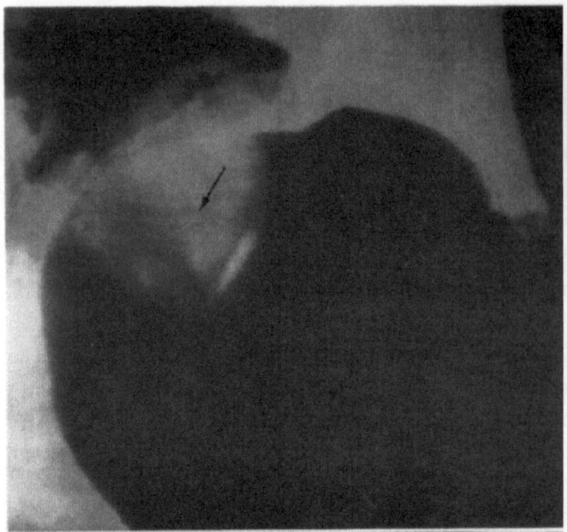

72d

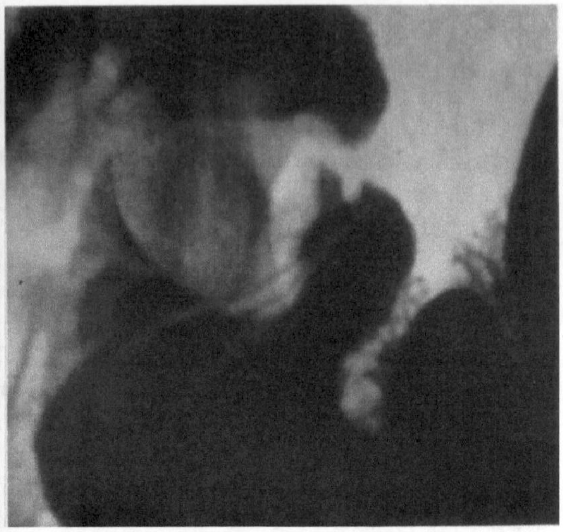

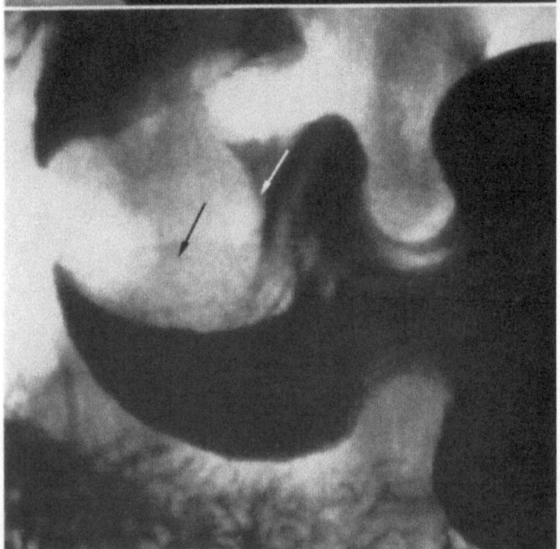

72e

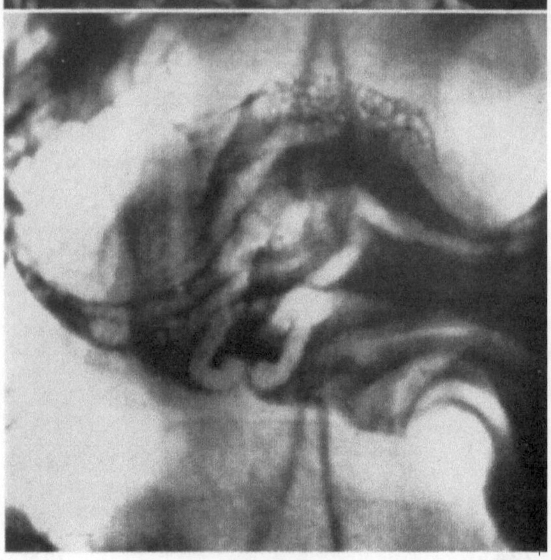

72f

Figs. 72c–e Upright, compression studies.

Fig. 72c Low degree of compression. A hemispherical, broad-based tumor is seen.

Fig. 72d Moderate degree of compression. Note the flat protrusion with a smooth surface, measuring from 2 to 3 cm in diameter.

Fig. 72e Proper degree of compression.

Fig. 72f Supine, double-contrast study (with a small amount of air). The flat protrusion has relatively sharp borders and looks spherical. The folds go around the protrusion.

72g

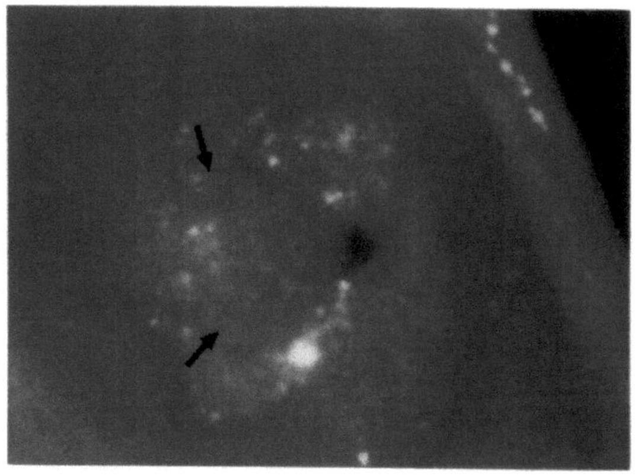

72h

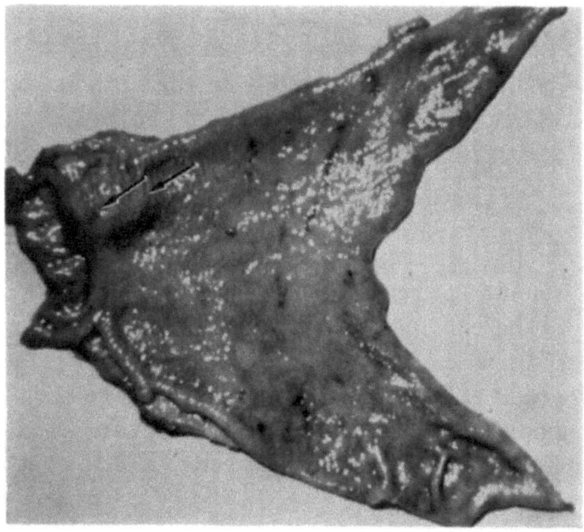

72i

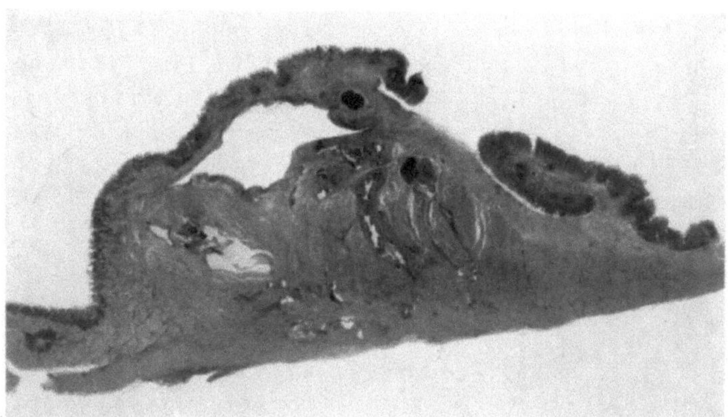

Fig. 72g Endoscopic picture. Note the spherical, smooth protrusion with a central depression in the prepyloric region. No difference is noted in the color of the surface mucosa and the surrounding area. These findings reveal it to be a submucosal tumor.

Fig. 72h Resected stomach. The tumor is located on the anterior wall of the prepylorus, with a central ulceration (marked with an arrow). The tumor measures 3.0×2.8 cm in diameter.

Fig. 72i Histopathological findings. Histologically the tumor consists of smooth muscle tissue.

b. Neurogenic tumor

Neurinoma (schwannoma) is the most common type of neurogenic tumor. Neurogenic tumors are subdivided as follows: neuroma, glioma, neurinoma, neurofibroma.

Both neurofibroma and neurinoma are often single. About 60 per cent of the cases are in the submucosal layer. The second most prevalent location is found in the subserosal layer, while they rarely occur in the muscular layer. Any type of neurogenic tumor can be found in any part of the stomach. The ones located in the gastric body account for half of the cases, and the rest are located in the antrum and the fundus. They are more frequently present on the lesser curvature than on the greater curvature and more often on the posterior wall than on the anterior wall. About 42 per cent are under 5 cm in diameter. About half have central ulcerations, with incidences no higher than those of myomas.

Case 8

c.c.: Epigastric discomfort.

71 year-old female.

The barium filled studies in the upright position (Fig. 73 a) and in the prone position (Fig. 73 b) revealed no abnormalities of the gastric contour.

A double-contrast study in the supine position (Fig. 73 c) showed an oval filling defect, measuring 2–3 cm in diameter, and two bridging folds on the anal side of the posterior wall of the corpus. With the aid of double-contrast pictures in the first oblique position (Figs. 73 d, e) as well as a compression study (Fig. 73 f) in the second oblique position, a high protrusion with a smooth surface was shown with no central ulceration.

The endoscopic photograph (Fig. 73 g) showed the same findings as the x-ray picture of the stomach. The tumor was more likely to be submucosal, because the mucosa of the surface did not differ much from that of the neighbouring areas. In this case, scopic biopsy was not required to obtain a histological diagnosis of this tumor, as the gross specimen (Fig. 73 h) was sufficient to diagnose it correctly. Histological examinations (Fig. 73 i) revealed it to be a neurofibroma.

73a 73b 73c 73d

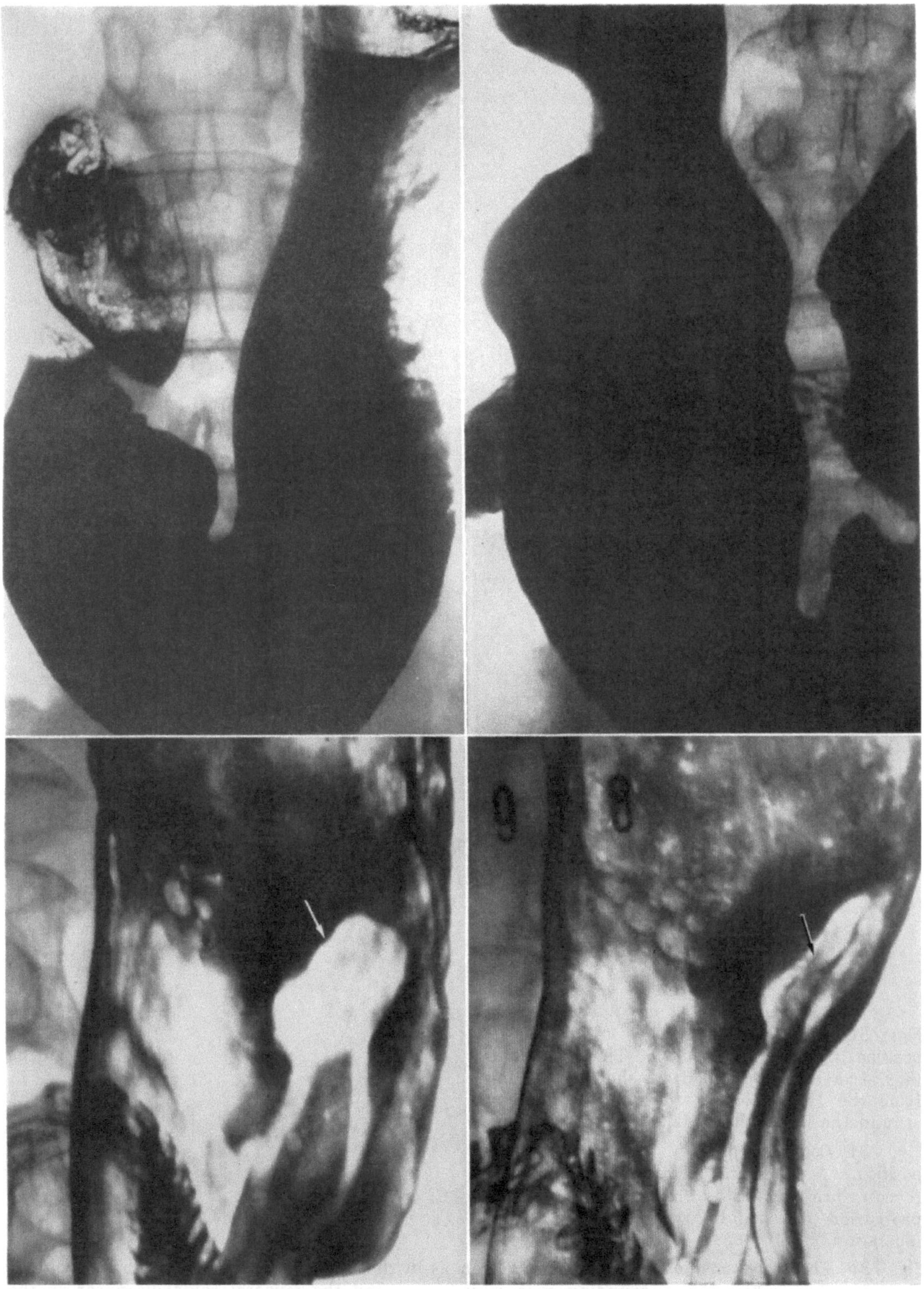

Figs. 73a, b Barium-filled studies in the upright and prone positions. There are no remarkably abnormal contours.

Figs. 73c, d Double-contrast studies in the supine position. On the posterior wall of the gastric body, there is an oval filling defect, measuring 2–3 cm in diameter, with two mucosal folds, which converge on the anal side of the defect and disappear on the surface of the defect. These mucosal folds are so-called bridging folds characteristic of submucosal tumors. Other pictures from various directions (Figs. 73d, e) reveal the bridging folds more clearly.

73e

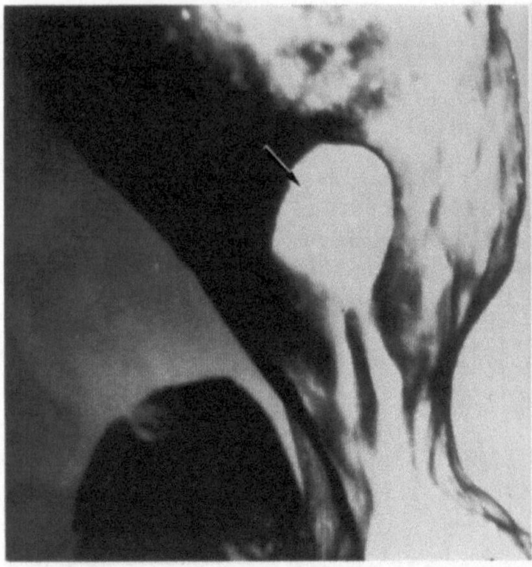

73f

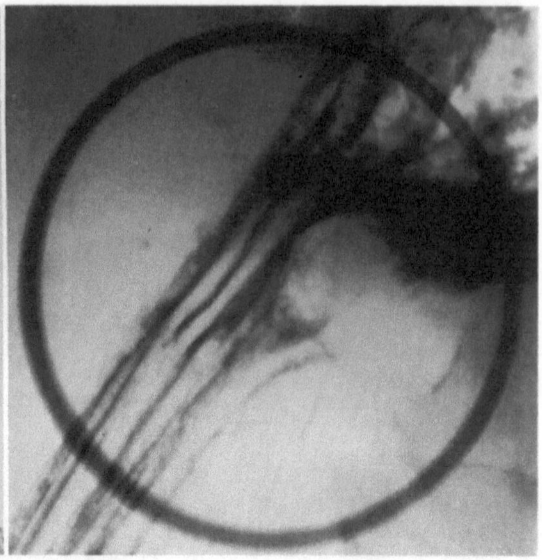

73g

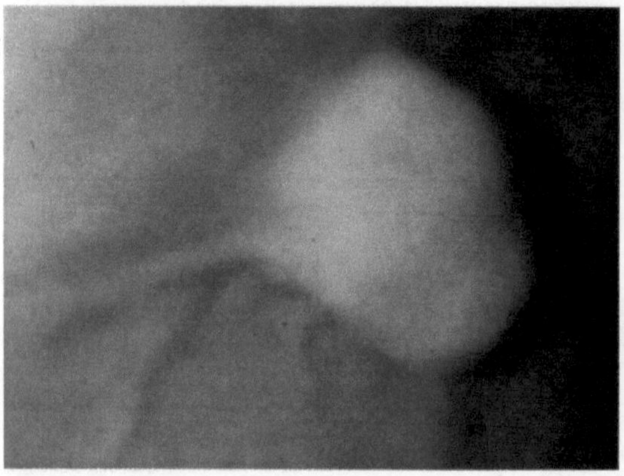

73h

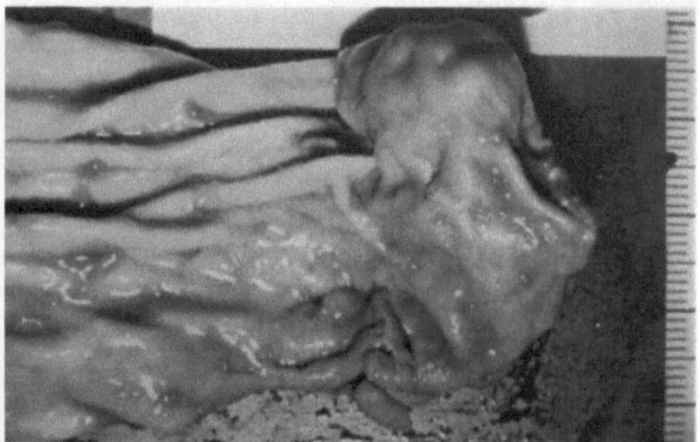

73i

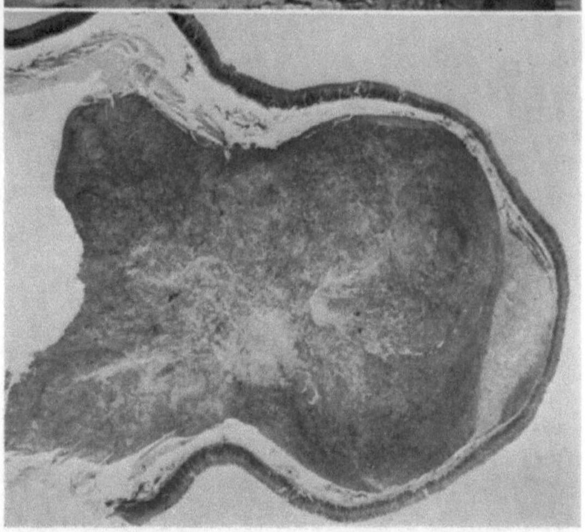

Fig. 73e Double-contrast study in the supine position (right oblique position). The same findings as in Figs. 73c and d are shown. Judging from the thick layer of the contrast medium around the tumor, it is a fairly high protrusion.

Fig. 73f Compression study in the left oblique position. A moderate degree of compression reveals bridging folds. The surface of the protrusion is smooth without any central ulceration.

Fig. 73g Endoscopic picture. The same protrusion as in the x-ray picture is seen. The mucosa of its surface resembles the surrounding mucosa in color, and the mucosal folds disappear on the surface. These findings indicate that the protrusion is a submucosal tumor.

Fig. 73h Resected stomach. The surface of the tumor is smooth. As we expected from radiological and endoscopic findings, it is a submucosal tumor.

Fig. 73j Histopathological findings. Histologically, the tumor is a neurofibroma.

5. Polypoid early gastric cancer (Type I)

This type of lesion arouses great clinical interest in relation to the problem of malignant degeneration of benign polyps. In 1929, STEWART *et al.* described the malignant change of a benign intestinal tumor. Many papers stress the importance of malignant degeneration of benign polyps, but it is not so easy to prove degeneration through clinical observation.

Even when we meet a case with an apparently malignant degeneration, we must at first resolve the problem of how to define the developement of polypoid cancers. Histopathologically, the growth of a polypoid cancer is thought to be upwards but without branching of the muscularis mucosa as in a benign polyp. This is very different from the appearance of the mucosal muscular layer of an adenomatous polyp. The fact that the frequency of cancer differs according to the size of the lesion might be suggestive of some relationship between the growth of a polyp and malignant degeneration. We realize that malignant degeneration has been a problem since early times and is still a difficult one to solve.

Case 9

c. c.: No subjective complaints. Checked by gastric mass survey.

52 year-old male.

A picture of the barium filled stomach in the upright position demonstrated a niche-like protrusion at the angle (Fig. 74 a). A prone picture under adequate compression showed a double-headed protuberance with an uneven surface on the anterior wall of the antrum. The surrounding mucosal folds of the tumor made a detour running along its elevated surface. A double-headed, pedunculated protuberance was observed in the supine, double-contrast studies (Figs. 74 d and e), identical with the one seen in the prone compression studies (Figs. 74 b and c).

A reddish, lustrous protuberance with a stem was observed endoscopically on the greater curvature of the antrum (Figs. 74 i and j). However, since roentgenological findings of the lesion suggested the possibility of malignancy, a biopsy was carried out under direct vision. The biopsy showed a partial tubular adenocarcinoma. Gross inspection of the resected stomach (Fig. 74 k) showed findings identical with the endoscopic and roentgenological findings of the antral lesion. Histopathologically, it was diagnosed as a papillar or tubular adenocarcinoma of the stomach (Fig. 74 l). Unexpectedly, carcinomatous infiltration was located not only on the head of the polyp but also around the stem, both of which were colored similar to the surrounding mucosa. The polypoid protuberance was finally diagnosed as a type I early gastric cancer in which carcinomatous invasion was limited to the submucosal layer.

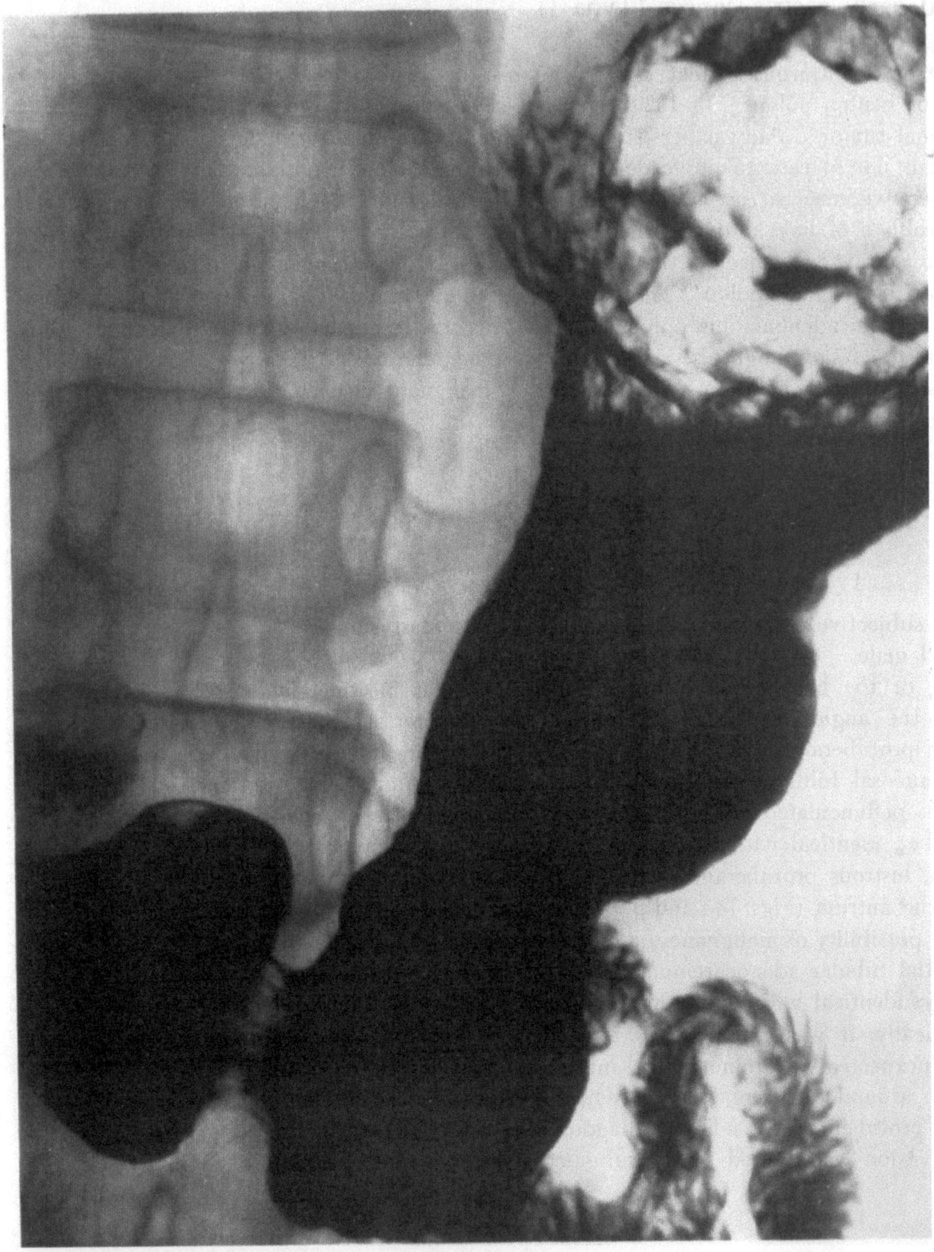

74a

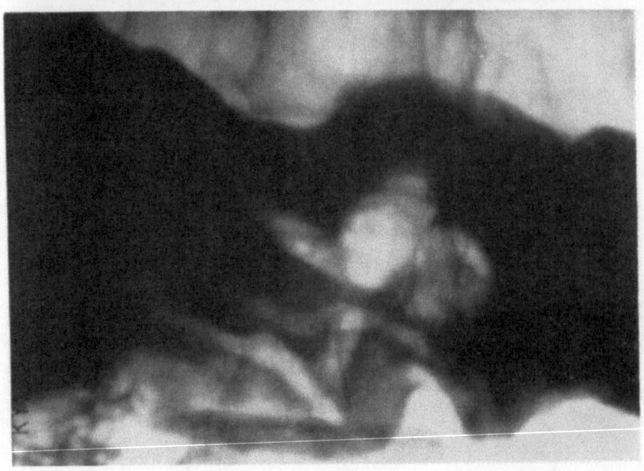

74b

Fig. 74 a Barium filled stomach in the upright position. The picture shows no abnormal finding except a slight irregularity at the angle.

Fig. 74 b Prone position study. A double-headed globular protuberance is seen on the greater curvature of the antrum. The surrounding mucosal folds make a detour running along the elevated area.

74c
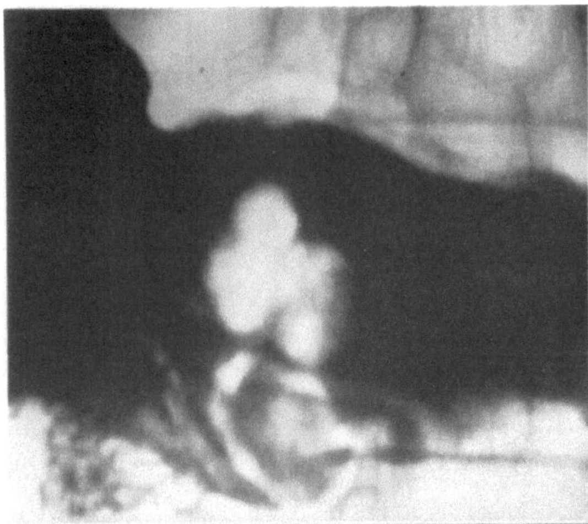

74d
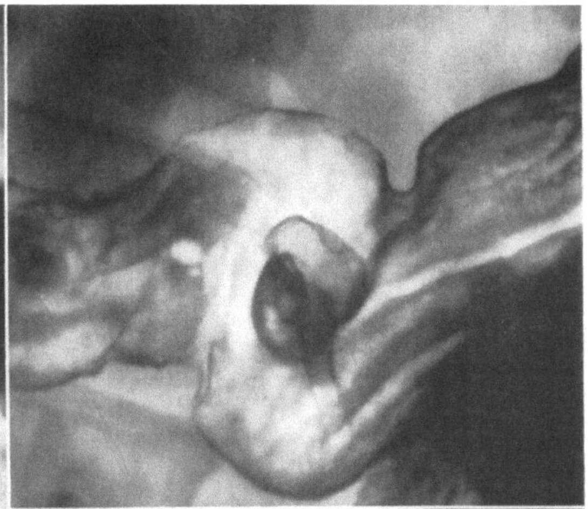

74e
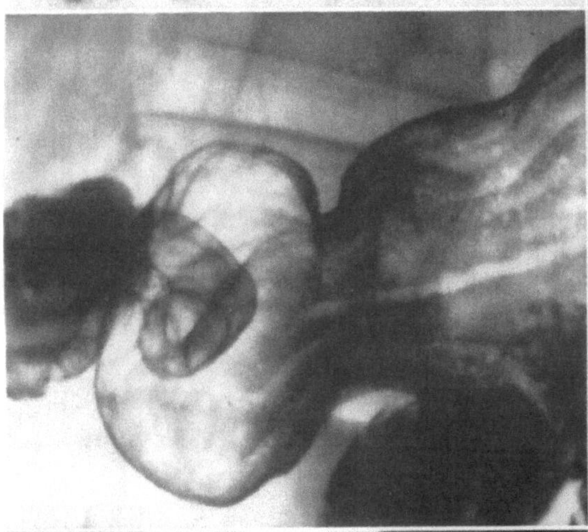

74f
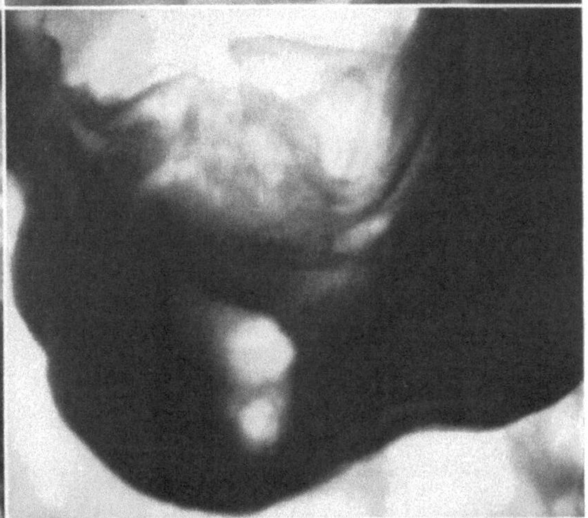

74g
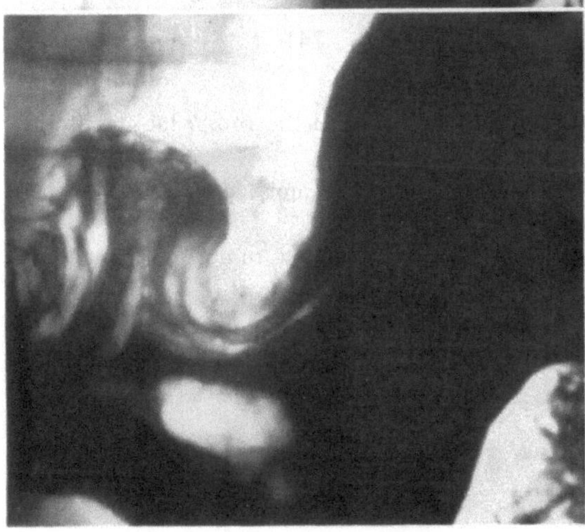

74h
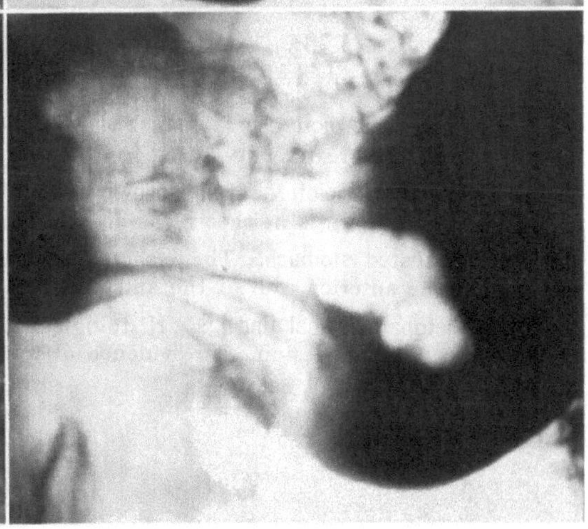

Fig. 74c Prone position study. A complete view of the pedunculated protuberance is shown.

Fig. 74d Double-contrast study in the supine position. The top and the edge of the protuberance are overlapping.

Fig. 74e Double-contrast study in the supine position. The surface of the lesion shows an uneven irregularity.

Fig. 74f Faint compression study. Only a part of the irregularity is shown.

Fig. 74g Compression study. The edge and the head of the protuberance are seen to be parallel to the x-ray film.

Fig. 74h Compression study. The fine, nodular, granular surface of the protuberance is clear, but it is difficult to give a complete view of the lesion with only one compression study.

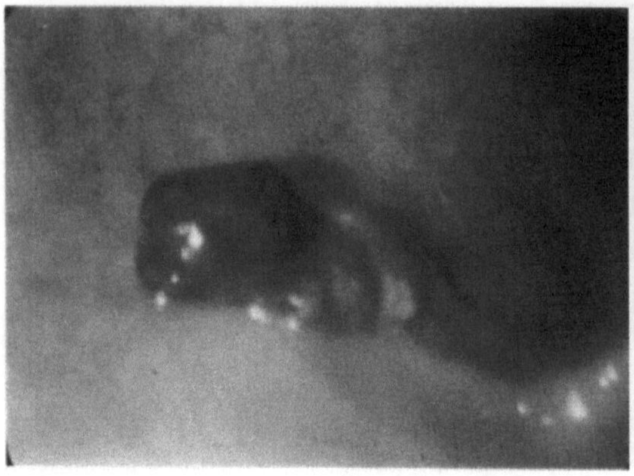

74i

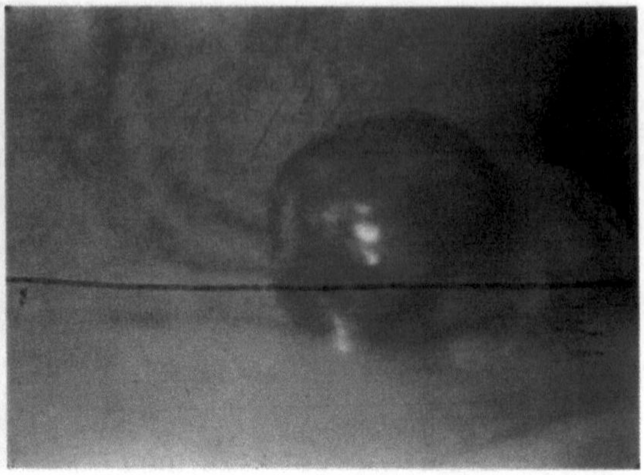

74j

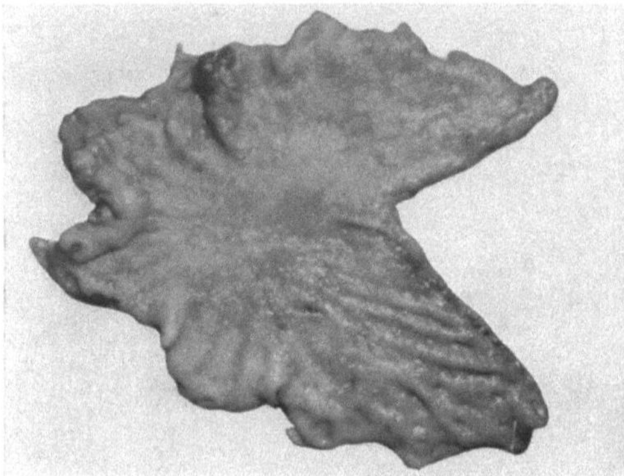

74k

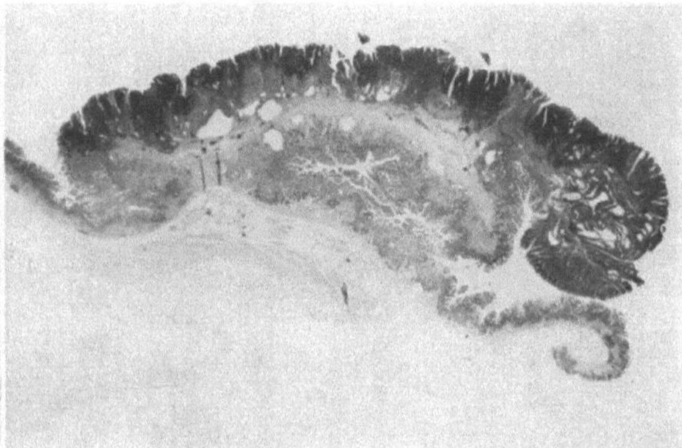

74l

Fig. 74i Endoscopic picture of a distant view. The head and the stem of the tumor look as if they are placed on the greater curvature.

Fig. 74j Endoscopic picture of a close-up view. The surface of the tumor shows reddening and slight rigidity. There is neither bleeding nor erosion.

Fig. 74k Resected stomach. The resected stomach shows a pedunculated tumor with a reddish summit on the anterior wall of the antrum.

Fig. 74l Histopathological findings. Histologically, an adenocarcinoma is seen on the head of the stalk of the polypoid lesion. No evidence of malignant degeneration of a benign gastric polyp is seen.

Naturally it is necessary for the clinicians to understand the merits and demerits of each type of examination: radiology, endoscopy, scopic biopsy, and cytology. Then in order to make a differential diagnosis, each lesion must be considered according to the following five points.

1) Ascertain whether or not the lesion protrudes into the lumen of the stomach.

2) Identify the protrusion of the stomach as epithelial or nonepithelial (submucosal). Endoscopic examinations are very useful to differentiate between these two.

3) Determine whether the lesion is benign or malignant. Differential diagnosis to determine whether the tumor is benign or malignant depends on the shape of the base in a profile view and the size measured by x-ray photographs.

4) Determine which layer of the gastric wall the lesion invades (the forecast of the degree of depth). The key points of the diagnosis depend on the size, the shape of the base in a profile view, and the degree of irregularity of the surface in a frontal view.

5) Determine what kind of submucosal tumor it is histologically. Usually it is possible to differentiate whether the submucosal tumor is benign or malignant, but it is sometimes impossible to diagnose its histology preoperatively; for instance, whether they are leiomyomas or lipomas, etc.

Above all, it must be emphasized that we must be careful to have x-ray and endoscopic photographs good enough to enable us to read the above-mentioned five basic points of the diagnosis from the x-ray photographs.

B. Indistinguishable cases

1. Prolapsing gastric polyps

We have already stated how to make differential diagnoses of some polypoid lesions in our introduction of typical cases. However, cases we frequently see in our clinic cannot always be easily differentiated according to type. There are series of obstacles in obtaining a correct diagnosis. The first and most frequent is the incorrect or incomplete reading of gastric x-ray films, but attention to the basics of x-ray and endoscopic examinations can certainly overcome this. The second obstacle is the hesitation in diagnosis if the case is presented under unusual conditions even though it is fairly well described and is a comparatively typical case.

Case 10

c. c.: Fullness of the epigastrium.

58 year-old female.

In the barium filled stomach in the upright position (Fig. 75 a), the prepyloric area was not well filled. A soft shadow defect could be seen confluent with the pyloric ring on the picture of the barium-filled stomach in the prone position. The double-contrast study in the supine position (Fig. 75 b) revealed a lobulated, soft-surfaced, spherical polypoid lesion with a stalk, measuring 2.0 cm × 1.0 cm. As seen under fluoroscopy, this tumor was prolapsed into the duodenal cap (Figs. 75 c, d). With the adoption of a moderate manual compression method in this case, this tumor gradually passed through the pyloric ring and prolapsed easily into the duodenal cap (Fig. 75 g).

The surface of the lesion was soft, uneven, and coarse. Because of its irregularity it was judged to be a spherical, sessile polypoid lesion. These findings indicated that the tumor was epithelial, and its size showed it to be negative for cancer.

Endoscopic examination (Fig. 75 h) showed a reddened gastric polyp hanging from the anterior wall of the antrum, clearly distinguishable from its stalk which revealed no difference in color from the surrounding mucosa. Histopathological findings of the resected stomach demonstrated it to be an adenomatous polyp.

Cases of pedunculated polyps prolapsing into the duodenal cap are not very rare, and the frequency is not related to the length of the stalk. When the pyloric antrum area shortens due to peristaltic movement of the stomach, the pyloric ring approaches the tumor. Observing the rough, submucosal tissue at the fringe of the polyp, we found the motility of the gastric mucosa much greater than expected. When a polyp prolapses into the duodenal cap, it is common to find that the lesion itself can not always be well observed.

Sometimes peristalsis is strong enough such that the contracted gastric wall appears as a pseudopyloric ring which can hide a polyp. Therefore, it is necessary to be careful not to conclude that there are no lesions in the stomach even if they cannot be observed endoscopically. To distinguish endoscopically between a real pyloric ring and a pseudo-pyloric ring, it is frequently necessary to administer large doses of spasmolytic drug to the patient. Clinically, this condition is called a "Ball-valve syndrome" and is sometimes accompanied by the obstruction symptoms of paroxysmal abdominal pain.

75a

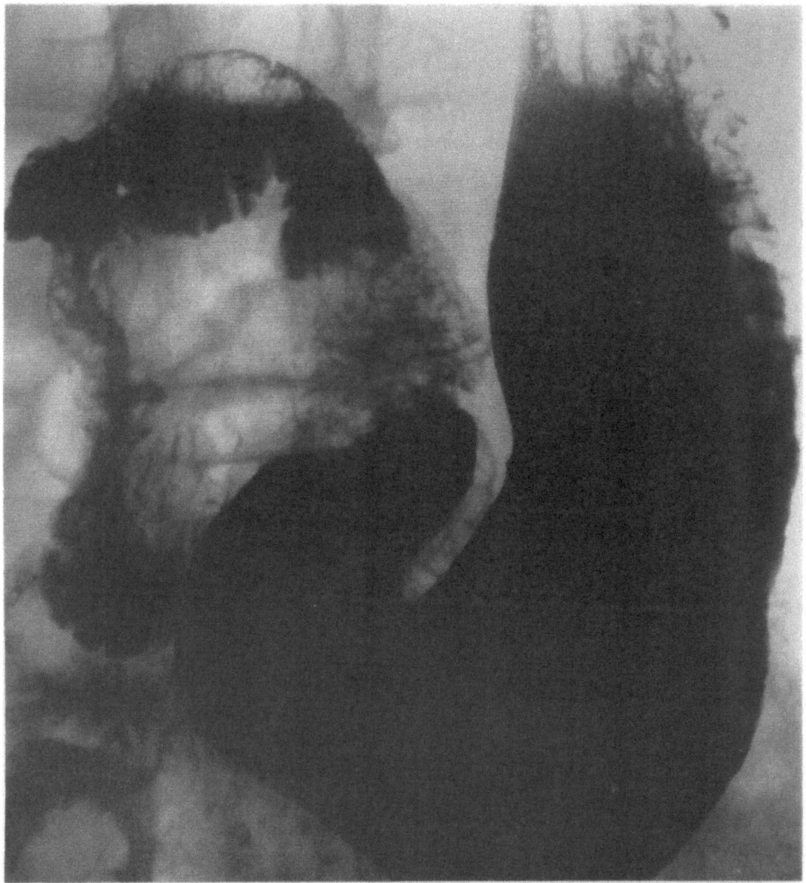

75b

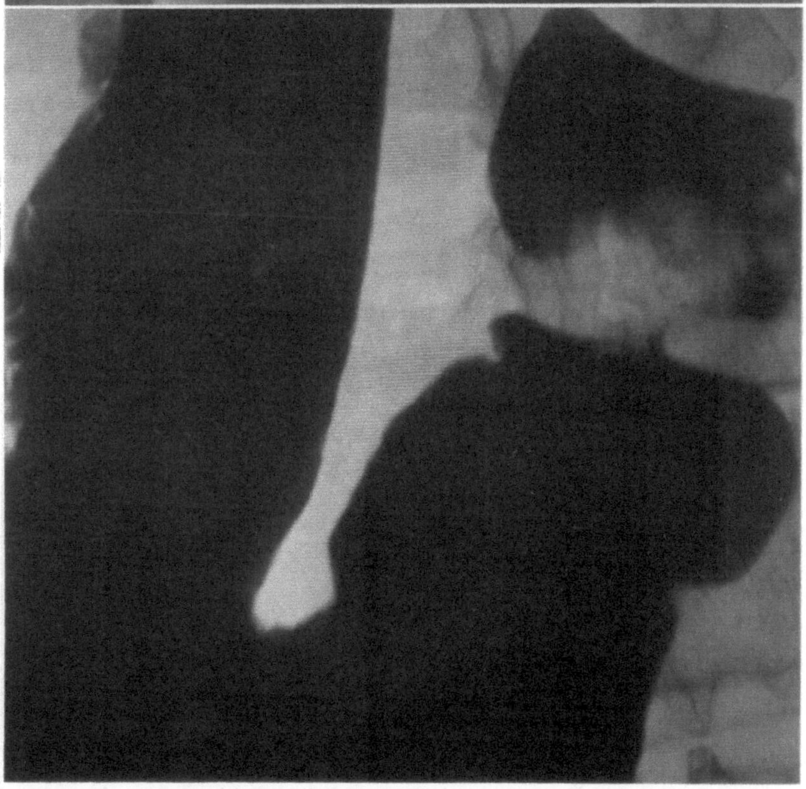

Fig. 75a Barium-filled stomach in the upright position. The pyloric antrum is not well filled. It is difficult to decide whether this is merely an incomplete filling or a defect of the shadow.

Fig. 75b Barium-filled stomach in the prone position. A soft defect of the shadow can be observed confluent with the pyloric ring.

75c

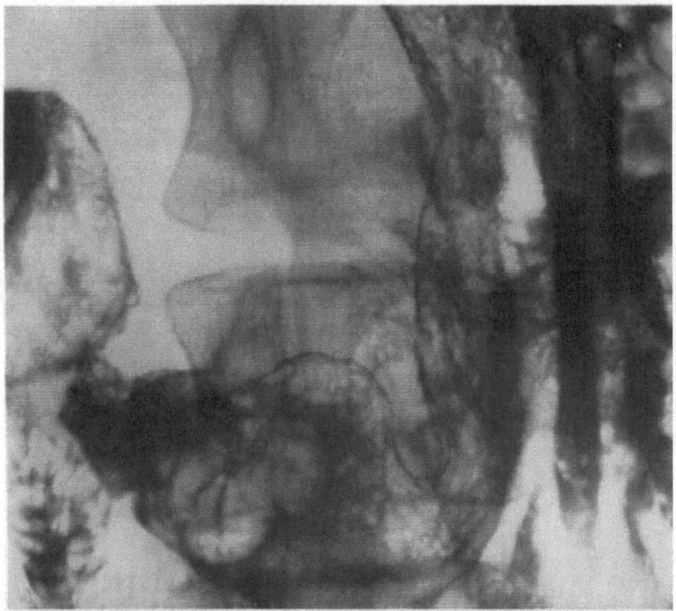

75d

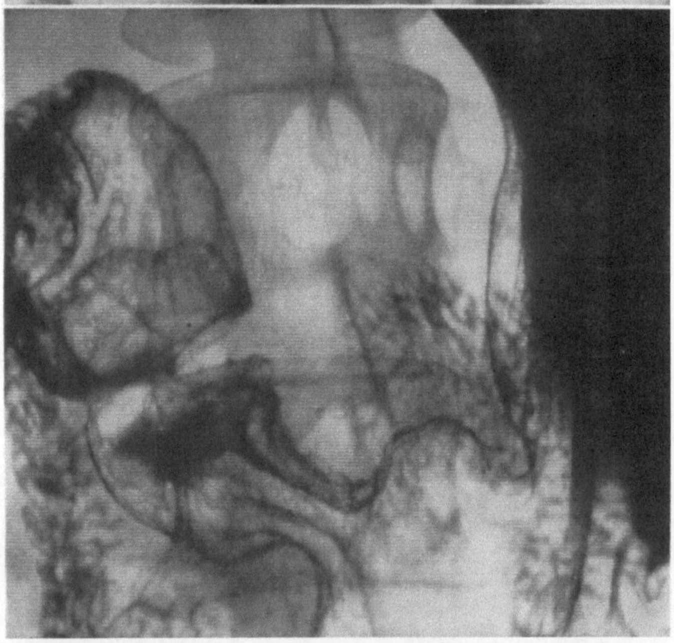

75e

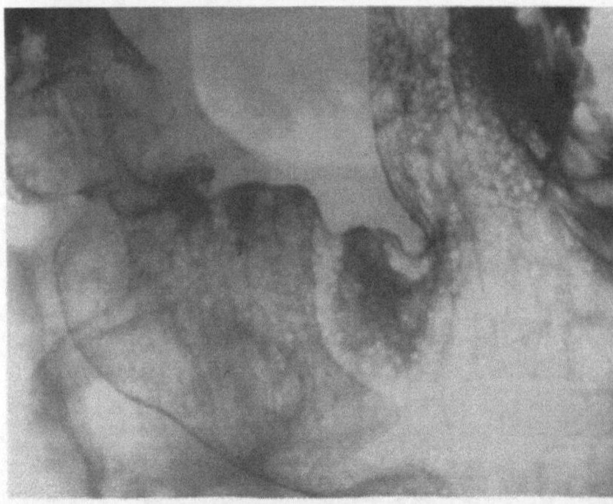

75f

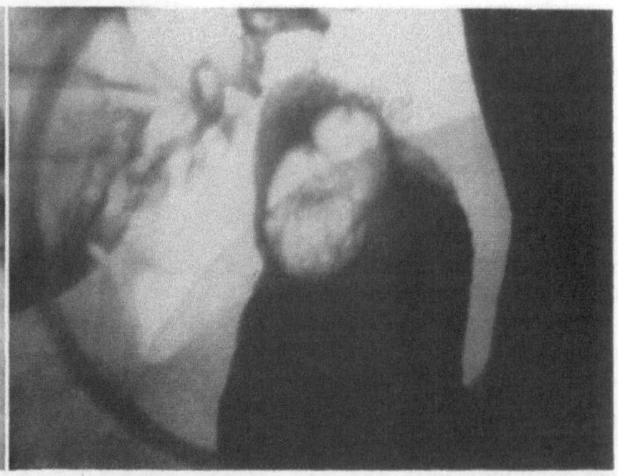

Fig. 75c **Double-contrast study in the supine position.** A lobulated and soft, pedunculated, polypoid lesion, measuring 2.0×1.0 cm in diameter, can be seen in the prepyloric region.
Fig. 75d **Double-contrast study in the supine position.** A pedunculated polyp can be seen at the pyloric antrum prolapsing into the duodenal cap.
Fig. 75e **Double-contrast study in the supine position.** The polyp with its stem located at the prepylorus completely prolapsed into the duodenum.
Fig. 75f **Proper compression study.** In this phase, this pedunculated polyp is still seen just in front of the pyloric ring.

75g

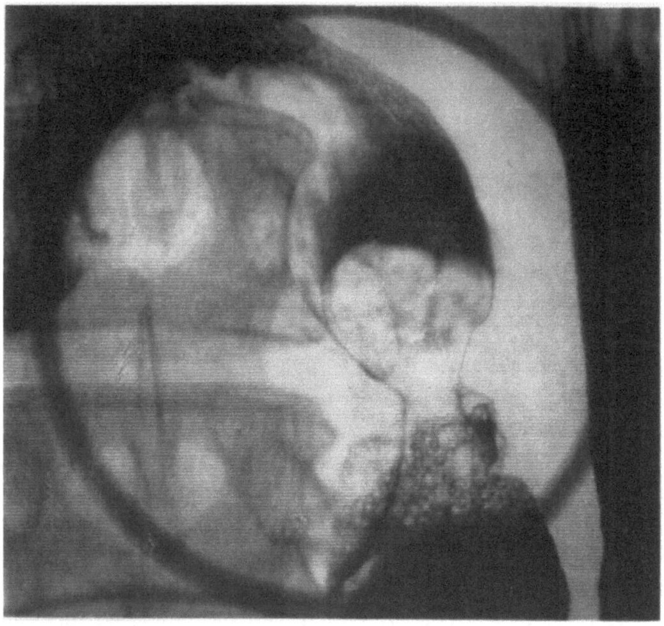

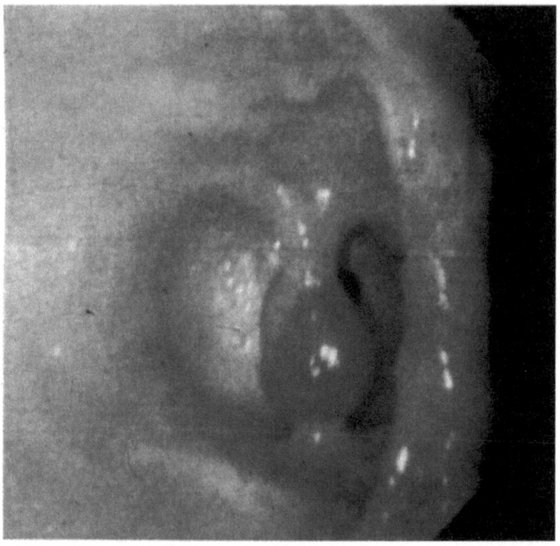

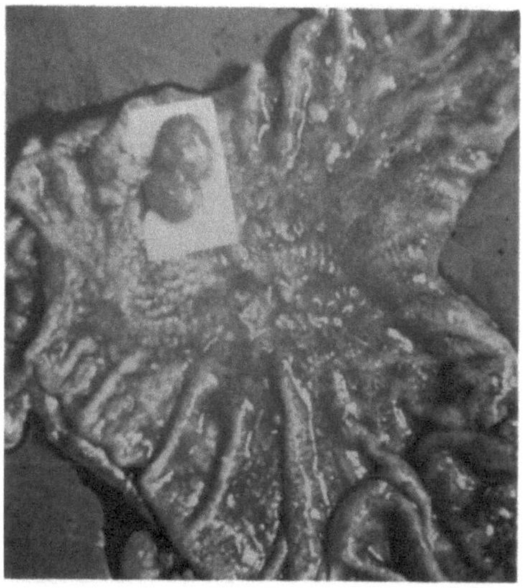

75h

75i

Fig. 75g Compression study. The polyp is completely prolapsed into the duodenum. The pyloric ring widens because of the stalk of the polyp. A soft, uneven, and coarse gastric area is observed on its surface, suggesting that it is an epithelial polyp of the stomach.

Fig. 75h Endoscopic picture. A reddened gastric polyp hanging from the anterior wall of the antrum can be observed. A long stalk of the same color as that of the surrounding mucosa is clearly demarcated from the head of the polyp.

Fig. 75i Resected stomach. A lobulated polyp is seen on the anterior wall of the antrum. Histopathologically, it is an adenomatous polyp.

2. Leiomyoma prolapsing into the duodenal cap

Case 11

c. c.: Precise examination was needed after a gastric mass survey.

66 year-old female.

There was no abnormality observable at the marginal line of the barium filled stomach in the upright position (Fig. 76 a). In the double-contrast study in the supine position (Figs. 76 b–d), a hemispherical tumor, measuring 2.4×2.2 cm in diameter, was visibly elevated from the surrounding gastric mucosa at the pyloric antrum.

A coarse area was present on the surface of the lesion. In a relief pattern in the prone position (Fig. 76 c), the stalk of the tumor was visible with its top bent. The barium filled stomach (Fig. 76 f) also resulted in a diagnosis of a pedunculated and probably epithelial polyp prolapsing into the duodenal cap. It was diagnosed as "epithelial" because of the finding of a small, coarse, uniform gastric area as seen in Figures 76 b–d. Furthermore, since the authors' statistical studies indicated that cancer was present in most cases of tumors over 3 cm in diameter, the possibility of cancer could be dismissed.

Endoscopically (Fig. 76 g), a somewhat reddened, pedunculated, polypoid lesion was seen on the anterior wall of the prepyloric region. This finding coincided with that of radiography. The most remarkable findings of the resected stomach (Fig. 76 h) were that this polyp had a small, coarse, granular mucosal surface compared with the surrounding mucosa, but showed no discoloration or other changes.

Histologically (Fig. 76 i), it was unexpectedly diagnosed as a leiomyoma. Careful note should be made that the tumor looked pedunculated and yet was prolapsed into the duodenum. Our endoscopic misdiagnosis was caused by misjudging the inadequately lighted tumor as a reddened lesion.

76a

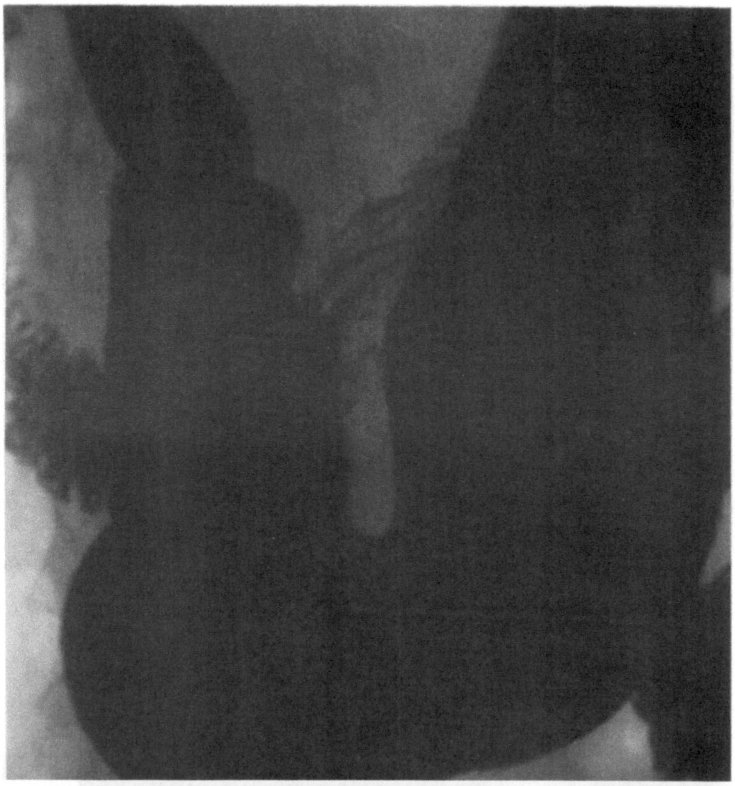

76b

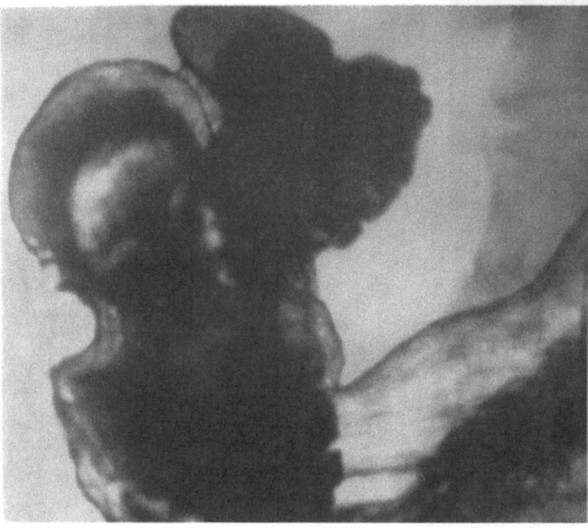

76c

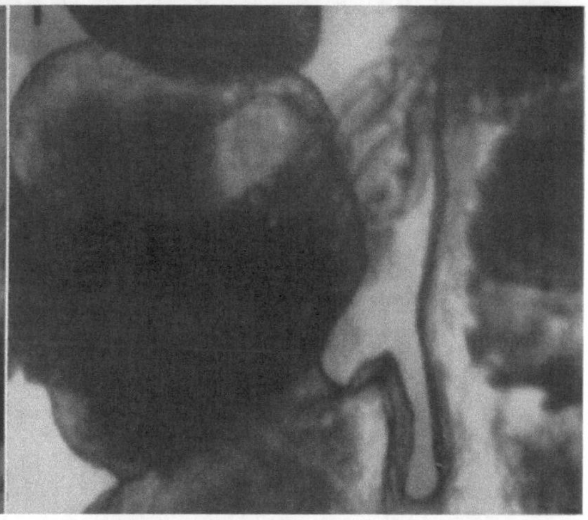

76d

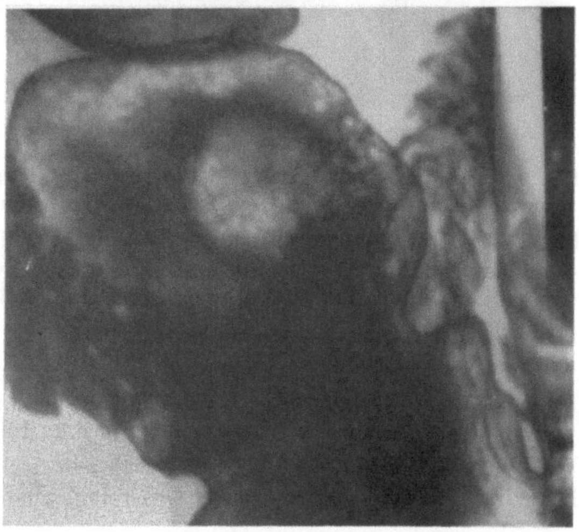

Fig. 76a Barium filled stomach in the upright position. There is no remarkable change at the margin of the stomach.

Figs. 76b–d Double-contrast studies in the supine position. It is somewhat difficult to read the radiograph because of the superimposition of duodenal and gastric shadows; but judging from the three sheets of film taken with position changes, a spherical and pedunculated tumor, measuring 2.4×2.2 cm in diameter, is located at the pyloric antrum elevated from the surrounding mucosa. A coarse gastric area is recognized on its surface.

76e

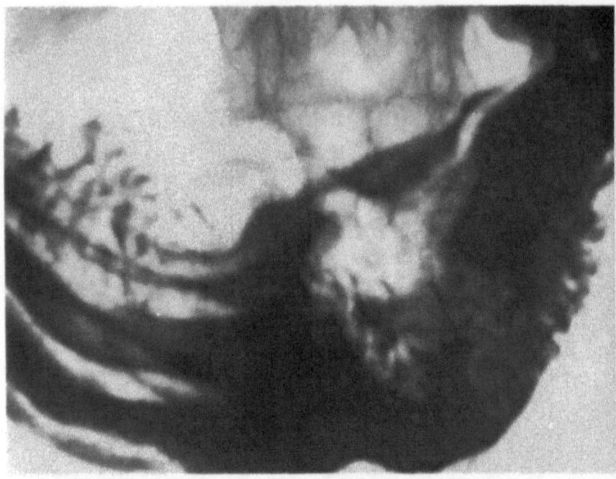

76f

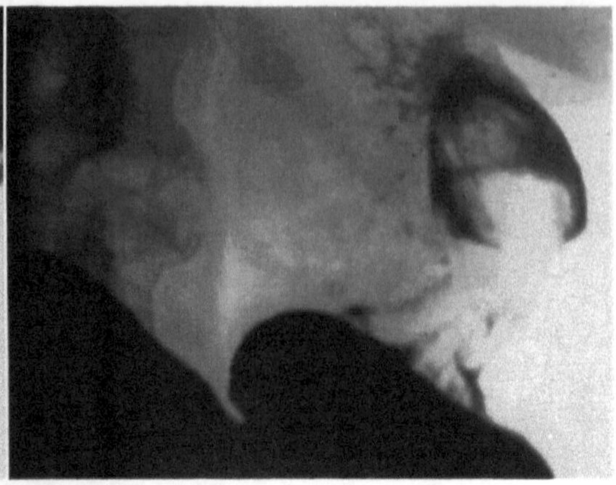

76g

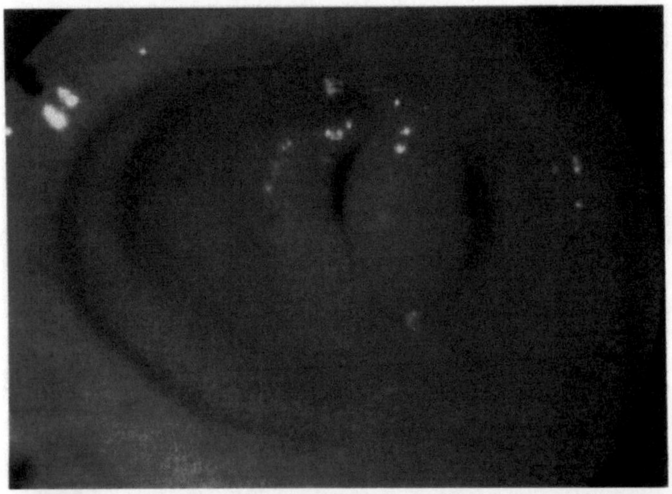

76h

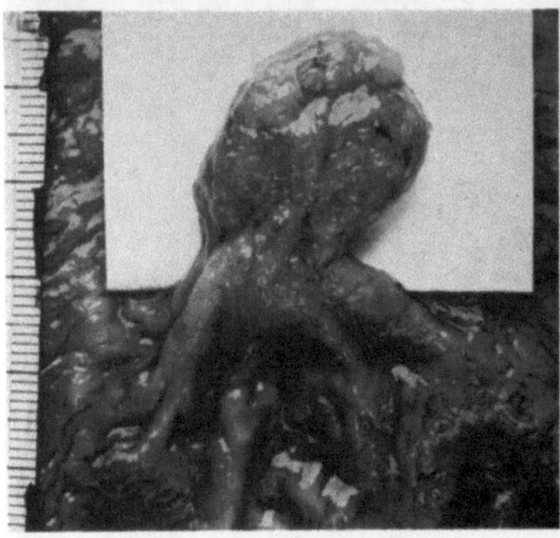

76i

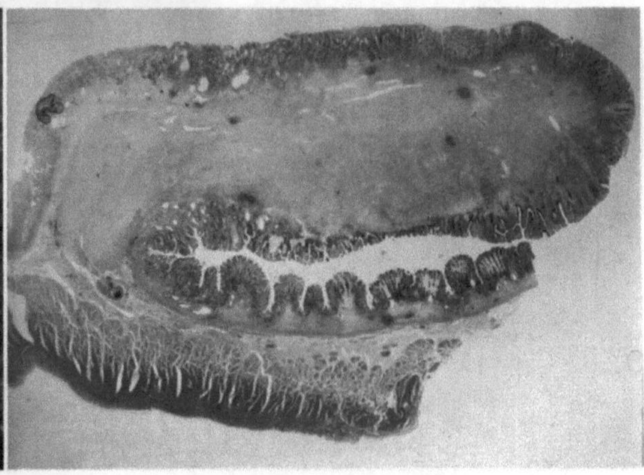

Fig. 76e Mucosal relief study in the prone position. There is a large tumor of the antrum with a somewhat-uneven surface toward the cardiac region. The lesion is shown to have a stalk.

Fig. 76f Barium filled stomach in the prone position. The top of the tumor prolapses into the duodenal cap, and its stalk is located at the prepylorus. Judging from these findings, it is diagnosed as a pedunculated and probably epithelial polyp.

Fig. 76g Endoscopic picture. A pedunculated and slightly reddened polypoid lesion is seen on the anterior wall of the prepylorus.

Fig. 76h Resected stomach. The lesion is pedunculated and its surface shows some coarse and granular mucosa, but there is no significant difference in color or properties from that of the surrounding area.

Fig. 76i Histopathological findings. Histologically, it is a leiomyoma.

X-ray pictures of gastric tumors prolapsing into the duodenum

In 1926 ELIASON *et al.* reported a case of gastric polyp prolapsing into the duodenum. Since then the possibility of a prolapsing polyp was a commonly recognized fact. SHORT *et al.* state that about 50 percent of the adenomas occur at the antrum, and about 40 percent of them are pedunculated and possibly prolapse into or obstruct the pyloric ring. However, there have been only 30 cases of prolapsing tumors of the stomach reported in English until 1968. In Japan also, not many of these occur cases in spite of the high frequency of gastric polypoid lesions.

Recently in both x-ray and endoscopic examinations, antispastic injections have been frequently used as premedication. The functional changes, such as the prolapsed state of gastric tumors, may be overlooked more than frequently expected. The sizes of prolapsing tumors are 1–2 cm in most cases, but cases with maximal diameters of more than 7.5 cm have been reported. The shape is generally spherical or oval, most commonly pedunculated, but sessile types are also common. Even submucosal tumors, not only pedunculated but also the sessile type, can prolapse into the duodenum if the fringe or surrounding mucosa of the tumor has enough mucosal motility. Our cases of tumors of the gastric body appear on the greater curvature where the submucosal layer is not rigid and mucosal motility is high.

Histologically, more than half of the prolapsing tumors are adenomatous polyps. Occasionally, though very rarely, a submucosal tumor or a tumor forming type of gastric cancer is reported. SHORT *et al.* have reported 10 cases of prolapsing tumors, 6 of which were of adenomas, 3 of which were leiomyomas, and 1 was a neurosarcoma. We experienced 4 cases, including the cases described here, out of 250 cases of stomach polyps, excluding cases of cancer. They are adenomatous polyps, leiomyomas, schwannomas, and early gastric cancer of the type I.

X-ray findings of prolapsing tumors are: 1) round or semiround shadow defects in the duodenum; 2) changes of the marginal line in a barium filled stomach, such as irregular peristalsis, abnormal contraction or irregularity of the wall, which are seen at the originating part of the tumor or the part closer to the pylorus; 3) abnormal shadows in the stomach made by the stalk of the tumors or by contracted mucosal folds. When a short, pedunculated tumor located in the gastric body or in the cardiac region prolapses into the duodenum, the most characteristic x-ray findings are a strong deformity of the stomach accompanied by an apparent contraction at the lesser curvature and the appearance of two different types of abnormal reliefs along and against the lesser curvature. If these findings and duodenal tumors are identified, they may be diagnosed as prolapsing or incarcerated cases of gastric tumors. As antispastic injections are usually given during endoscopic examination of the stomach, there are few opportunities to observe prolapsing tumors. When a lesion of the gastric body prolapses into the duodenum, a string-like contracted mucosa composed of several gastric folds, and a slackening of the lesser curvature by the contraction are observed. As mentioned above, a prolapsing tumor can be either epithelial or nonepithelial, benign or malignant. Their characteristics must be clearly understood so that they may be correctly identified.

3. Exogastric compression

Case 12

c. c.: Anorexia.
61 year-old male.

Compression of the gastric wall with exogastric tumors caused a considerable deformity of the intragastric wall. Variations of the posture and respiratory phase made them more easily distinguishable. In a double-contrast study in the supine position (Figs. 77 a, b), a smooth, wide shadow defect was seen. A submucosal-like tumor was observable on the posterior wall of the upper gastric body. There was observed some irregularities of the gastric wall, but they were not as constant as those of gastric cancer. The margin was very sharp. Tumors growing inside the stomach do not show such a sharp line of demarcation.

In adequately compressed studies (Figs. 77 c, d), mucosal folds ran smoothly on the tumor. In Figure 77 e, the tumor could barely be distinguished, so that a diagnosis of a submucosal tumor became more doubtful.

The location of the tumor, the posterior wall of the gastric body, suggested it to be a pancreas impression. Compression by submucosal tumors and those by exogastric tumors all show the same changes in the gastric mucosa. A submucosal tumor is an endogastric tumor and never fails to give a finding of distending the mucosal surface from below. If x-ray findings are varied by changing the posture or the respiratory phase, the presence of an exogastric compression must be considered.

It is very difficult to differentiate pancreatic cancer from pancreatic cysts. By laparotomy (Fig. 77 f), a portion of the pancreatic body was swollen with an elastic, hard induration (Fig. 77 g). A histological examination of the resected portion of the pancreatic tissue revealed it to be a cyst of the pancreatic body.

77 a

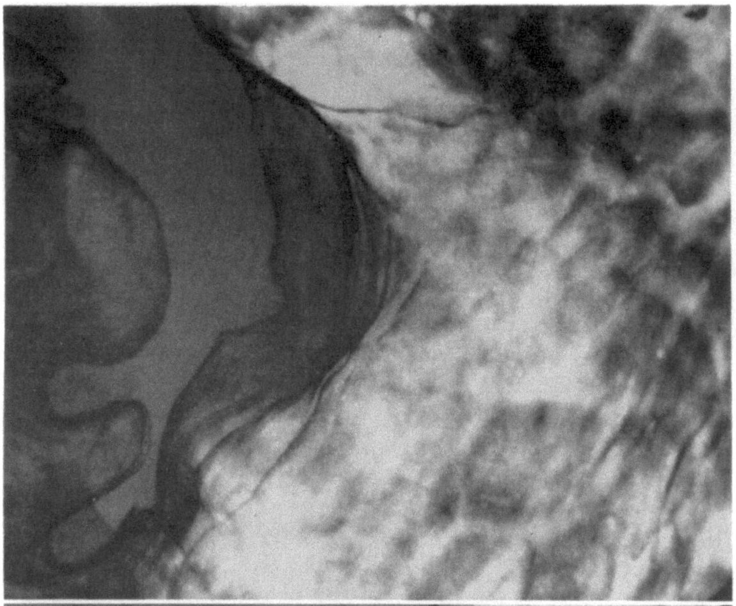

77 b

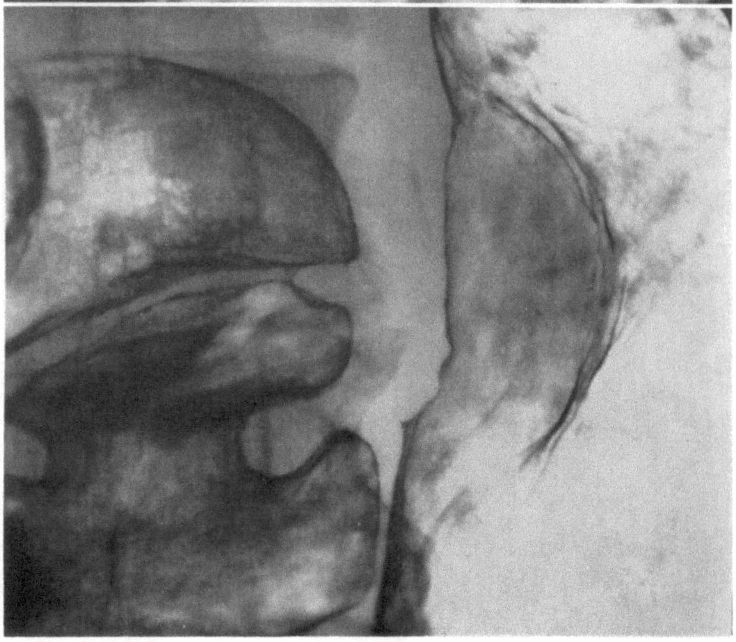

Fig. 77 a Double-contrast study in the supine position.

Fig. 77 b Double-contrast study in the supine position. A smooth, wide defect of the shadow is seen on the posterior wall of the upper gastric body. Although there is some irregularity of the wall, the stability of the shadow and the irregularity of the wall as seen in cases of gastric cancer are not observed in either picture. The margin is very clear.

77c
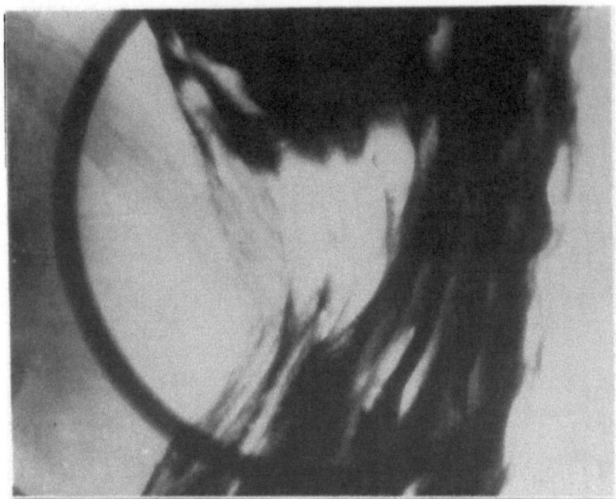

77d
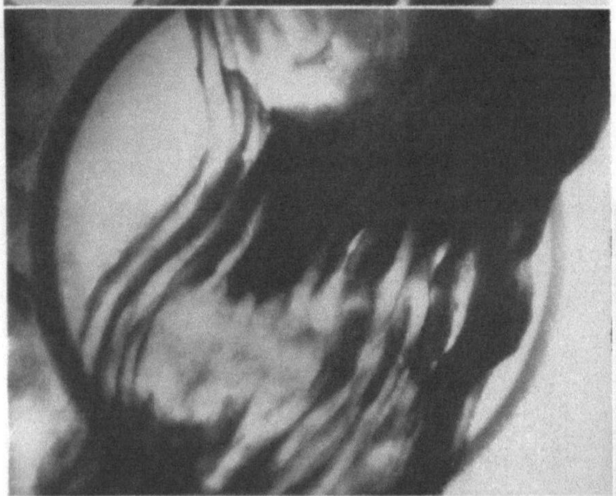

77e
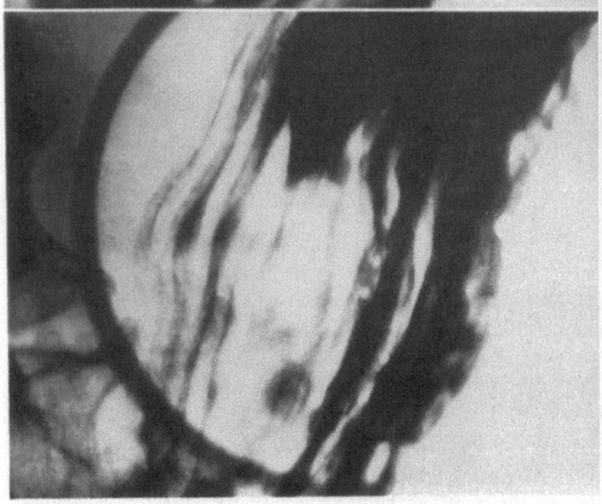

77f
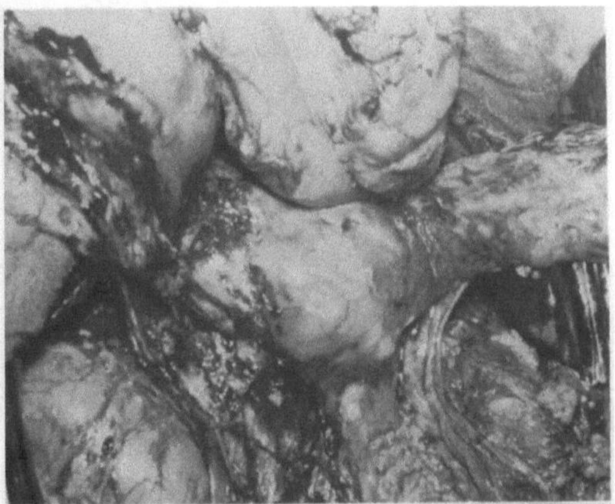

77g
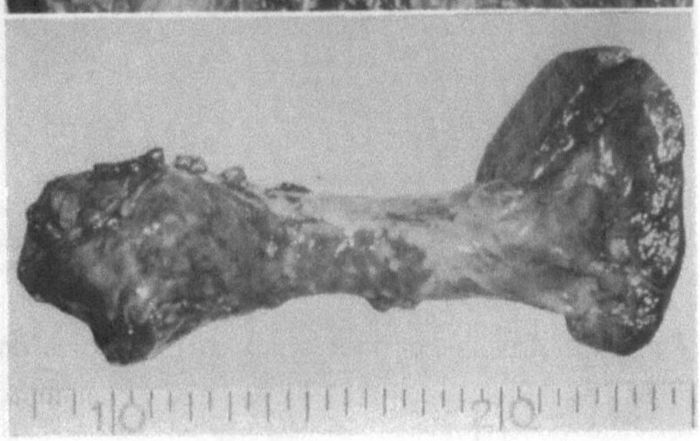

Figs. 77c–e Compression studies in a semi-upright position. Mucosal folds running smoothly on the tumor are observed in these three pictures in which the compression is gradually changed.

Fig. 77d Appears to be a mucosal tumor. The so-called bridging folds are seen from all directions. The changes as observed in this picture suggest an exogastric compression.

Fig. 77e Compression study in a semi-upright position. This barely shows the shadow of the tumor and suggests an exogastric compression.

Fig. 77f Finding at the time of laparotomy. A part of the pancreatic body swollen with an elastic, hard induration is observed in the center.

Fig. 77g Resected pancreatic tissue. Histologically, it was proved to be a cyst of the pancreatic body.

4. A typical neurogenic tumor

Case 13

c. c.: Epigastric discomfort.

43 year-old female.

In either the upright position (Fig. 77 a) or the prone position (Fig. 77 b), the radiograph of the barium filled stomach showed no abnormal contours. A double-contrast study in the supine position revealed a soft, club-like protrusion on the folds of the posterior wall of the gastric angle. Since the protrusion was surrounded by a thin layer of contrast medium, it was diagnosed as a flat or hemispheric tumor with a gently sloping surface. In the picture, its size measured 1 cm in diameter. Compression studies (Figs. 77 f, g) showed a club-like protrusion of the fold, which readily disappeared under their layer of the contrast medium with a light grade compression. Note that the area on the surface of the protrusion resembled that of the surrounding intact mucosa. Since the surface of the so-called hyperplastic polyps was rougher, the protrusion was suspected of being a submucosal tumor.

Endoscopically, the above-mentioned flat protrusion was located on the posterior wall of the gastric angle. Since the surface was slightly reddish and glossy, it was difficult to diagnose whether it was an epithelial or nonepithelial tumor. It could also be suspected of being an early gastric cancer of the Type IIa based on its shape and size.

From macroscopic findings of the resected specimen (Fig. 77 i), the lesion was diagnosed as a submucosal tumor. Histologically (Fig. 77 j), the tumor was a neurofibroma developing under the submucosal layer. Radiologically, this case was diagnosed as a submucosal tumor and endoscopically, as an epithelial one.

According to PALMER, the incidence of neurofibroma under 3 cm in diameter accounted for only 17 per cent of the total. YAMAGATA reported the incidence of cases under 3 cm in diameter as 24 per cent and those under 1 cm in diameter as 2 per cent.

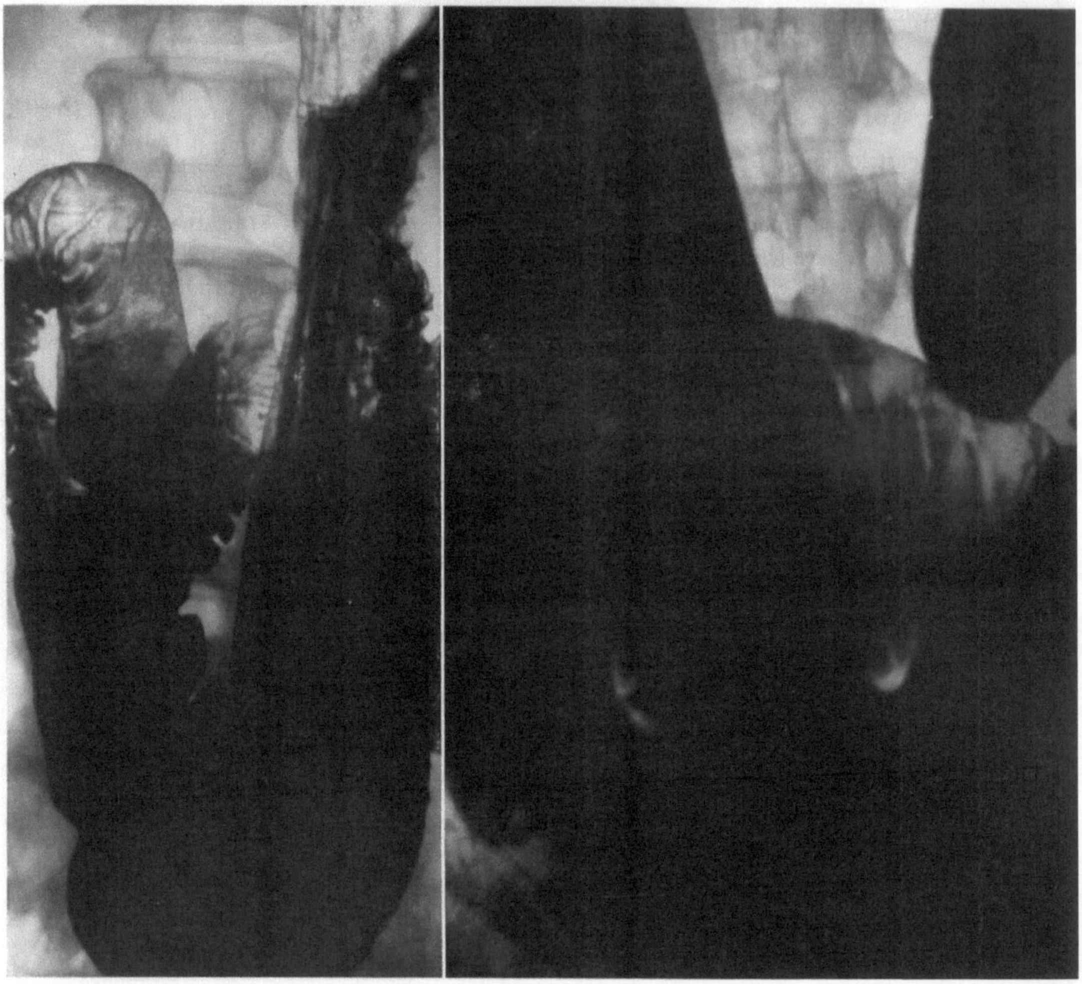

77a

77b

Fig. 77a Upright position.

Fig. 77b Prone position. Barium filled study shows no abnormality.

77c 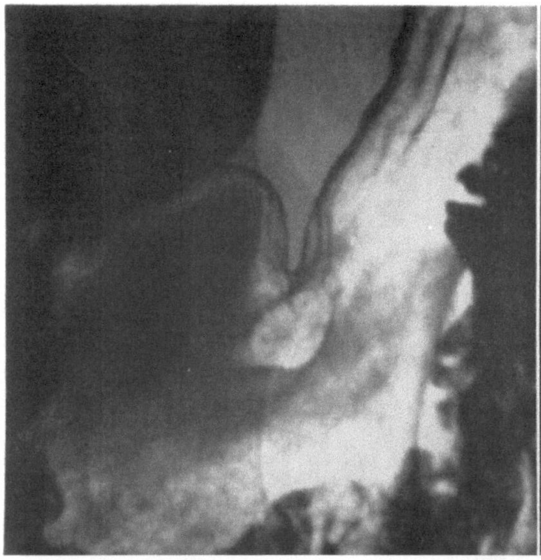 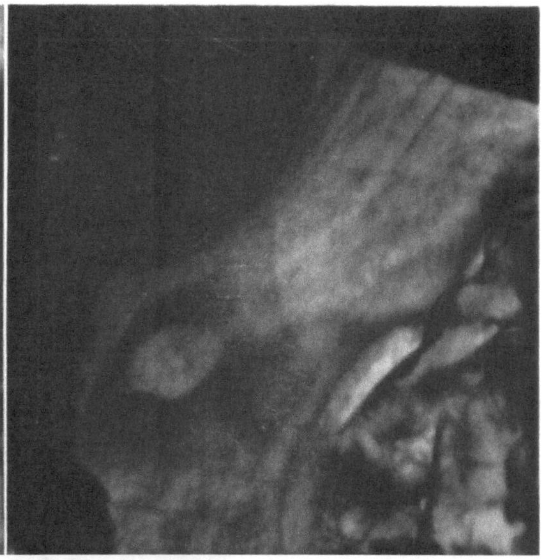 77d

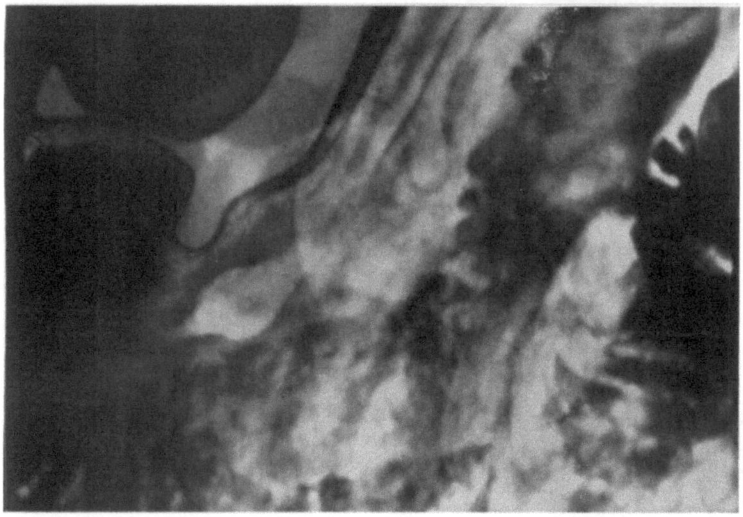 77e

77f 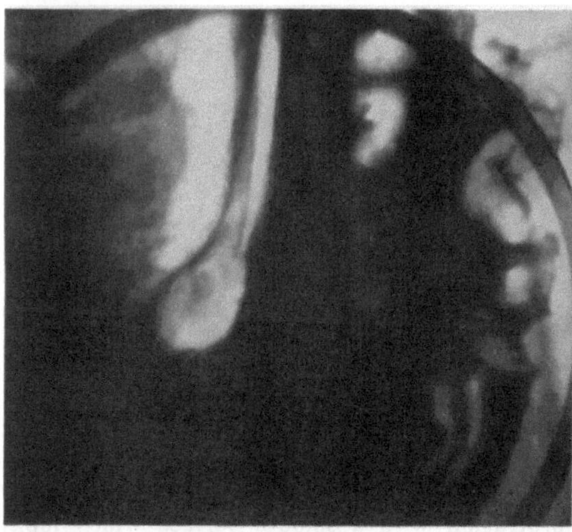 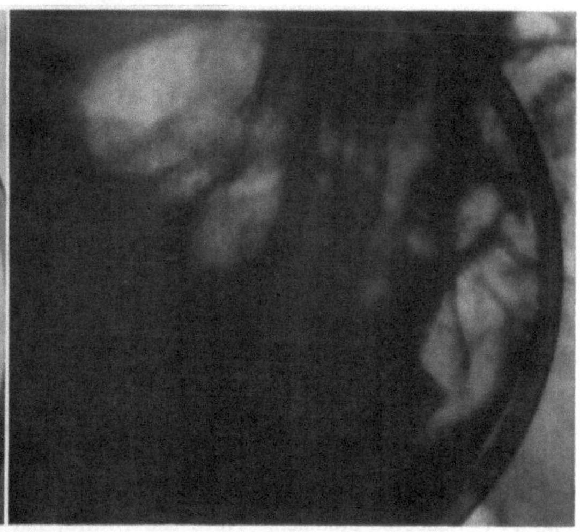 73g

Figs. 77c, d Double-contrast studies in the supine position.

Fig. 77e A soft, club-like protrusion on a fold on the posterior wall of the gastric angle. The protrusion surrounded by a thin layer of contrast medium is diagnosed as a type I or II polypoid lesion. This protrusion is flat or hemispheric in shape with a gently sloping surface. The surface of the protrusion appears rough, similar to that of the surrounding intact mucosa.

Figs. 77f, g Compression studies. Note the same findings as in the double-contrast method. The low, flat protrusion disappears into the contrast medium under a light grade compression.

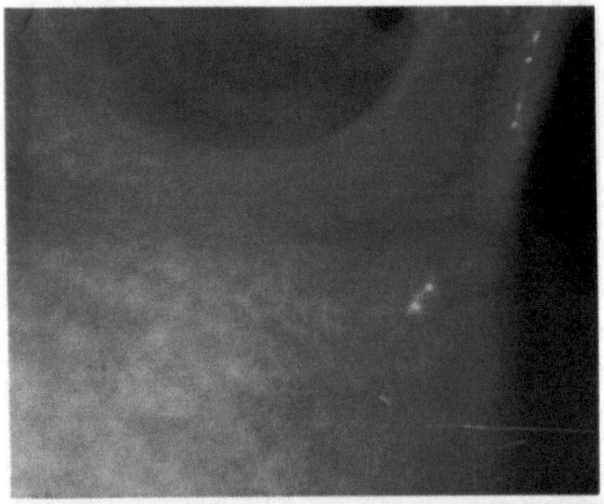

77h

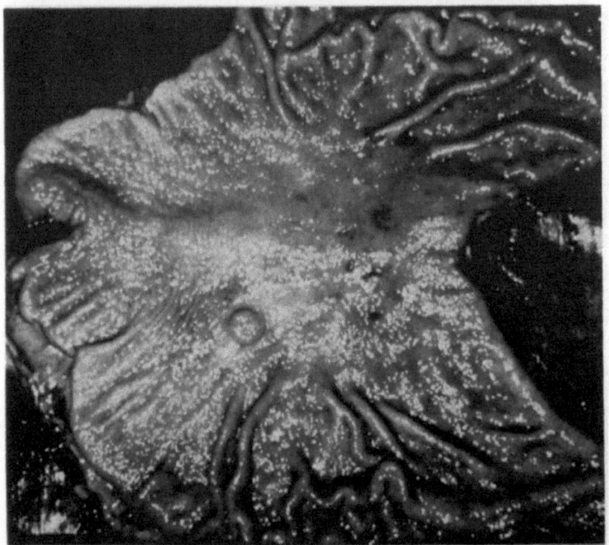

77i

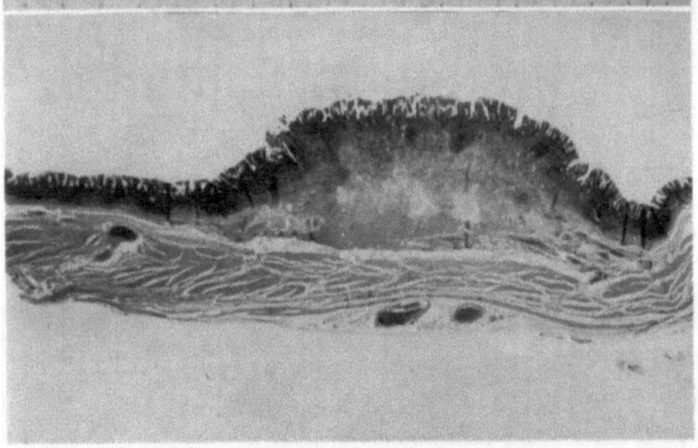

77j

Fig. 77h Endoscopic picture. The slightly reddish and glossy surface of the flat protrusion lead us to diagnose it as an epithelial tumor. An early gastric cancer, type IIa, is suspected though cancers of that type are generally indicated by discoloration.

Fig. 77i Resected stomach. Note the round, flat protrusion with a smooth surface which looks similar to the neighboring mucosa. The protrusion is located on the posterior wall of the gastric angle.

Fig. 77j Histopathological findings. The tumor is a neurofibroma growing in the submucosal layer.

5. Adenoma and cyst

Ususally adenomas are nodular, sometimes histologically showing polypoid or papillary structures. Occasionally, an adenoma forms a cystic structure because of a secretion stasis due to underdevelopment of excretory glands.

Cysts are classified as follows by PALMER:

1) congenital 2) echinococcal 3) mechanical
4) neoplastic 5) miscellaneous

The roentgenographic appearance of a cyst is almost identical to that of a submucosal tumor. Endoscopic examination shows the lustrous surface of the cyst.

Case 14

c. c.: Epigastric discomfort.

61 year-old female.

A picture taken under adequate compression demonstrated two connected filling defects clearly outlined on the posterior wall of the body. However, a supine, double-contrast study showed a hill-like protuberance, measuring 1.5×1.3 cm, which was confirmed as a hemispherical form of polypoid lesion. It was diagnosed as a submucosal tumor.

Gastrofiberscopy revealed a reddish, lustrous, low, mucosal elevation. There were black hemorrhagic flecks on top of the mucosal elevation. From these endoscopic findings of a mucosal elevation of epithelial origin, an early gastric cancer of the type IIa or localized hyperplasia could not be differentiated.

In some cases, roentgenologic and endoscopic diagnoses do not agree. The patient was operated on with his permission. Gross findings of the resected stomach revealed a low, mucosal elevation with a reddish surface. Histologically, it was diagnosed as an adenoma developing in the submucosal layer like a cyst.

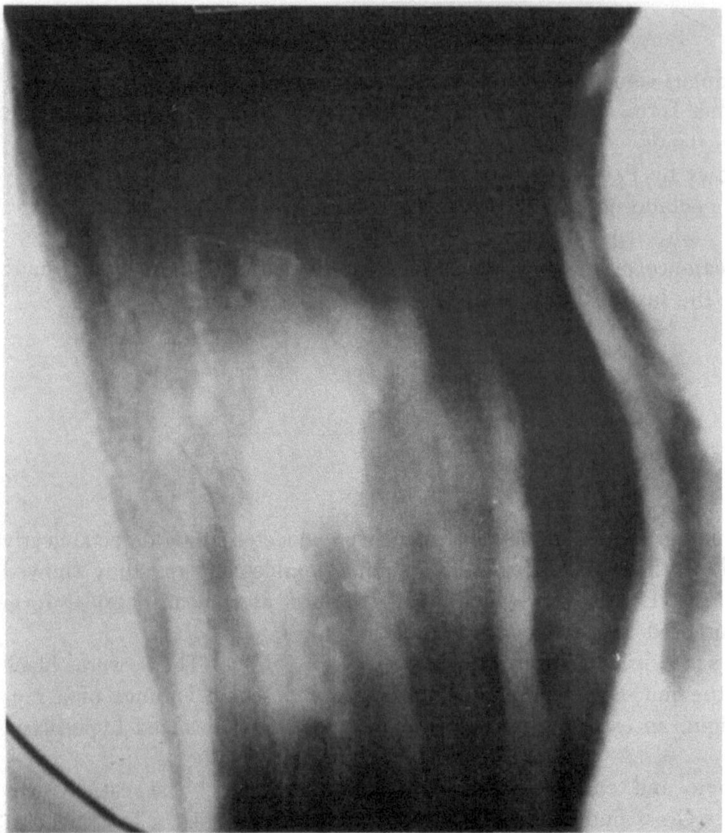

79 a

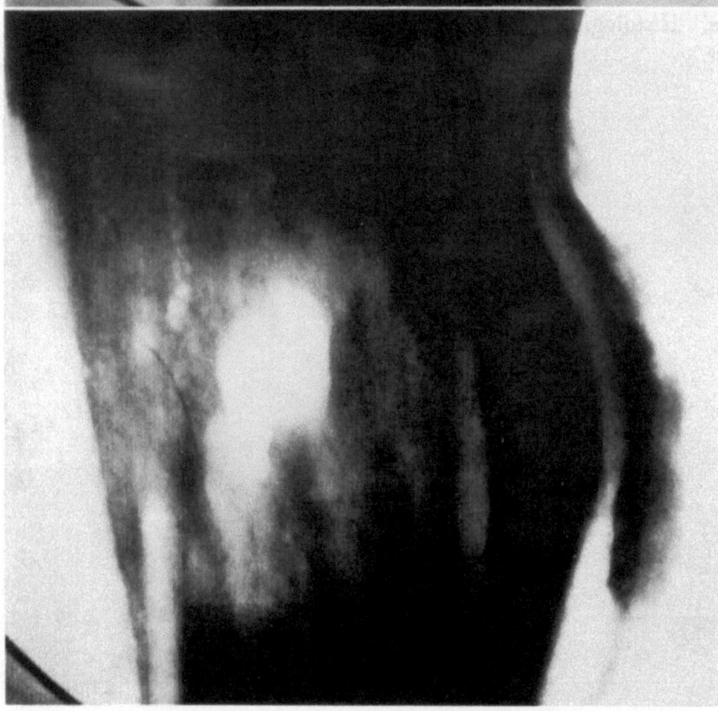

79 b

Figs. 79 a and b Compression studies (adequate and deep compression). A slightly elevated lesion is connected with two bean-sized filling defects.

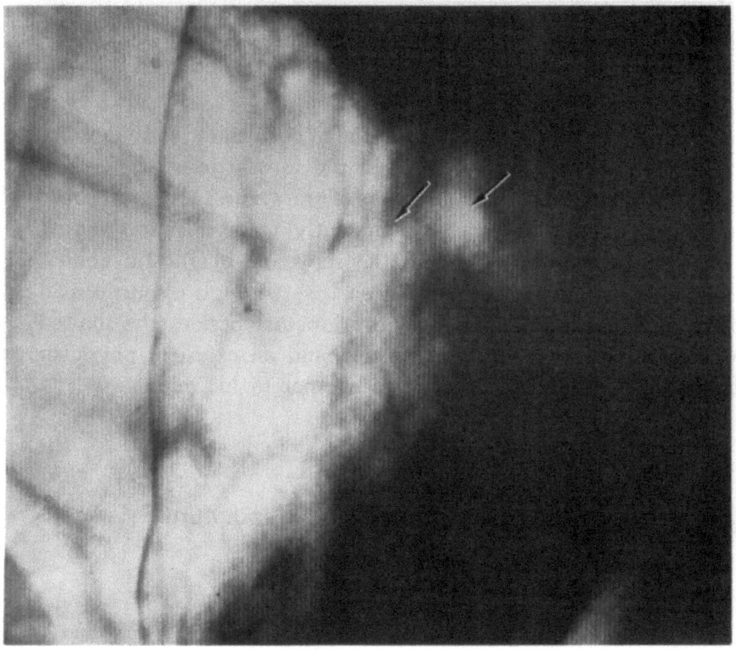

79c

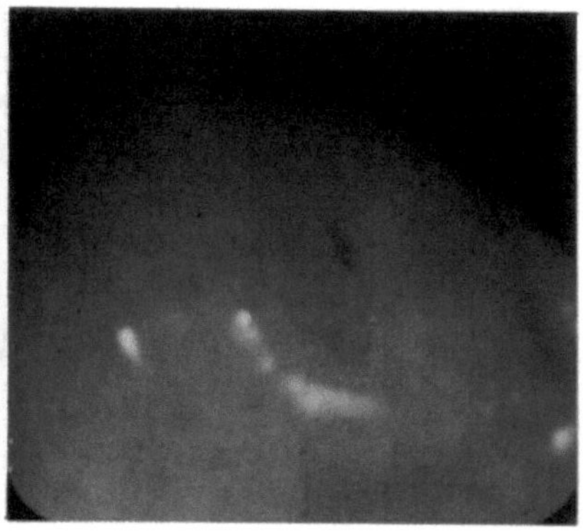

79d

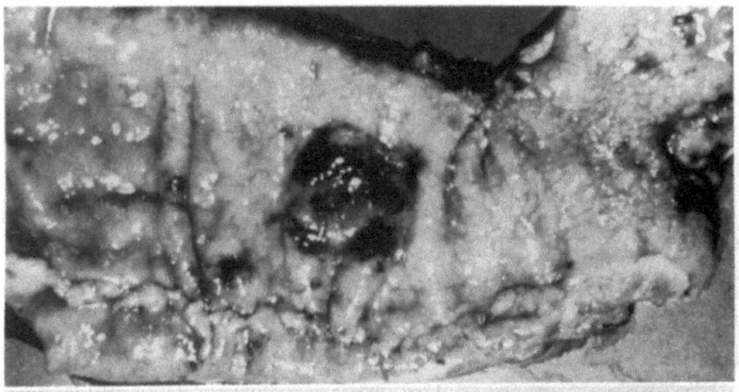

79e

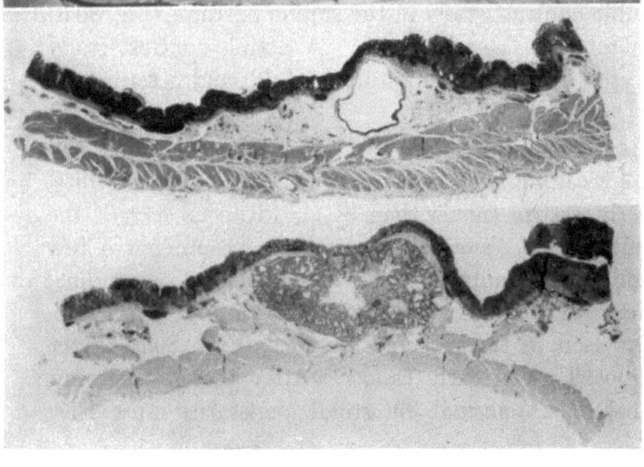

79f

Fig. 79c **Double-contrast study in the supine position.** Connected protrusions measuring 1.5×1.3cm are seen.

Fig. 79d **Endoscopic picture.** A reddish, lustrous, low, mucosal elevation with a central hemorrhage is revealed. With these endoscopic findings, we cannot rule out an early gastric cancer of the type IIa nor a polyp due to localized hyperplasia.

Fig. 79e **Resected stomach.** Gross inspection of the resected stomach reveals a low, elevated lesion with an erythematous mucosa.

Fig. 79f **Histopathological findings.** Histologically, it is an adenoma developing in the submucosal layer like a cyst.

C. Rare cases

The first and second problems in diagnosing protruding lesions have been stated with descriptions of some misleading, indistinguishable, or not typical cases in previous articles. The third problem is encountered in rare cases. When the characteristics of rare cases of protruding lesions in the stomach have been learned, diagnoses can be confidently made. Understanding and remembering the distinctive features of rare cases widens the scope of diagnostic ability. The most important thing is to find the questionable points in each case through discussions in a small group. It is important to know of cases diagnosed by other doctors besides the limited cases of one's own experience. Medicine is experimental diagnostics, and an excellent physician has the features of rare and difficult cases classified in an orderly manner in his mind.

1. A case of type I early gastric cancer invaginated into the duodenum

Case 15

c. c.: Complaints of anemia and diarrhea with tenesmus.

62 year-old male.

A barium filled study in the upright position (Fig. 80 a) exhibited a giant filling defect, measuring 4.5×4.0 cm, in the pyloric region. Slight marginal rigidity was noted. A barium filled study in the prone position (Fig. 80 b) exhibited antral peristalsis and a few longitudinal folds running towards the tumor which was prolapsing into the duodenum. A double-contrast study in the supine position (Fig. 80 c) and the other double-contrast method revealed not only the superficial irregularity of the tumor, but also the longitudinal fold formation of the antrum. Although marginal rigidity was not very remarkable in the double-contrast method, superficial irregularity of the tumor placed it in Grade IV.

It was diagnosed as a duodenal relapse of a gastric tumor because such remarkable changes were not observed in duodenal tumors. A double-contrast study in the supine position (Fig. 80 d) demonstrated the duodenal bulb filled with the relapsing gastric tumor. A double-contrast study in the prone position (Fig. 80 f) exhibited the crossing sign of longitudinal folds and a transverse one on the anterior wall of the antrum.

Much experience is required to read these x-ray pictures accurately. The size and superficial irregularity of the tumor suggested a diagnosis of a carcinomatous tumor. Because of its mobility, it seemed more proper to diagnose it as an early gastric cancer than as an advanced one of the fungating type. Endoscopically, the tumor could not be observed under direct vision, but a few longitudinal folds and a remakable contraction of the antrum were detectable. Longitudinal folds including an erosion with slight bleeding were suspicious of carcinomatous infiltration. Biopsy proved it to be an adenocarcinoma. As seen in the resected stomach (Figs. 80 h, i), the pedunculated, spherical protuberance was diagnosed as an early cancer. After the gastrectomy, the complaints of diarrhea with tenesmus abated. Abnormal intestinal peristalsis must have caused the diarrhea with tenesmus in this case.

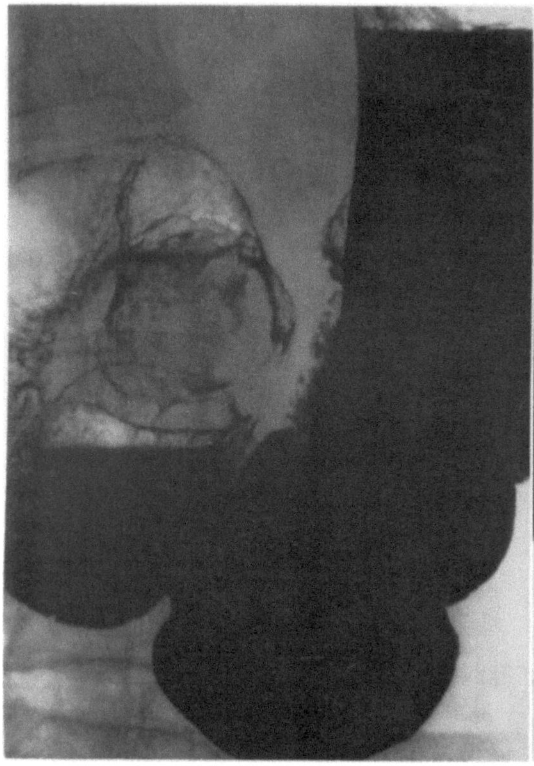

80a

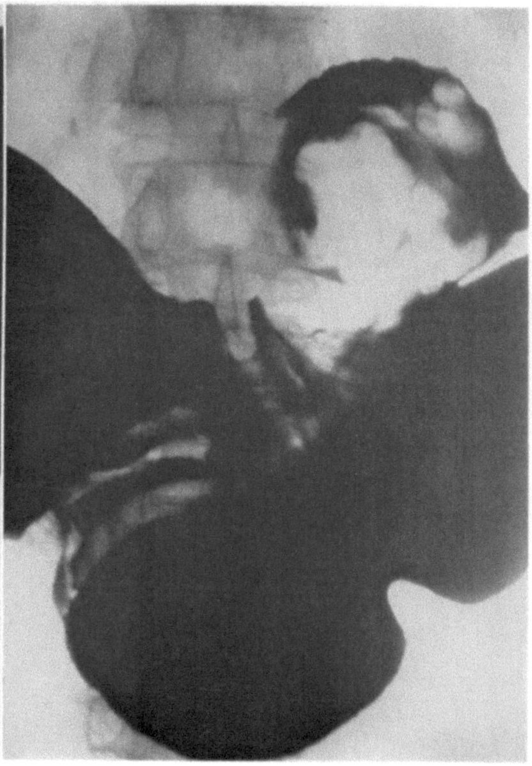

80b

80c

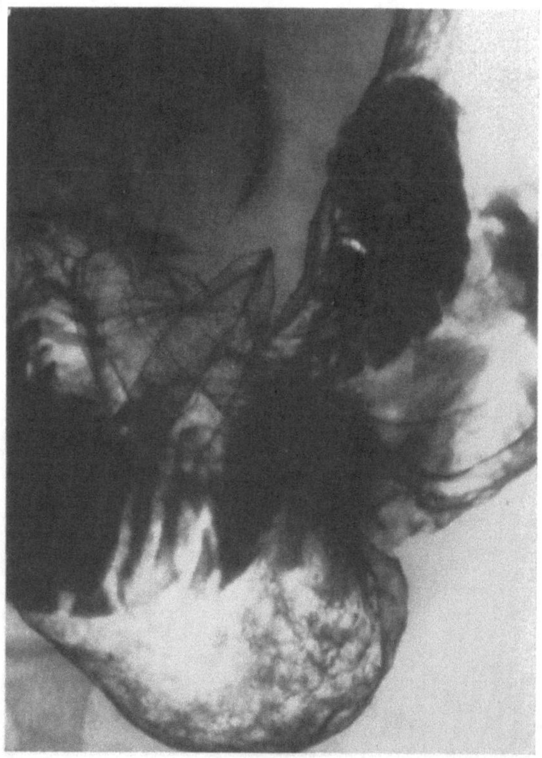

Fig. 80a Barium filled stomach in the upright position. A giant filling defect, measuring 4.5× 4.0 cm, is observed in the duodenal bulb. Marginal rigidity is not markedly noticeable.

Fig. 80b Barium filled stomach in the prone position. An irregular, giant filling defect is seen in the duodenal bulb. Antral peristalsis and a few longitudinal folds are seen running towards the tumor.

Fig. 80c Double-contrast study in the supine position.

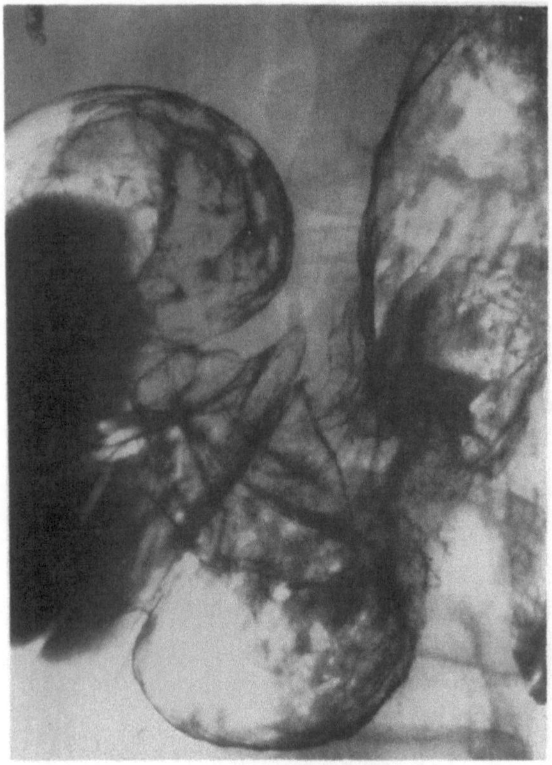

80d

Fig. 80d Double-contrast study in the supine position. Not only superficial irregularity but also longitudinal folds of the contracting mucosa are shown.

Fig. 80e Double-contrast study in the supine position. A crossing sign of the longitudinal and transverse folds is seen.

Fig. 80f Double-contrast study in the prone position.

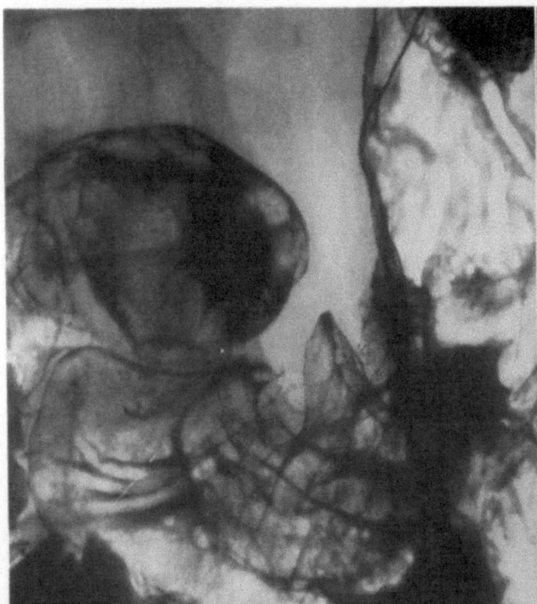

80e

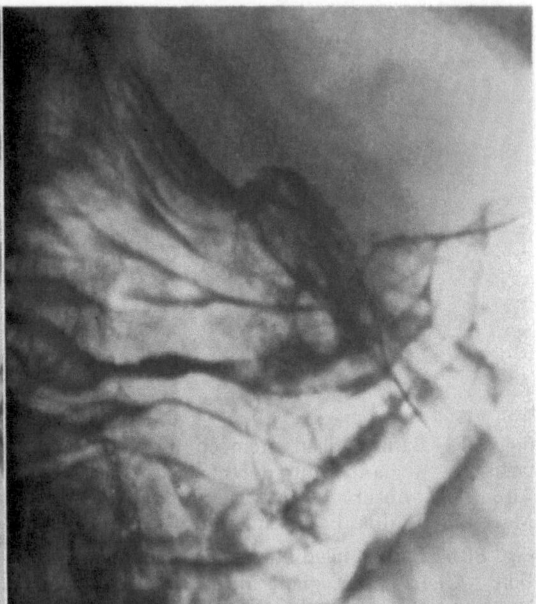

80f

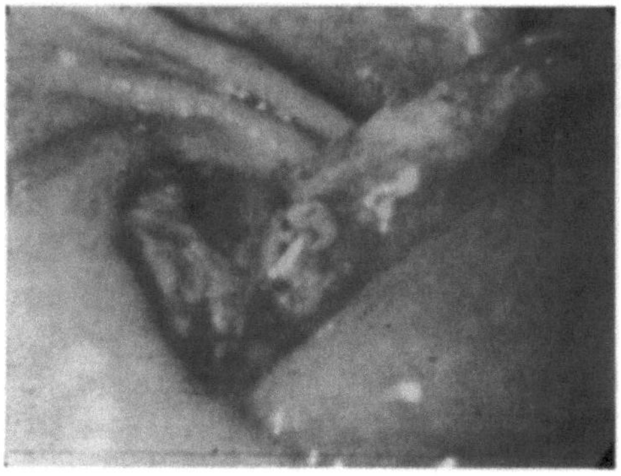

80g

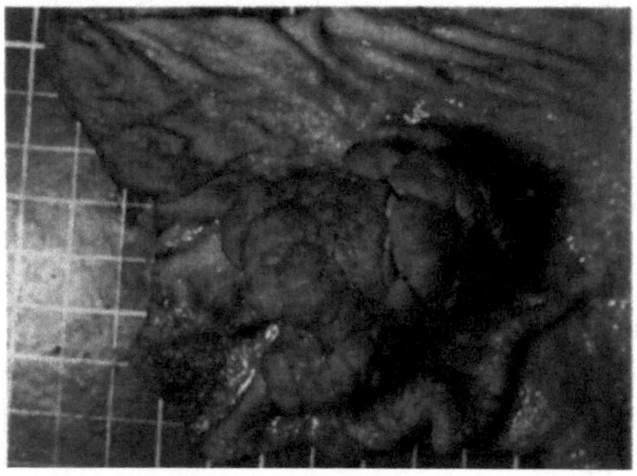

80h

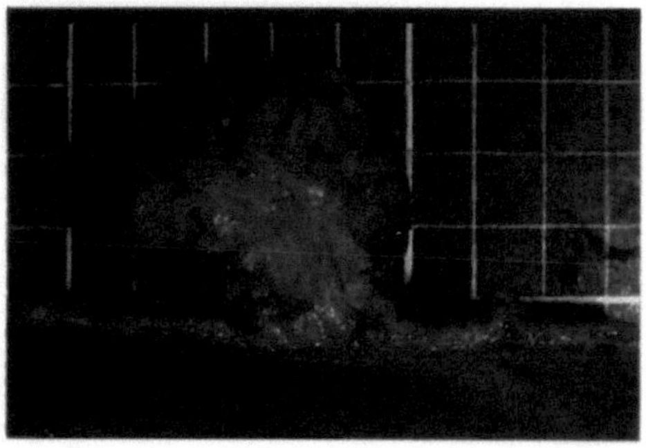

80i

Fig. 80g Gastrofiberscopic picture. Multiple erosions and irregular bleeding are seen at the base of this prolapsed, polypoid lesion.

Fig. 80h Resected stomach. A pedunculated, globular protuberance with a nodule is seen in the prepyloric region.

Fig. 80i Cut section. Histologically, the tumor is diagnosed as an early gastric cancer of type I. Carcinoma cells are seen on the surface and also on the edge of the tumor.

2. Polyposis

"Polyposis" means a multitude of polyps, as against multiple polyps. Polyps or multiple polyps are often located on the greater curvature of the antrum. The disposition of polyposis, however, differs from other polyps.

Case 16

c.c.: Epigastric distress.

56 year-old female.

A barium filled study in the upright or prone position demonstrated smooth and hemispherical filling defects crowded in the gastric body. They showed no marginal irregularities. These roentgenological findings were also seen in the double-contrast method. Numerous pea-or bean-sized protuberances were seen in the pictures (Figs. 81 c, d). The most interesting finding was that the polypoid lesions were not located in the antral region. There were no polypoid lesions observed in the antrum by endoscopic examinations (Figs. 81 e, f).

Crowded polyps were visualized in the body by the retroflexion technique. Their surfaces were almost completely smooth except for partial erosions. They showed no bleeding and no discoloration. The polyps were shaped hemispherically or were elevated like hills. Seventy polypoid lesions of various sizes were seen in the resected stomach, placed on the transitional zone from the fundic to the pyloric glands (Fig. 81 g). Histologically, carcinoma cells were not observed (Figs. 81 h, i).

Polyposis differs widely from the pedunculated, adenomatous polyps as seen in multiple polyps. It has not been determined whether polyposis is a precancerous stage. The polyps of this case belonged to type II of Nakamura's classification. Remarkable hyperplasia of the gastric mucosa was seen.

81a

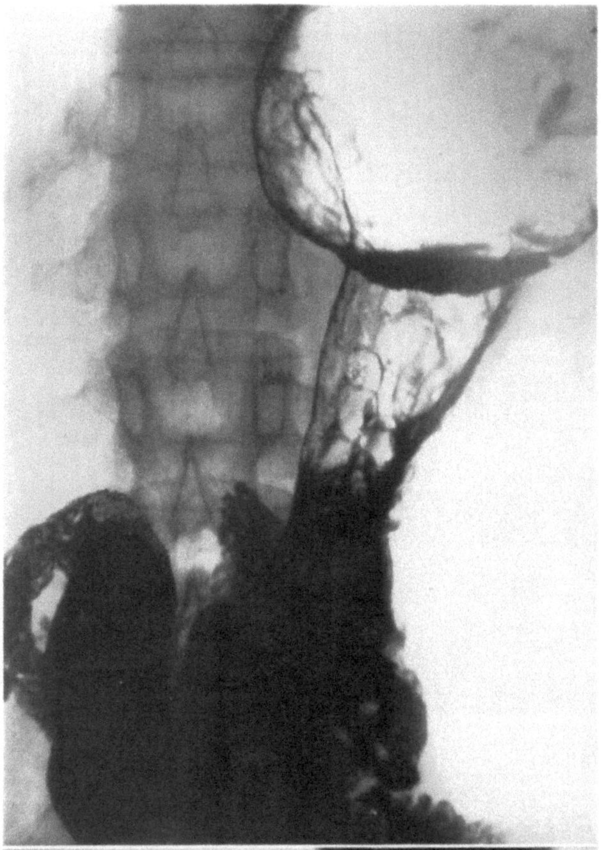

81b

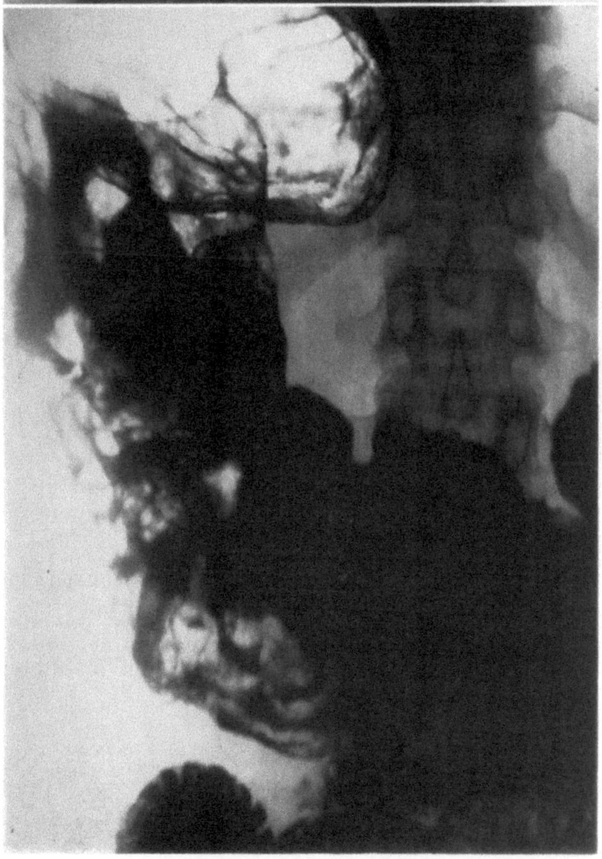

Fig. 81a Barium filled stomach in the upright position.
Fig. 81b Stomach half filled with barium in the prone position. Many hemispherical filling defects are crowded on the gastric body.

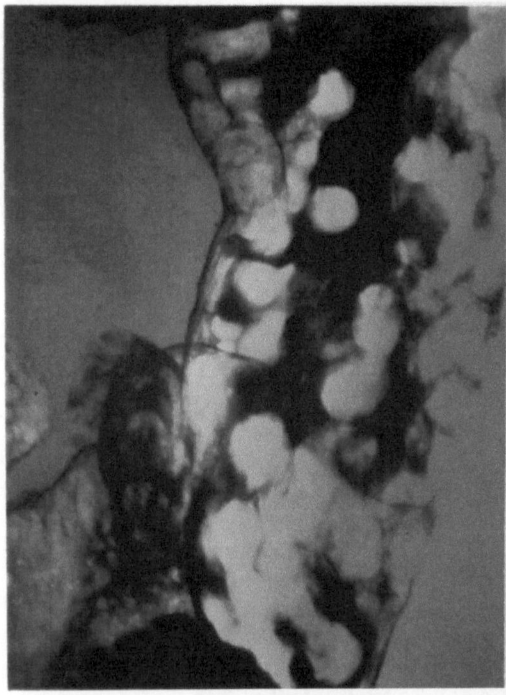

81c

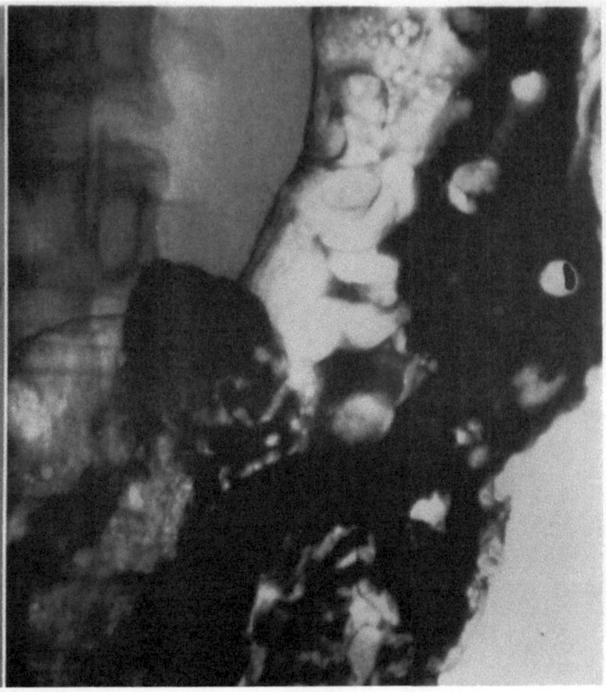

81d

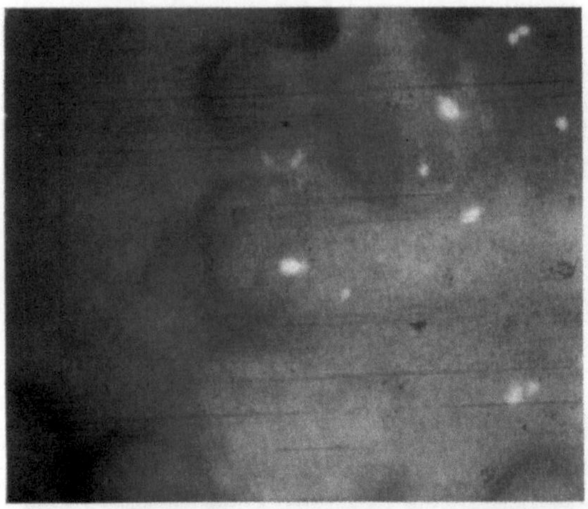

81e

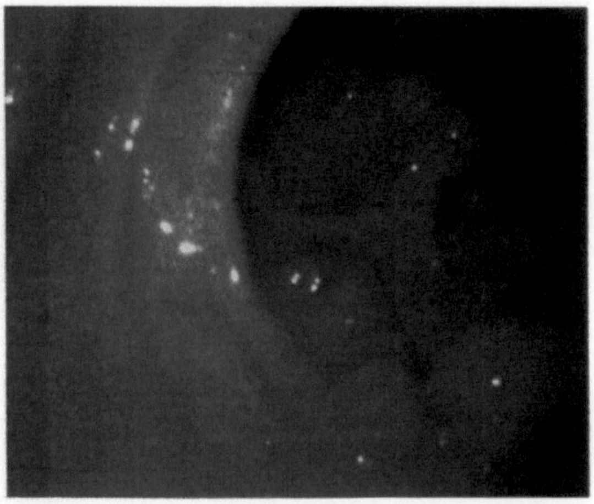

81f

Figs. 81c, d Double-contrast method in the supine position. Many pea- or bean-sized protuberances with a wide base are located on the gastric body.

Figs. 81e, f Endoscopic picture. Elevations of hemispherical forms with smooth surfaces are crowded and connected on the gastric body. Neither bleeding nor dirty discoloration are noticed on their surfaces, except for apical erosions.

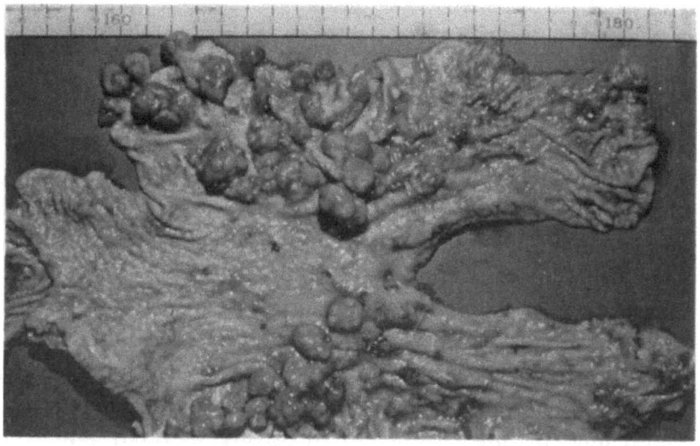

81g

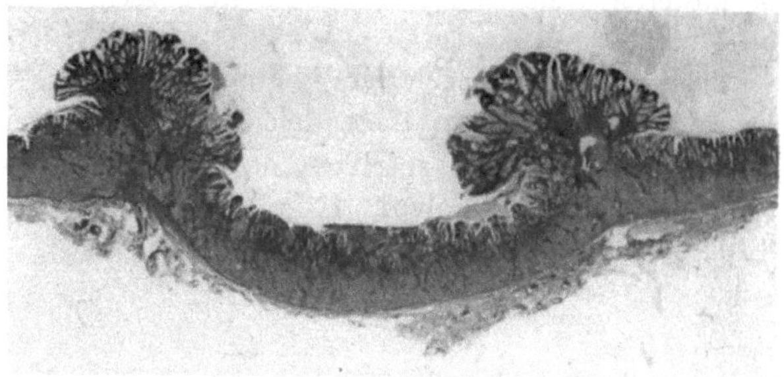

81h

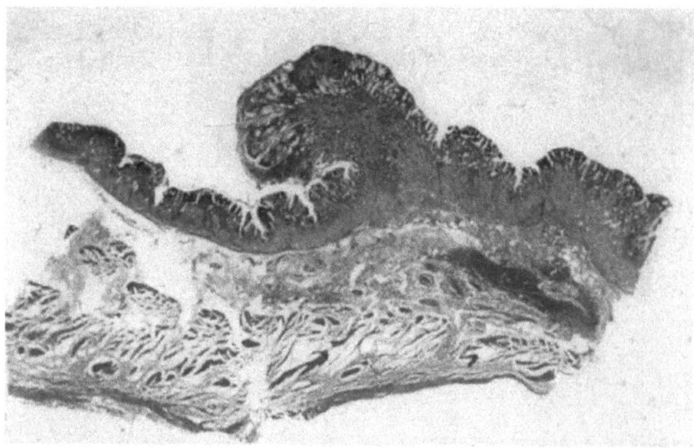

81i

Fig. 81g Resected stomach. Seventy polypoid lesions of various sizes are seen from the transitional zone of the fundic glands to the pyloric glands.

Fig. 81h Histopathological findings. The cut section of a spherical polypoid lesion shows hyperplasia of the gastric mucosa and a partial thickening of the pseudo-pyloric glands. Gastric cancer was not established.

Fig. 81i Histopathological findings. An adenoma surrounded by a deeply stained columnar epithelium looks like an onion.

Case 17

c. c.: Epigastric fullness.

62 year-old female.

In the upright, barium filled study a widespread, irregular margin of the lesser curvature and a small, radioluscent area were demonstrated in the lower gastric body (Fig. 82 a). No particular change, however, was seen along the lesser and greater curvature of the antrum (Fig. 82 b). In the supine, double-contrast study, spherical, stalkless, grouped protuberances, measuring about 1 cm in diameter, were noticed above the angle (Figs. 82 c, d).

The mucosal folds near the greater curvature were slightly hypertrophic. In the three compression studies (Figs. 82 e–g), seven polypoid prominences were widely spread above the angle. Each of the seven protuberances was less than 1 cm in diameter and was hill-shaped or hemispherical in elevation, varying in height and arranged in a necklace-like configuration. In the endoscopic picture (Fig. 82 h), relatively elevated polyps with no stalks on either the anterior or posterior walls above the angle were seen. Neither bleeding flecks nor granular surfaces were seen.

The resected stomach showed grouped, mucosal elevations in the borderline area, which could be considered similar to those demonstrated by previous cases (Fig. 82 i). Judging from such growing forms and the specificity of their origin, it seemed necessary that polyposis be differentiated from multiple polyps. Histologically, no polyp had been proven to be a carcinoma (Fig. 82 j).

82 a

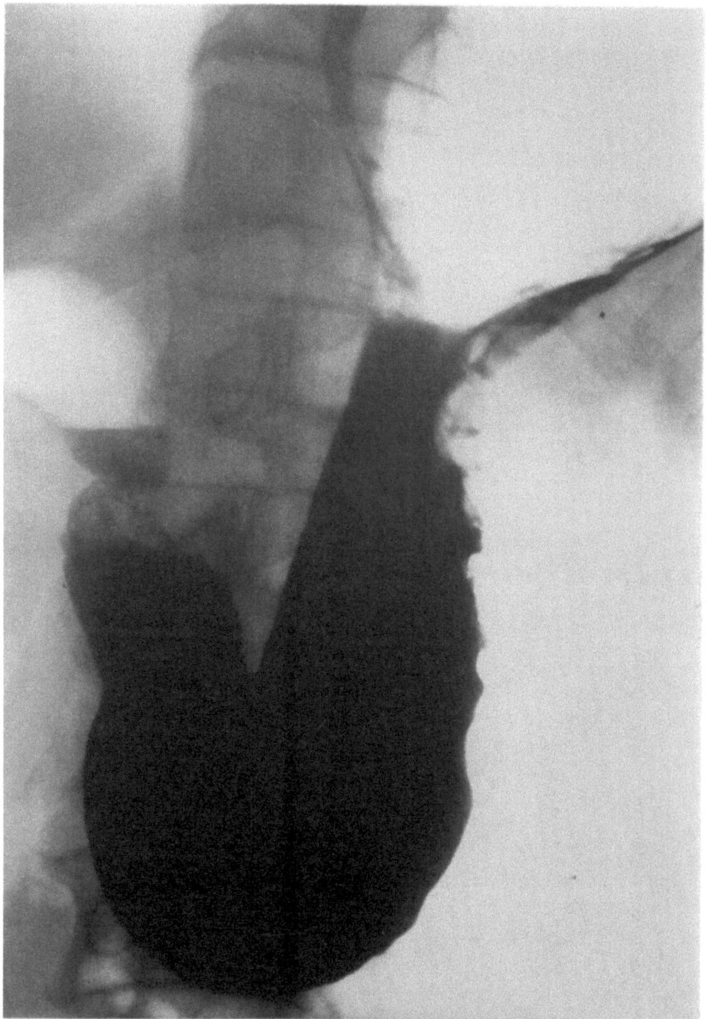

82 b

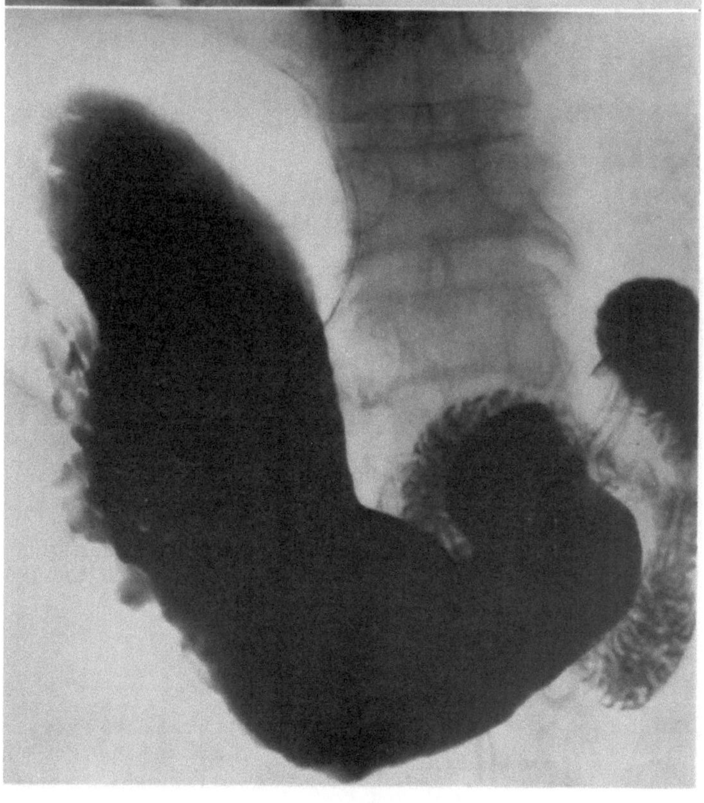

Fig. 82 a Upright, filling study. The irregular margin of the lesser curvature can be seen on the lower gastric body. No other definite change is seen.

Fig. 82 b Prone, filled study. A slight irregularity or small niche is detected above the angle.

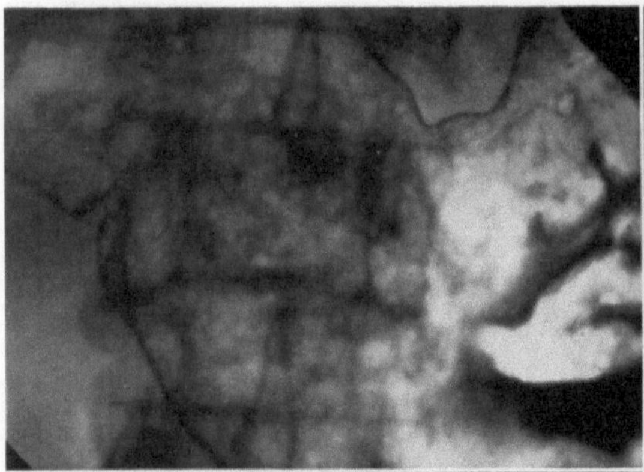
82c

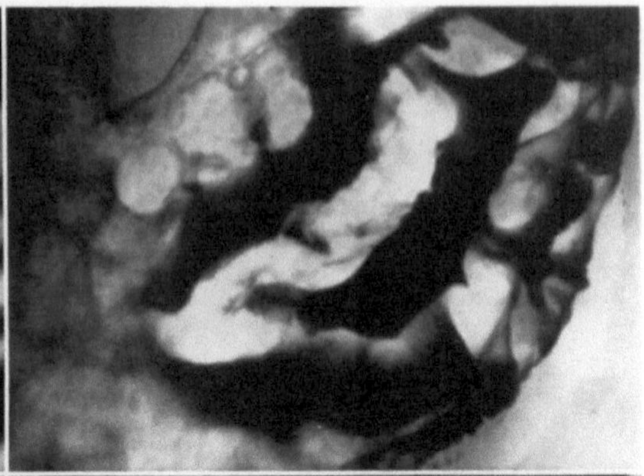
82d

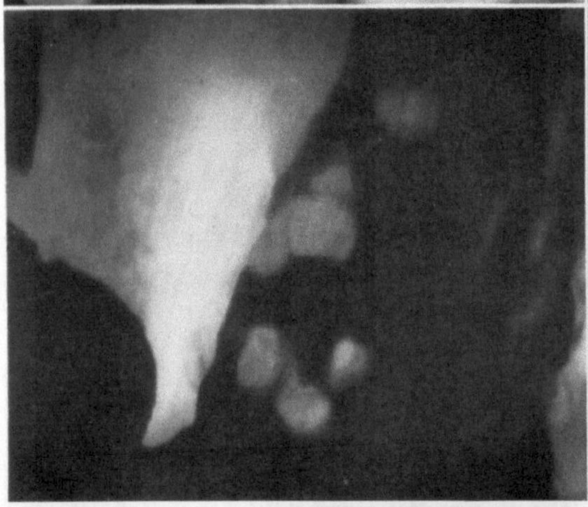
82e

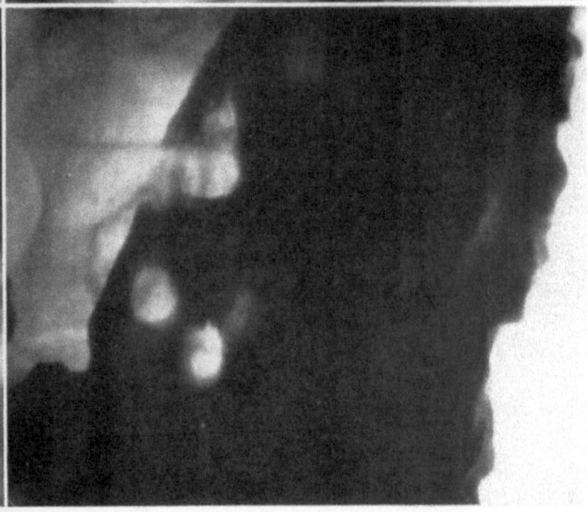
82f

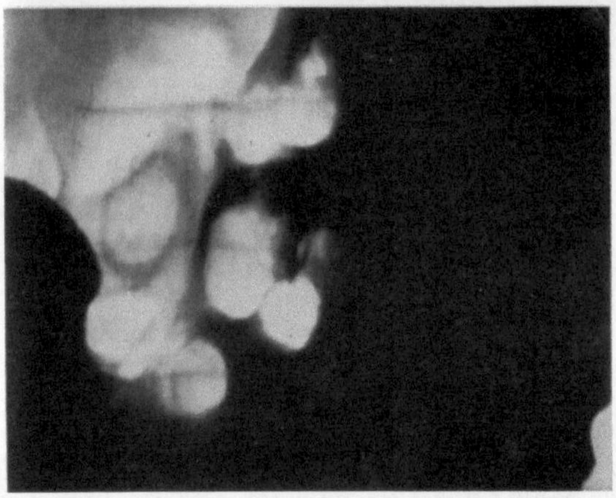
82g

Fig. 82c Supine, double-contrast study. Lesions are not noticed in the antrum.

Fig. 82d Supine, double-contrast study. Hypertropic mucosal folds near the greater curvature and hill-shaped or hemispherically grouped elevations are apparent above the angular portion.

Fig. 82e Upright, compression study.

Fig. 82f Upright, compression study.

Fig. 82g Upright, compression study. By various compression methods, fairly well-outlined, grouped elevations are made apparent in the lower portion of the gastric body.

82h
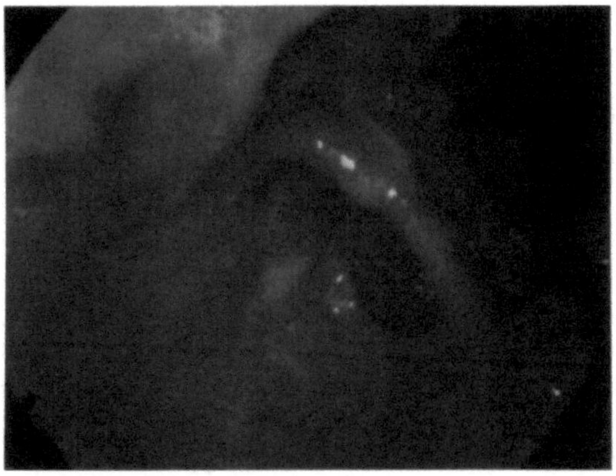

82i
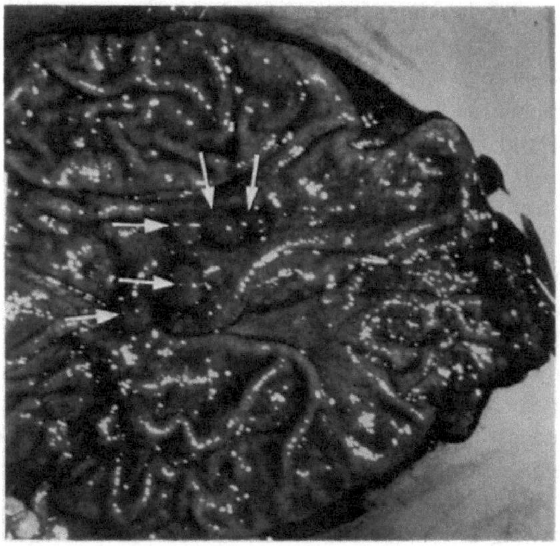

82j
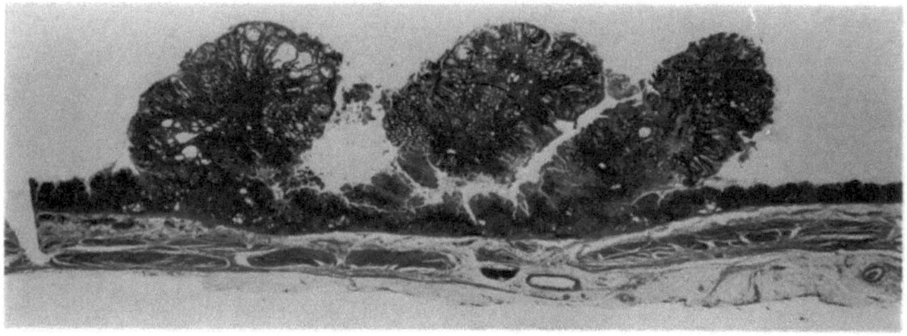

Fig. 82h Endoscopic picture. Several elevations are seen in the lower portion of the gastric body, whereas in the antrum no elevations are noticed.

Fig. 82i Resected stomach.

Fig. 82j Histopathological findings. Histologically, epithelial polyps resulting from gastric hyperplasia and proliferation of pseudo-pyloric glands are detected. No malignancy is seen.

3. Polyp accompanied by leiomyoma

Case 18

c. c.: Comprehensive examination of the stomach.

54 year-old male.

No particular lesion was seen along the margin in the upright, filled study (Fig. 83 a), nor in the prone, filled study (Fig. 83 b). But the prone, double-contrast study showed a little fingertip-sized elevation, lobulated, and spherical with a stalk in the granulated area on the antral anterior wall. The polyp with its stalk was demonstrated by adequate compression studies (Figs. 83 d, e). Its size was 2.3×1.8 cm in diameter.

It was probably an adenomatous polyp, but a carcinomatous polyp could not be ruled out. In this case, it was important that a rice grain sized, spherical elevation was unexpectedly observed on the double-contrasted fornix in the prone, filled study.

Usually when one lesion can be satisfactorily demonstrated by fluoroscopy, an accompanying lesion is often left unseen. Careful study in this case saved us from misdiagnosis. By the U-turn technique of gastrofiberscopy, a small, soft, hemispherical elevation without discoloration was observed in the fornix (Fig. 83 g). It was diagnosed as a small leiomyoma by histological examination of the resected stomach (Figs. 83 i, j).

Palmer reported that lesions with diameters of less than 2 cm were proved in 9% of 139 cases to be leiomyomas. Also according to Yamagata, smaller lesions measuring less than 1 cm in diameter were detected in 2 out of 74 cases.

Since many gastroenterologists have recently become more familar with finer techniques, more reports of small lesions will probably increase. However, it should be kept in mind that protuberances which are apparently epithelial polyps are sometimes diagnosed as submucosal tumors. To avoid this confusion, gastric elevations should be named " polypoid lesions " rather than " polyps ", which have the nuance of being " epithelial ".

It is necessary that lesions throughout the entire stomach be demonstrated by a routine radiographic study. It is apparent that the fluoroscopic technique is excellent for the purpose of demonstrating lesions in the stomach, yet the pathogenesis of all lesions cannot be established only by this method.

83a

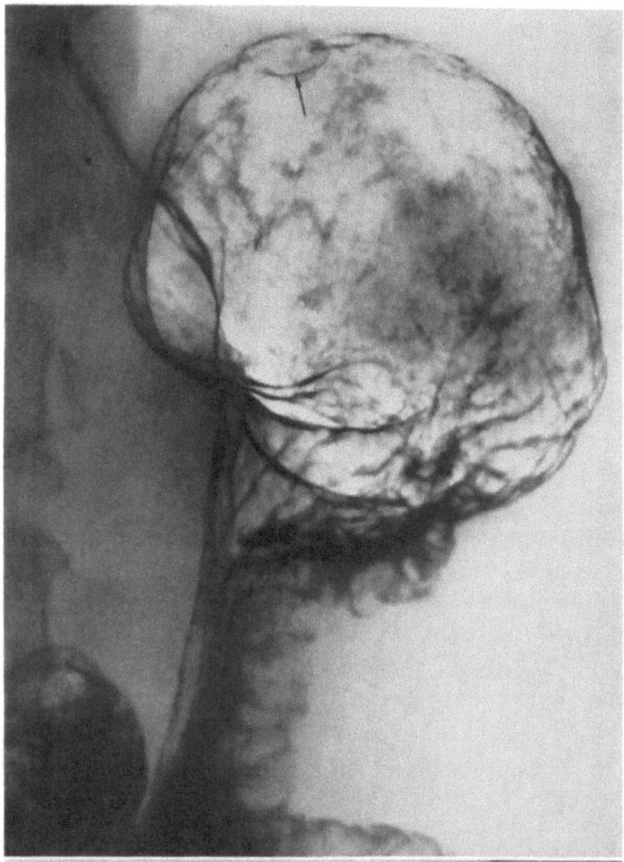

83b

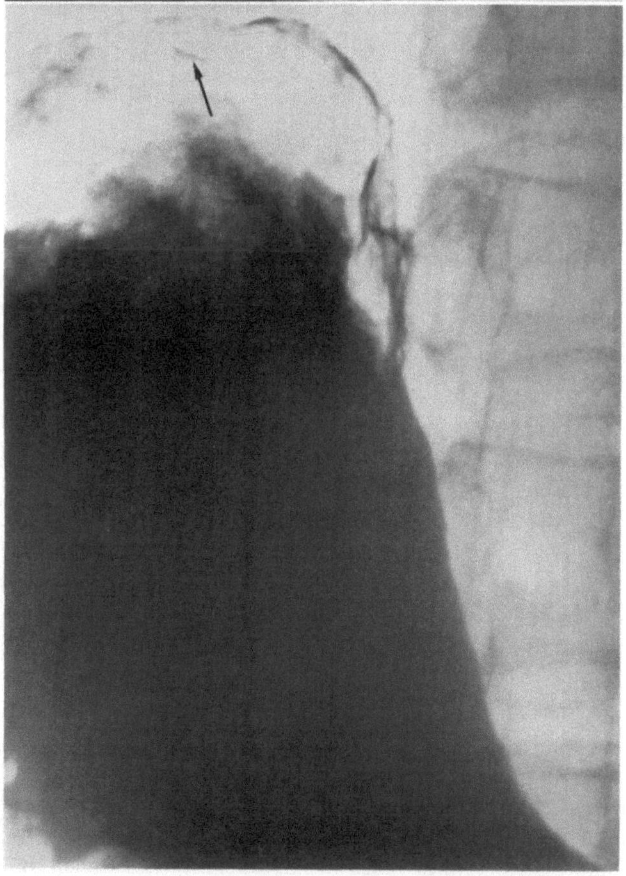

Fig. 83a Upright, filled study. No abnormality is detected in the filled photograph along the margin of the stomach, but a sharply outlined hemispherical elevation in the fornix is demonstrated in each picture taken after the infusion of large amounts of air.

Fig. 83b Prone, filled study. No particular change is noted at the margin in the prone, filled picture. This elevation in the fornix is observed by chance. All changes, however, must be demonstrated by a routine examination.

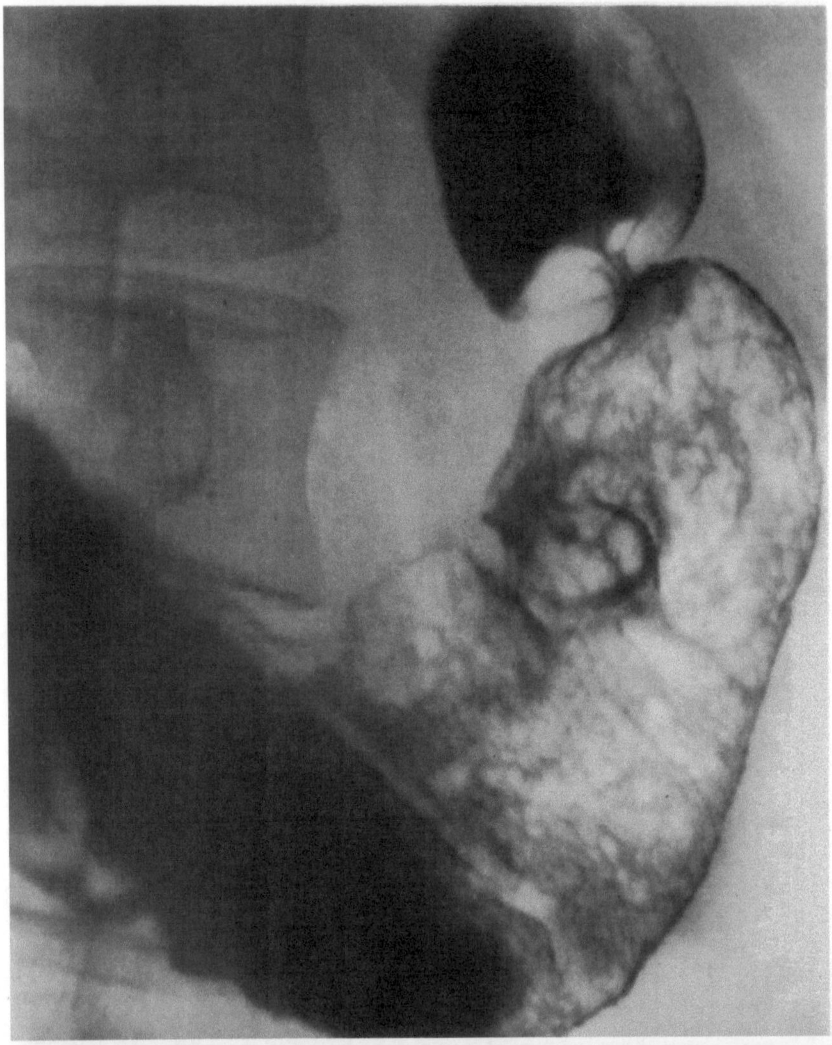

83c

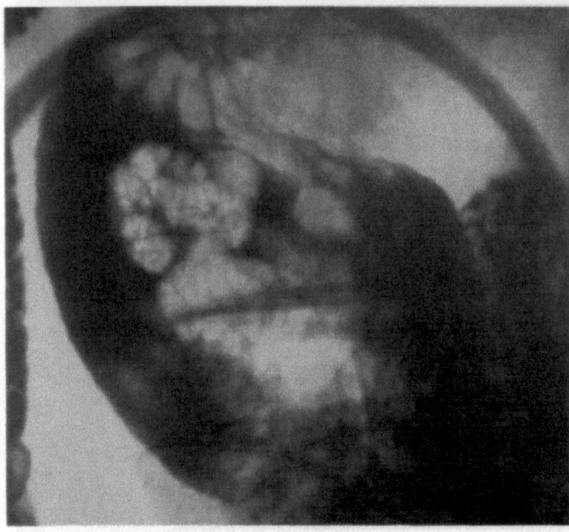

83d

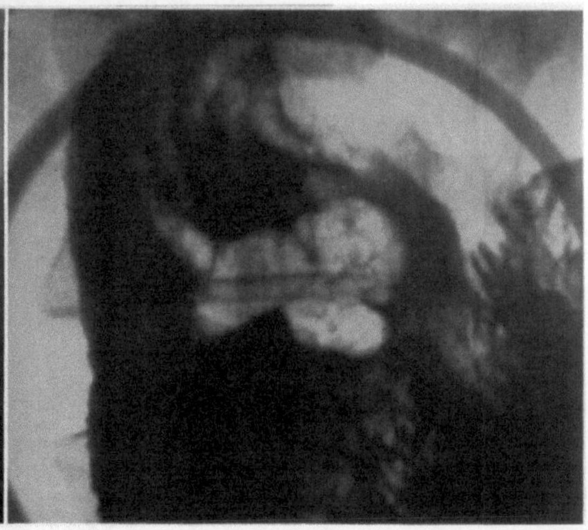

83e

Fig. 83c Prone, double-contrast study. An obviously outlined, little finger-sized, protruding lesion with a lobulated surface is apparent in the antrum. It is thought probably to be a polyp with a stalk. The surrounding mucous membrance is fairly granulated.

Figs. 83d, e Compression study. Different parts of the head of the tumor are noticed by two adequate compression studies taken from different directions. It is considered to be a spherical elevation with a long stalk, 2.3×1.8 cm in diameter. Its irregular and lobulated surface is well demonstrated.

83f

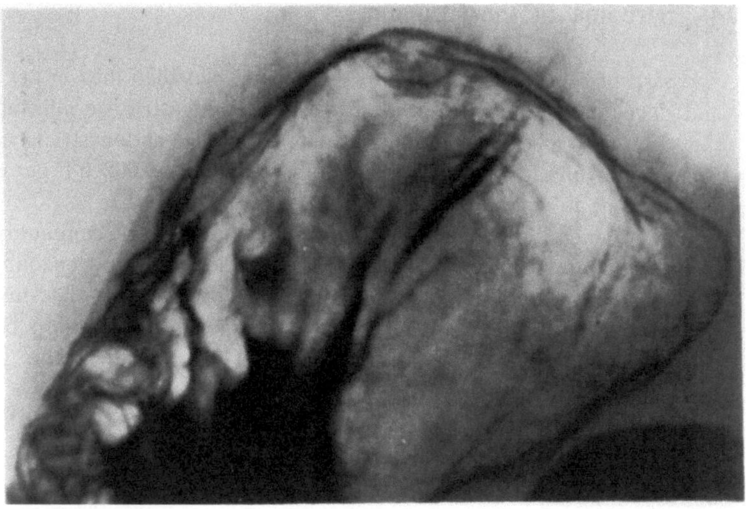

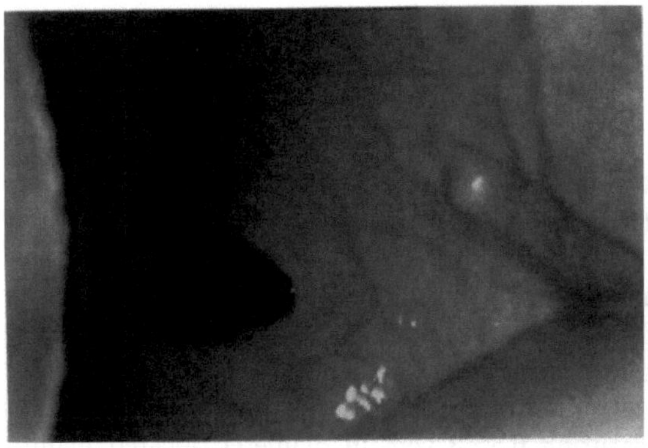

83g

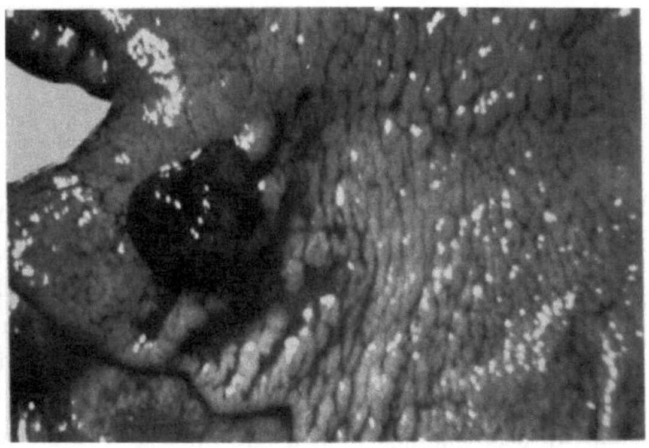

83h

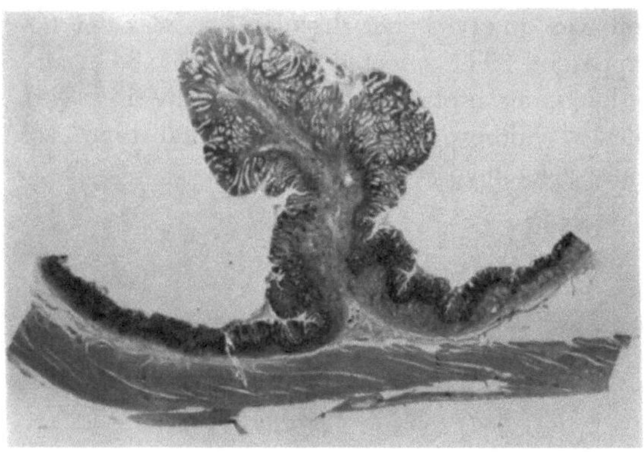

83i

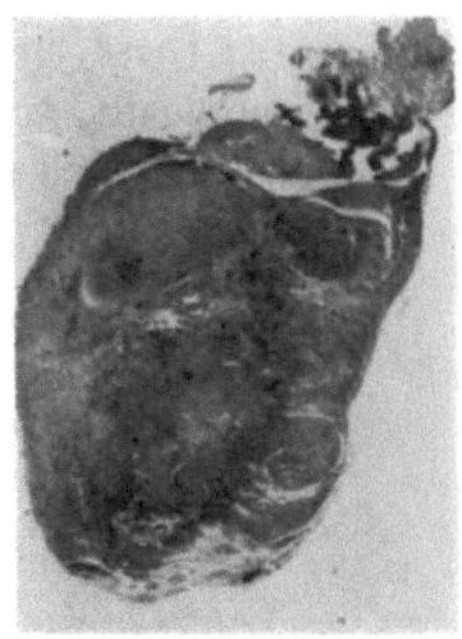

83j

Fig. 83f Prone picture. Beside the antral lesion, a rice grain sized protuberance is noticed in the fornix. It was a hill-shaped protuberance with a smooth surface.

Fig. 83g Endoscopic picture. By the U-turn technique of the gastrofiberscope, a small, hemispherical elevation without discoloration is demonstrated in the fornix.

Fig. 83h Resected stomach. A lobulated polyp with moderate discoloration is noticed on the antral anterior wall.

Fig. 83i Histopathological findings of the polypoid lesion in the antrum. Histologically, it was diagnosed as a benign adenomatous polyp.

Fig. 83j Histopathological findings of the elevation in the fornix. The lesion was diagnosed as a small leiomyoma by a histological study.

4. Sarcoma of the stomach

Sarcomas of the stomach are genetically classified into either primary or secondary sarcomas and developmentally into either exogastric, endogastric, or infiltrating types. On the other hand, they are, also classified into localized (exogastric-endogastric), diffused, and transitional types. Frequencies of sarcomas have been reported to be 0.002–0.1 per cent in autopsy cases and 0.17–7.4 per cent in surgically resected cases.

It is generally assumed that central ulcerations are commonly encountered in most cases of intragastric sarcomas; however, central ulcerations are also encountered in benign tumors. Therefore, central ulcerations of malignant tumors are not the determining factor.

As has been previously stated, regarding the relationship between the size of tumors and their malignancies, one of the standards in identifying tumors should be their size, namely, of more than 3 cm in diameter.

a. Leiomyosarcoma

Case 19

c. c.: Nausea.

57 year-old female.

A filling defect was observed along the antral lesser curvature in the upright, filled study (Fig. 84 a), but was seen with a relatively smooth margin along the greater curvature. In the antrum, a soft defect was noticed in the prone, filled study (Fig. 84 b). As seen in the prone, mucosal study (Fig. 84 c), the margin of the tumor was smooth and the mucosal folds kept clear of the tumor. In the supine, double-contrast study with a medium amount of air, the antral region was not extended satisfactorily. In the left oblique projection, the supine, double-contrast study demonstrated that the mucosal folds kept clear of this tumor and that the surface was smooth.

It was diagnosed as a submucosal tumor, measuring 6.5×3.3 cm in diameter, located mainly on the antral anterior wall. From the size of the tumor, it was highly suspected of being a localized sarcoma.

Endoscopically, a giant hemispherical elevation was observed, but discoloration was not noticed on its surface. No central ulceration was apparent. The resected stomach (Fig. 84 h) also presented these findings. On the serosal surface the tumor protruded hemispherically (Fig. 84 i). Macroscopically, this was a tumor of the so-called "endo-exogastric developmental type" as pointed out by SKANDALAKIS. This was histologically a leiomyosarcoma.

84 a

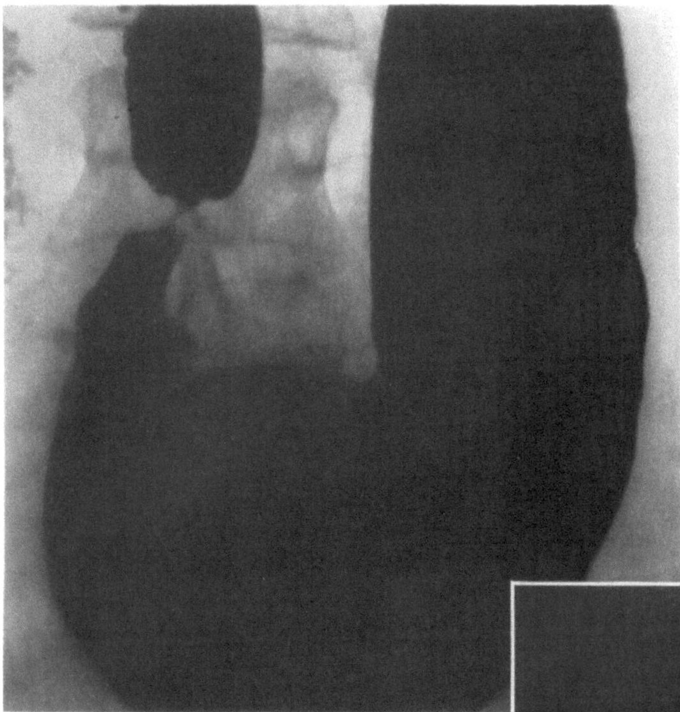

84 b

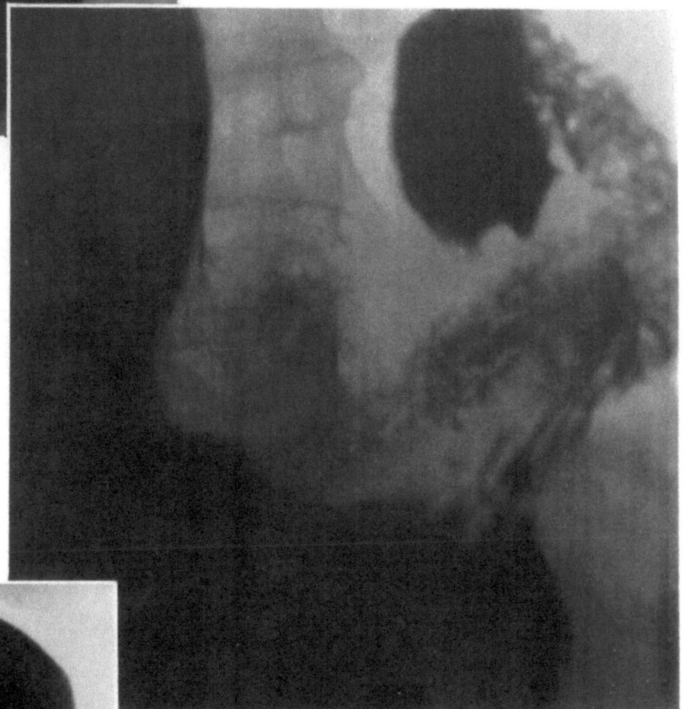

84 c

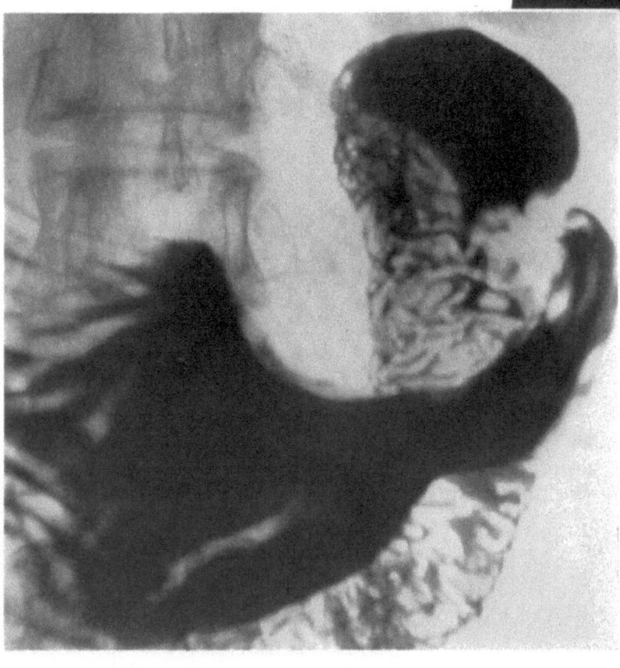

Fig. 84 a Upright, filled study. A filling defect is seen on the antral lesser curvature, but the margin of the greater curvature is relatively smooth.

Fig. 84 b Prone, filled study. A soft filling defect is noticed in the antrum.

Fig. 84 c Prone, mucosal study. On the antral lesser curvature, a sharply outlined, soft defect is present. The mucosal folds keep clear of the tumor.

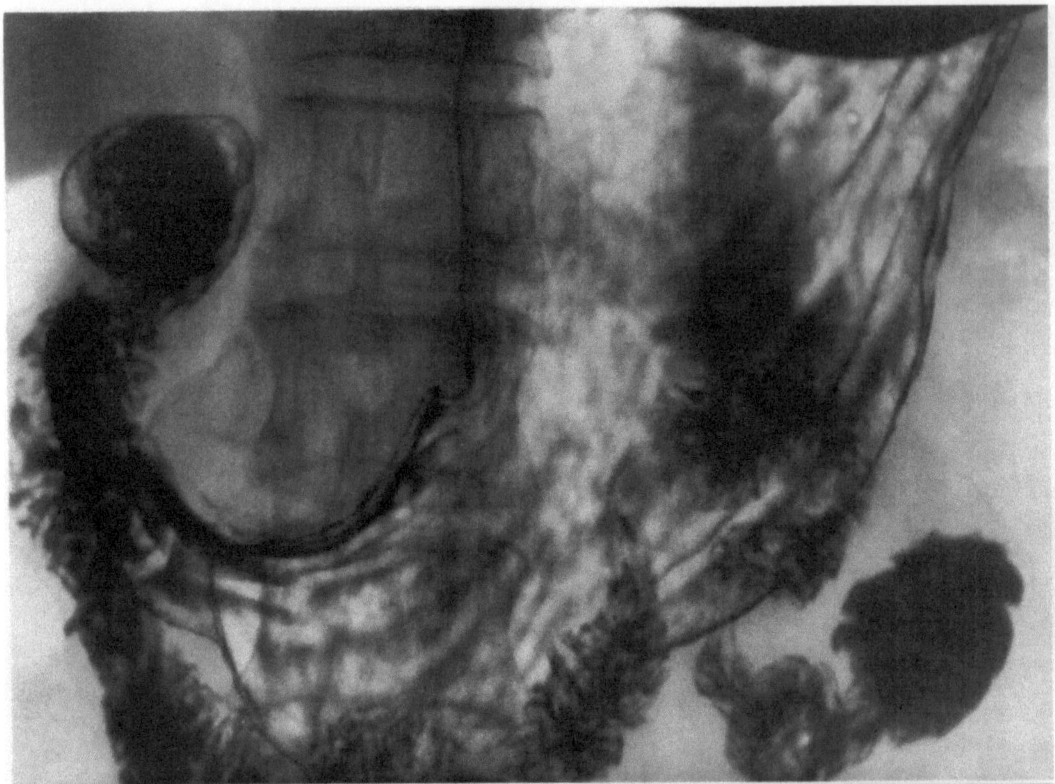

84d

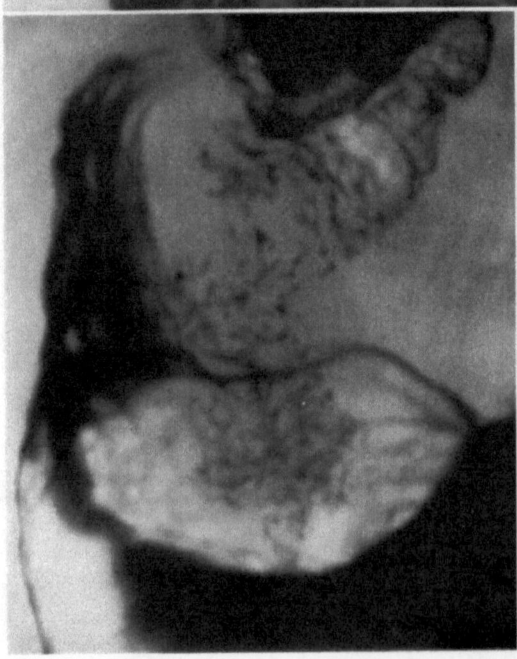

84e

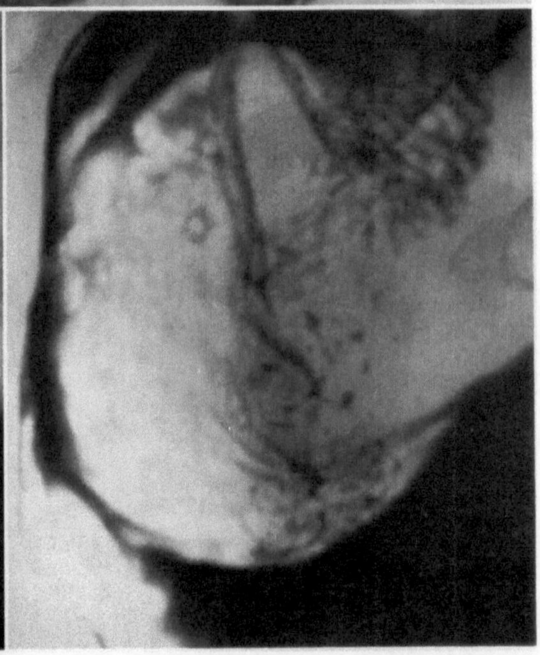

84f

Fig. 84d Supine, double-contrast study. The antrum could not be distended sufficiently with the infusion of a moderate volume of air, but the same filling defect as that in the supine, mucosal study is seen on the lesser curvature.

Fig. 84e, f Supine, double-contrast studies (left oblique projection). An oval shaped, radiolucent area is seen in the antrum. Its surface is relatively smooth, and the mucosal folds keep clear of the tumor. It is diagnosed as a submucosal tumor, located mainly on the anterior wall, measuring 6.5×3.3 cm in diameter.

84g

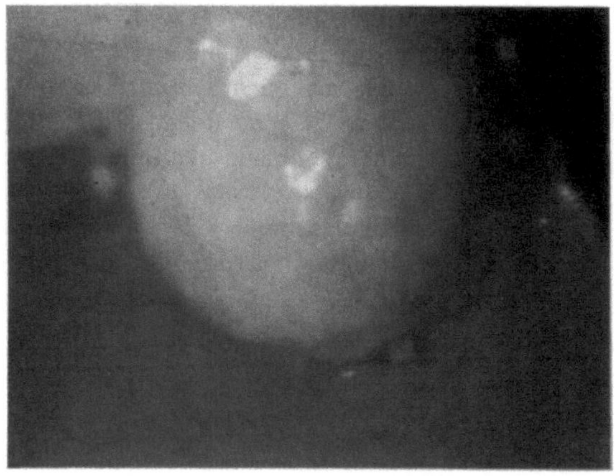

84h/84i

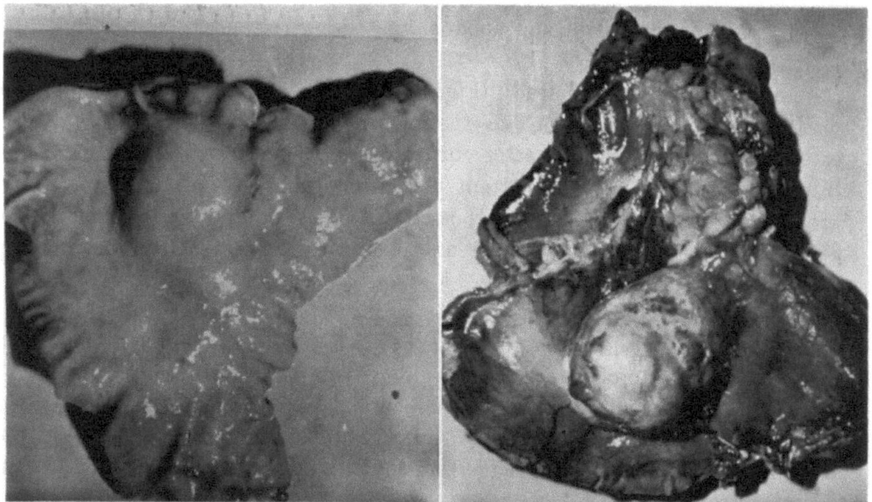

84j

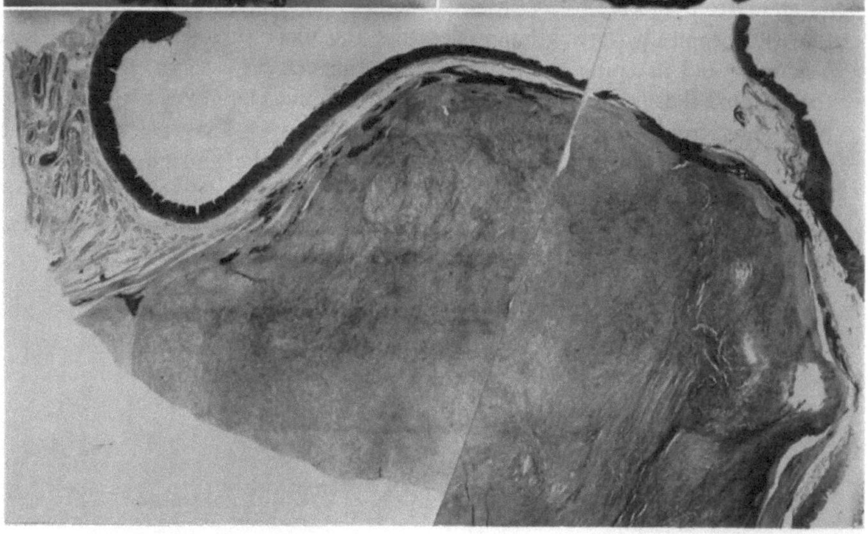

Fig. 84g Endoscopic picture. On the anterior wall of the antrum, a giant, hemispherical elevation with a smooth surface is observed. The color of the mucous membrane covering the surface of the tumor does not show any difference from that of the surrounding membranes.

Fig. 84h Resected stomach. A hemispherical submucosal tumor is observed, but no central crater is seen.

Fig. 84i Resected stomach (serosal surface). A hemispherical tumor, which has developed "endo-exogastrically" is seen on the serosal surface as well as on the mucosal surface.

Fig. 84j Histopathological findings. A leiomyosarcoma was demonstrated histologically.

b. Malignant lymphoma of the stomach

Along with myosarcomas, liposarcomas, and neurosarcomas, which undergo malignant change from benign tumors, malignant lymphomas, such as reticulum cell sarcomas, lymphocytic sarcomas, and HODGKIN's disease are regarded as diffuse gastric sarcomas. Lack of rigidity of the gastric wall, marked infiltration, and multiple ulcers in a normal mucosa are characteristic findings of these diseases. Multiple ulcers surrounded by a low, thin ulcer wall, and partially irregular, thickend mucosal folds are specific for the diagnosis. Furthermore, coexistent with these findings, the superficial depressed pattern, like the IIc of early gastric cancer, surrounded by abruption of mucosal folds near these ulcerations and the lack of stiffness of the gastric ulcer wall are commonly seen.

Case 20

c. c.: Epigastric pain and anemia.

22 year-old female.

In the upright, filled study (Fig. 85 a), the picture showed a slight rigidity of the gastric wall along the lower corpus to the pyloric antrum. Slight rigidity of the gastric angle and extensive rigidity of the greater curvature of the antrum were seen in the prone, filled study (Fig. 85 b). Much more important points were an irregular ulcer on the gastric angle and the broad marginal swelling around the lesion. These findings were remarkable in the picture (Fig. 85 c). The mucosal folds on the greater curvature ran irregularly, forming a part of the marginal swelling of the ulcer.

In a double-contrast study in the prone position, taken with a small amount of air (Fig. 85 d), the ulcer with its marginal swelling was markedly shown. Double-contrast studies (Figs. 85 e, f) showed a broad, marginal swelling from the gastric angle down to the antrum. Radiographic signs of infiltration into submucosal layers extended to the upper corpus, and multiple irregular erosions were seen. However, rigidity of the lesser curvature in the upright, filled study was not remarkable. This suggested some kind of malignant disease or infiltrative growth different from cancer.

Endoscopically, it was impressive that the ulcer surrounded by the broad marginal swelling was large and its crater looked remarkably uneven (Fig. 85 g). The biopsy material, taken from the base of the ulcer, showed a cluster of lymphocytes. We diagnosed the lesion as a malignant lymphoma from the x-ray and endoscopic findings. The resected stomach (Fig. 85 h) revealed two tumors on the anterior and posterior walls of the antrum, and an irregularly shaped ulcer with mucosal folds disappearing abruptly on the lesser curvature of the corpus could be seen. An irregular, uneven mucosa was present from the ulcer to the tumors. Histologically, this lesion was found to be a reticulum cell sarcoma (Fig. 85 i).

85a

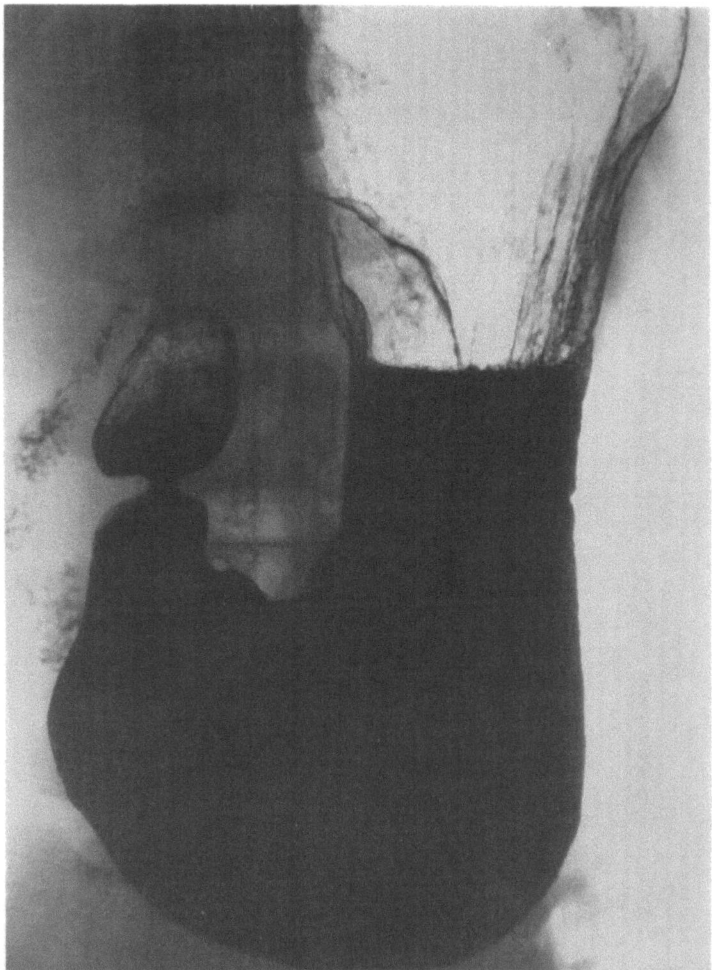

85b

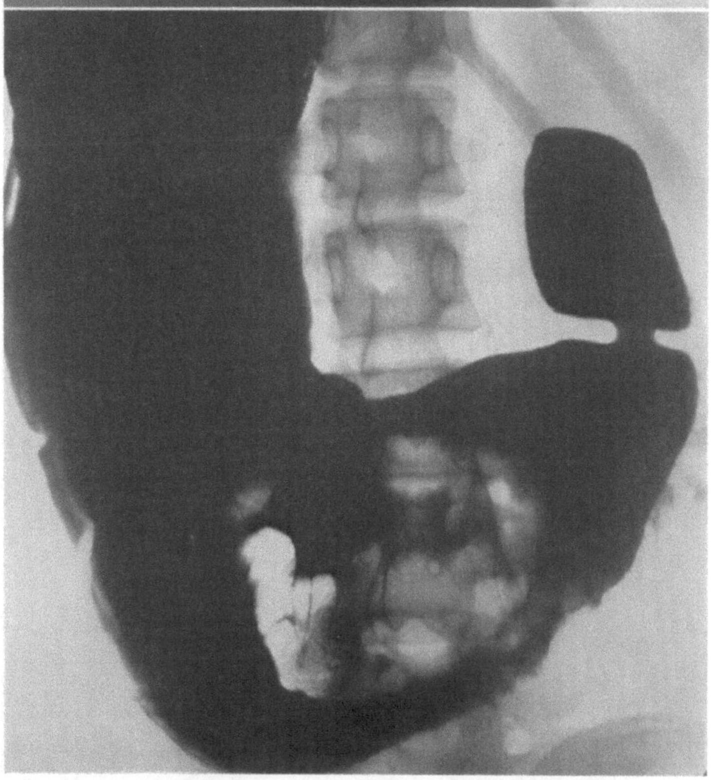

Fig. 85 a Upright, filled study. Slight rigidity of the gastric wall along the middle corpus down to the pyloric antrum is demonstrated. An irregular tumor shadow is seen on the lesser curvature of the upper corpus.

Fig. 85 b Prone, filled study. Slight rigidity of the gastric angle and a broad rigidity of the greater curvature of the antrum are seen. The most remarkable finding is an irregular ulceration surrounded by a broad marginal swelling on the gastric angle. It looks to be an advanced ulcerative carcinoma, but the swelling of this lesion is broader than those seen in carcinomas.

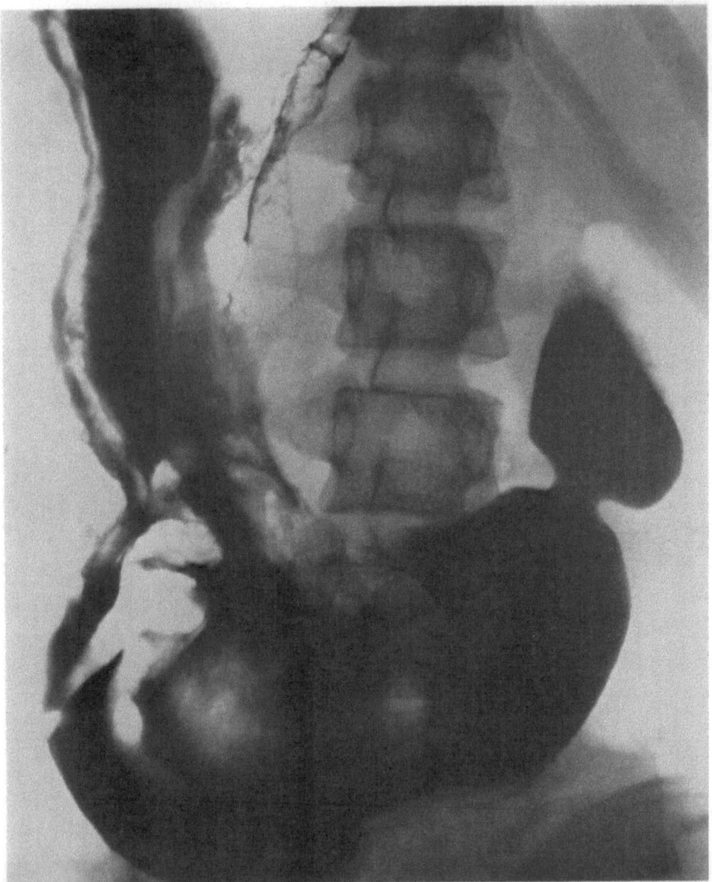

85 c

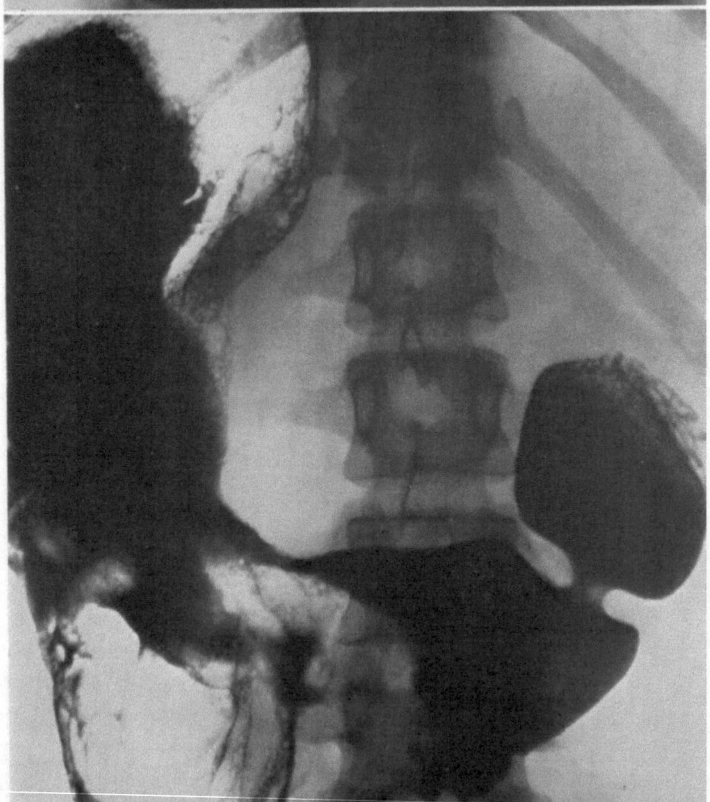

85 d

Fig. 85 c Mucosal relief study in the prone position. On the greater curvature of the lower corpus, mucosal folds run irregularly, and a barium filling defect is seen on the lesser curvature from the gastric angle to the antrum. Giant folds are comparatively specific for this disease and different in nuance from those of diffusive infiltration of scirrhous changes.

Fig. 85 d Mucosal relief study in the prone position. A broad, marginal swelling is seen surrounding an irregular ulcer.

85e

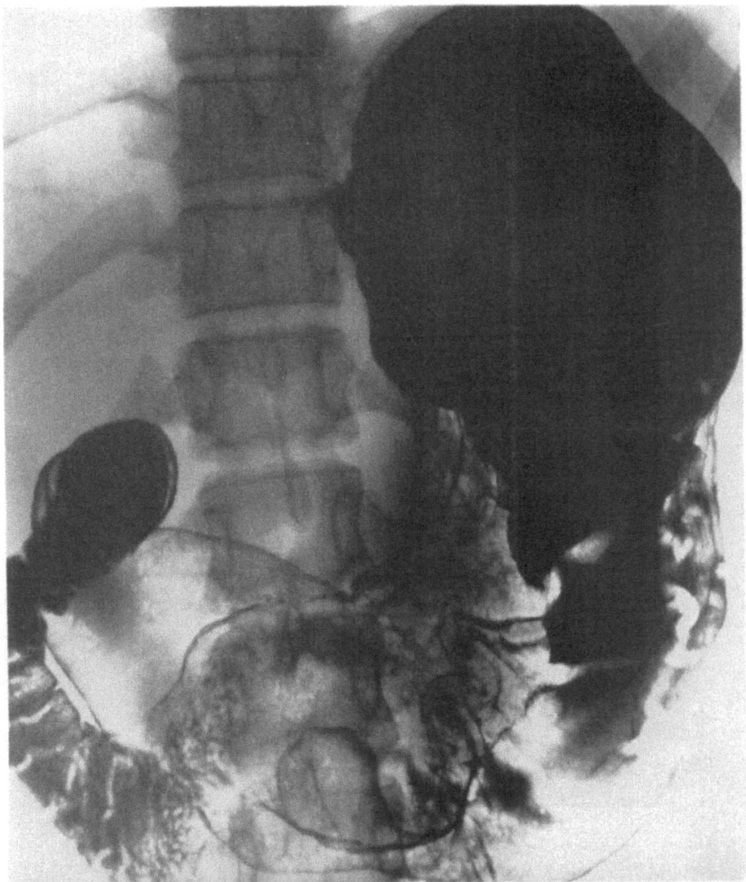

85f

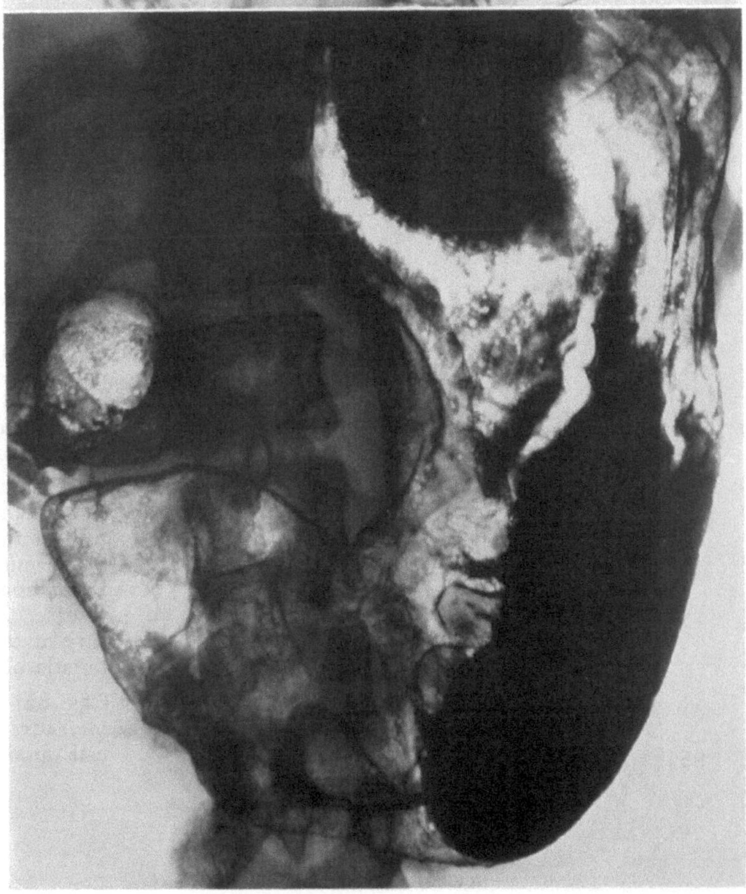

Fig. 85e Supine, double-contrast study. A broad, marginal swelling along the gastric angle to the antrum on the posterior wall is seen. The infiltration into submucosal layers extends to the upper corpus. Rigidity of the lesser curvature is not very remarkable, regardless of the size of the lesion.

Fig. 85f Double-contrast study taken in a half-upright position. Wide irregularity of the gastric contour and abrupt disappearance of the folds are seen along the lesser curvature of the corpus.

85g
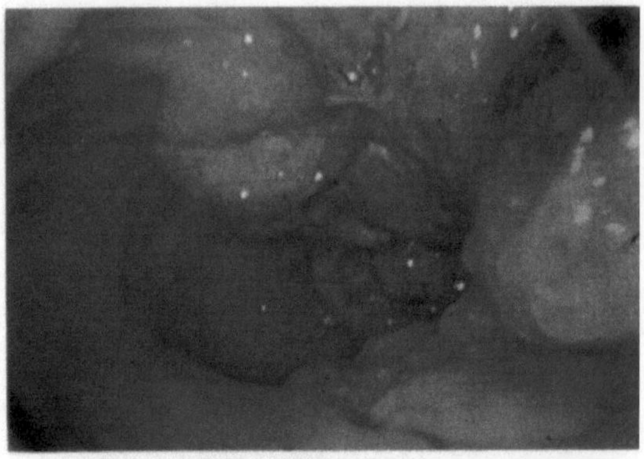

85h
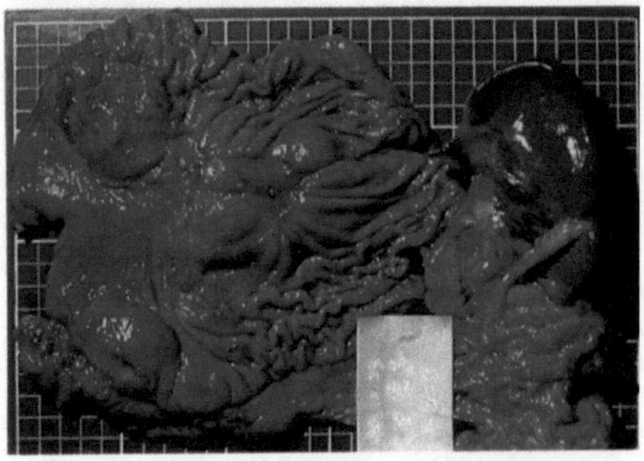

85i

85j
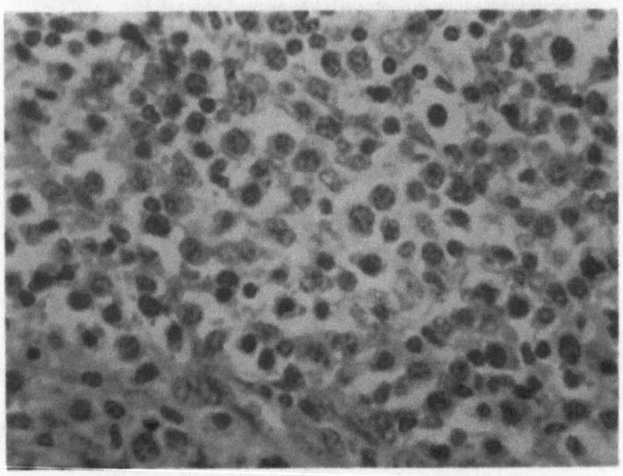

Fig. 85g Endoscopic picture. An irregularly shaped ulcer surrounded by a marginal swelling on the anterior wall of the antrum, a tumor on the posterior wall, and an infiltrative uneven mucosa are seen. The ulcer is sharply demarcated, and the marginal swelling is unexpectedly high. The lesion extends from the corpus to the pylorus on both walls.

Fig. 85h Resected stomach. There is a large tumor with central ulceration on the anterior wall of the antrum and an irregular ulceration with mucosal folds that disappear abruptly. Formation of multiple ulcers is specific to this disease. Infiltration of the gastric wall, a mixture of tumors and irregular ulcers are characteristic of malignant lymphomas.

Figs. 85i and j Histopathological findings. Histologically, this lesion proves to be a reticulum cell sarcoma.

5. Eosinophilic granuloma (Inflammatory fibroid polyp)

Eosinophilic granulomas are often seen on the gastric antrum as a tumor with a wide base, measuring 3 cm or less in diameter. There are parasitic and allergic theories as to the etiology of this disease. Rough proliferation of the connective tissue in the submucosa and cell infiltration by eosinocytes, lymphocytes, plasmacells, and eosinophilic histiocytes are specific to this disease. The lesion can be a pedunculated tumor and sometimes can form an ulcer.

Case 21

c. c.: Epigastric pain and diarrhea.

36 year-old male.

In the upright, filled study (Fig. 86 a), a slight contraction on the greater curvature of the antrum was seen, but there were no abnormalities in the prone, filled study (Fig. 86 b). In the supine, double-contrast study (Fig. 86 c), an enlarged fold was seen on the posterior wall of the antrum. The circumference of this round protrusion was not clear in the upright, compression study (Fig. 86 d). The picture with slight compression demonstrated a tumor that was not elevated. It was diagnosed as a submucosal tumor.

The endoscopic picture showed a low, hemispherical tumor with a smooth, slightly discolored surface. There was neither hemorrhage nor erosion on the surface. From an endoscopic point of view, such small protrusions seemed to suggest epithelial tumors. There were no remarkable changes in the resected stomach (Fig. 86 g). The histological findings showed an eosinophilic granuloma (Fig. 86 h).

86a

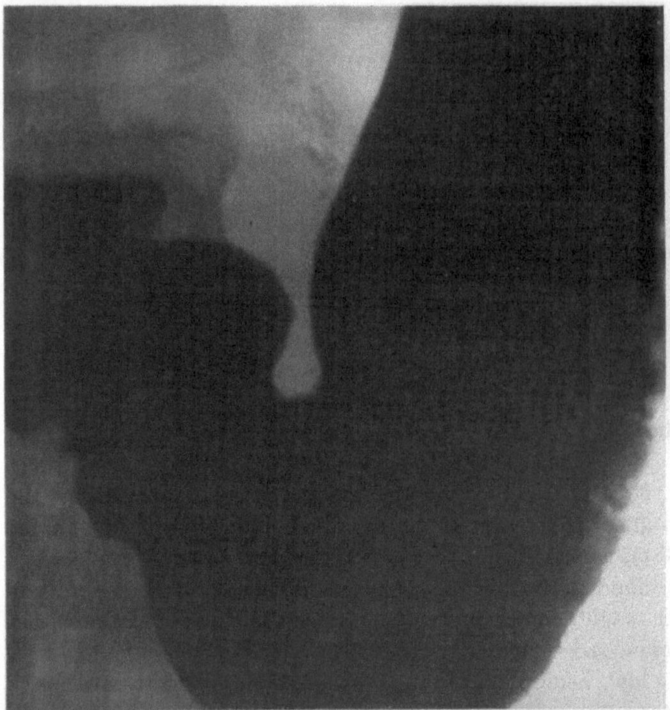

86b

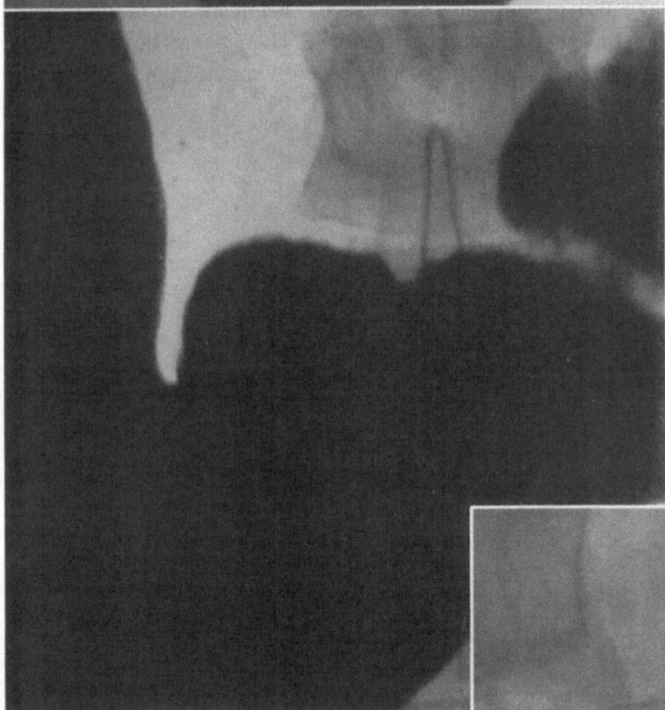

Fig. 86a Upright, filled study. There are no abnormalities except an irregular ulceration on the greater curvature of the antrum.

Fig. 86b Prone, filled study. No abnormal changes are seen on the stomach contour.

Fig. 86c Supine, double-contrast study. A small tumor shadow with enlarged ends of the mucosal folds is seen on the posterior wall of the antrum.

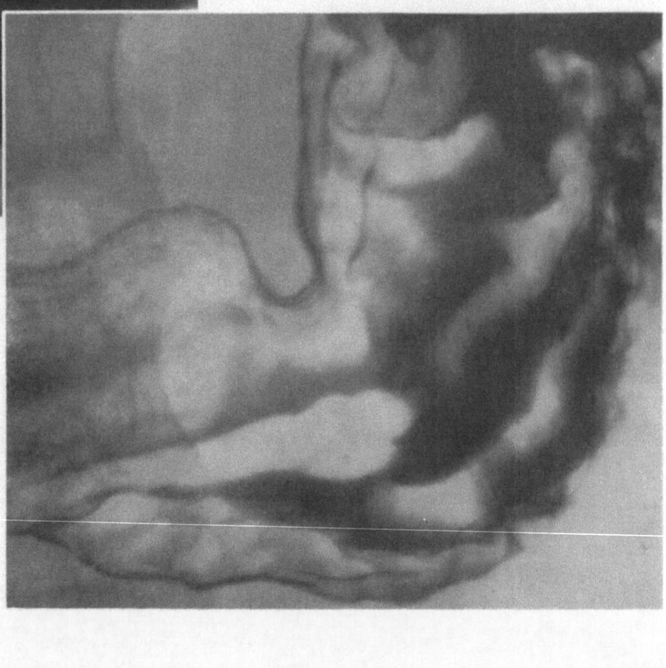

86c

86d
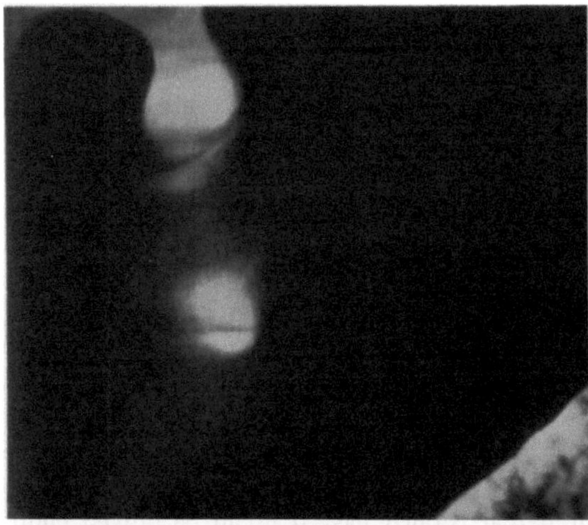
86e
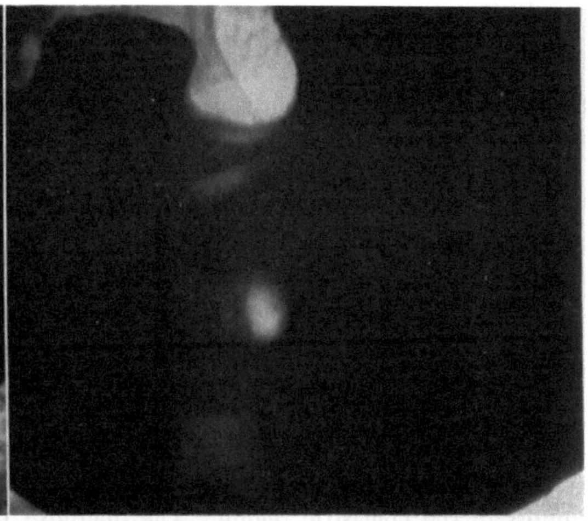
86f
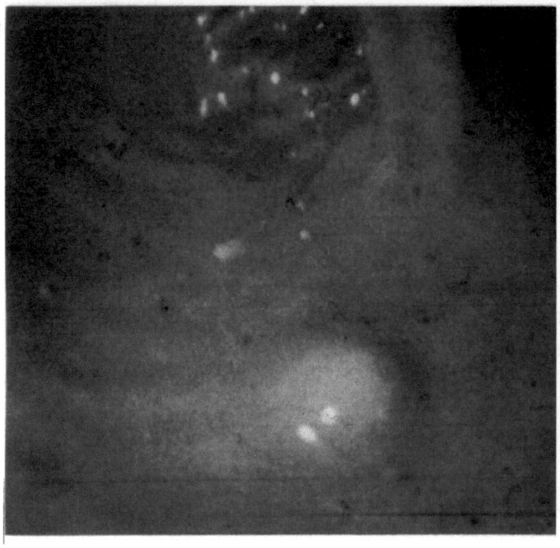
86g
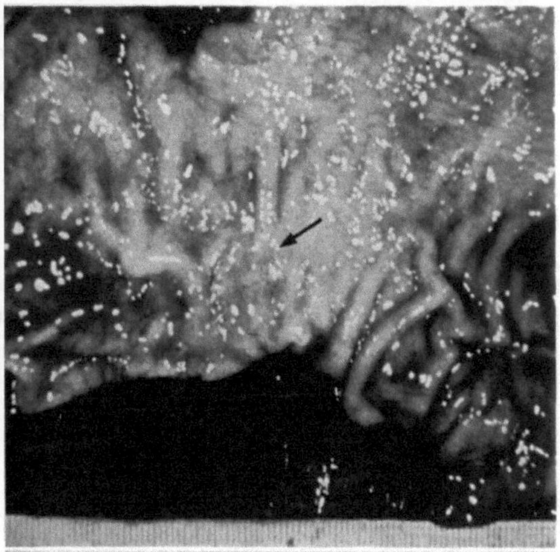
86h
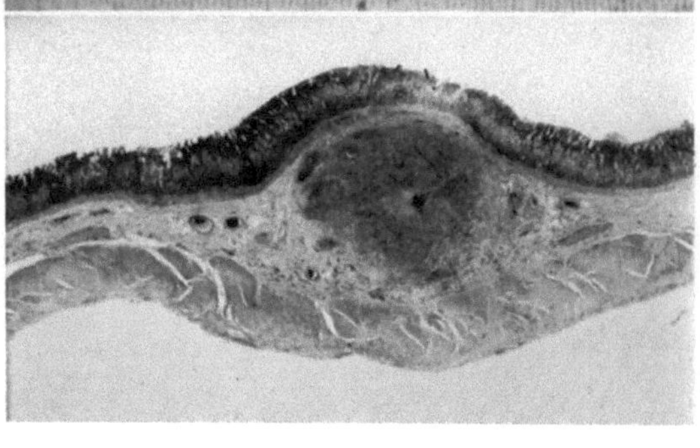

Figs. 86d, e Compression studies. These two pictures taken under strong and slight compression reveal a round protruding lesion. Its circumference is not definitely sharp. This tumor is not very high.

Fig. 86f Endoscopic picture. A slightly discolored, hemispherical tumor with a smooth surface is noted on the posterior wall of the antrum. Hemorrhagic erosions are scattered around the circumference of the lesion. Differential diagnosis from epithelial benign tumors is difficult.

Fig. 86g Resected stomach. The lesion is small and not very elevated. The border between this lesion and its surrounding mucosa is not clear. It is suspected of being a submucosal tumor.

Fig. 86h Histopathological findings. The lesion is an eosinophilic granuloma histologically.

6. Bezoar

A bezoar results from swallowed material under various intragastric conditions. According to its composition, a bezoar is usually classified into phytobezoar, trichobezoar, trichophytobezoar, medicamental bezoar, etc.

In Japan, almost all bezoars are phytobezoar, and trichobezoar is extremely rare. Phytobezoar is generally composed of vegetable fibers of persimmons, plums, raisins, celery, parsley, beets, tobacco, coconut, etc. Three fourths of the phytobezoars are the result of persimmons, which are said to be made by eating large numbers of persimmons on an empty stomach.

Manifestation of clinical symptoms of a bezoar is divided into two types, acute and chronic. Persimmon bezoars belong mostly to the former type. More than fifty per cent of the bezoar cases have the same symptoms as gastritis or gastric ulcer, such as epigastric pain, full sensation of the stomach, heartburn, nausea, and vomiting. As these symptoms are least helpful for a differential diagnosis of bezoar, it is important to ask the patient about his taste and the contents of his meals. About 10 per cent or less of the bezoar cases are palpable as movable tumors in the epigastric region. The diagnosis of bezoar is fairly easy if it can be proved endoscopically and radiologically that the tumor can be freely moved by hand or can change in position. However, when the tumor will not move owing to a strangulation into the pyloric antrum, isolation from the gastric wall by air infusion is necessary.

The shape of a bezoar is radiologically spherical, oval, or sometimes irregularly polygonal, with a smooth and clear margin. Unevenness of its surface is largely gentle. For final diagnosis, an endoscopic examination of the color of the tumor and a histological investigation by gastric biopsy are necessary.

The rate of coexistence of a gastric ulcer in bezoar cases is high. It is generally considered that the coexistent gastric ulcer is caused by the mechanical injury of a bezoar to the gastric mucosa. It is also possible that a gastric ulcer itself changes the gastric movement and other intragastric factors, which create suitable circumstances for the formation of a bezoar.

Case 22

c. c.: Epigastric pain.

32 year-old male.

At the beginning of this year, he overate rice cakes and persimmons (more than 10 dried persimmons a day). After that, he complained of a colicky epigastric pain. The pain was relieved by taking medicine, but slight, late post-prandial epigastralgia persisted. On his admission to our hospital, an apple-sized, globular, movable tumor was palpable on the left hypochondrium with slight tenderness in the epigastrium.

In the picture of the barium filled stomach in the upright position (Fig. 87 a), widening of the angle and shortening of the lesser curvature were noticed. Furthermore, an obscure filling defect in the antrum suggested an intragastric tumor. A shallow niche on the angle and a large filling defect were noticed (Fig. 87 b).

By the double-contrast method (Figs. 87 c, d), a large tumor was shown on the posterior wall of the sinus. Its contour was smooth, but many irregular barium flecks were seen on it suggesting an uneven surface. The tumor moved freely within the stomach. For example, sometimes it was located in the fornix in the semirecumbent position (Fig. 87 d); at other times, it was found at the height of the gastric angle in the double-contrast study in the prone position (Fig. 87 e). The tumor shadow was reversed from that in the supine position. On the lesser curvature of the angle, a niche with a linear barium fleck was noticed. From these x-ray findings, a bezoar and a gastric ulcer were diagnosed.

From an endoscopic point of view (Figs. 87 f, g), there were two long-oval ulcers arranged symmetrically against the axis of the lesser curvature of the angle. A large brown tumor was observed in the mucous lake, and on a closer view, it was proved to have a smooth but gently undulating surface. This tumor was easily moved during endoscopy with a change of position.

A bezoar, $8 \times 4.5 \times 3.7$ cm in size, 60 g in weight, was observed in the stomach. A linear ulcer, 2.5×0.7 cm in size, was found on the angle (Fig. 87 h). A persimmon seed was found in the brown, cut surface of the tumor (Fig. 87 i). Histologically, the sponge-like structure consisted of nets of the fiber bundles with light-brown pigment granules scattered among them.

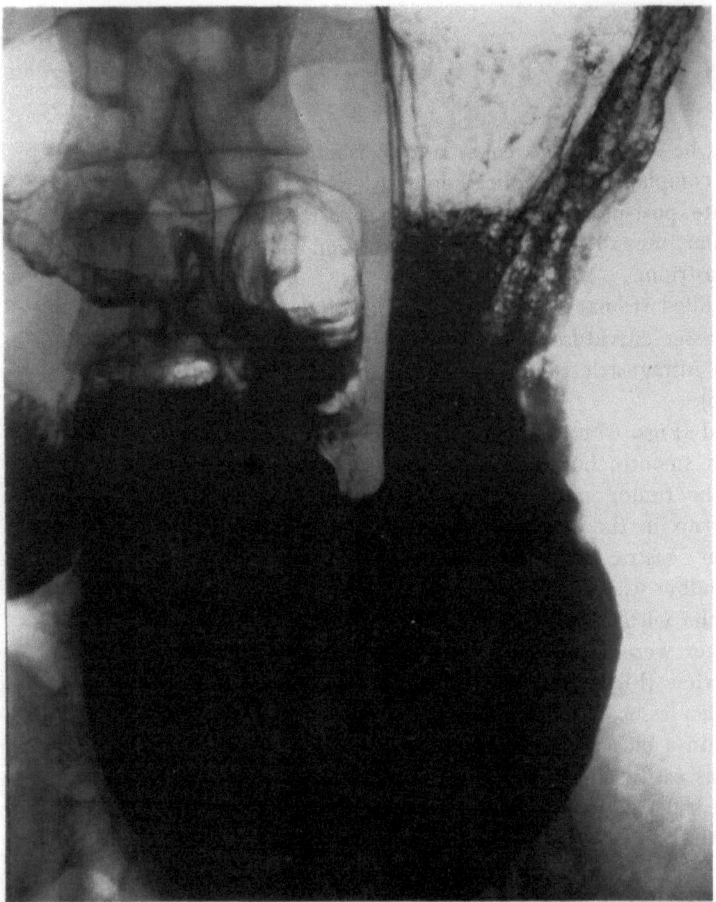

87 a

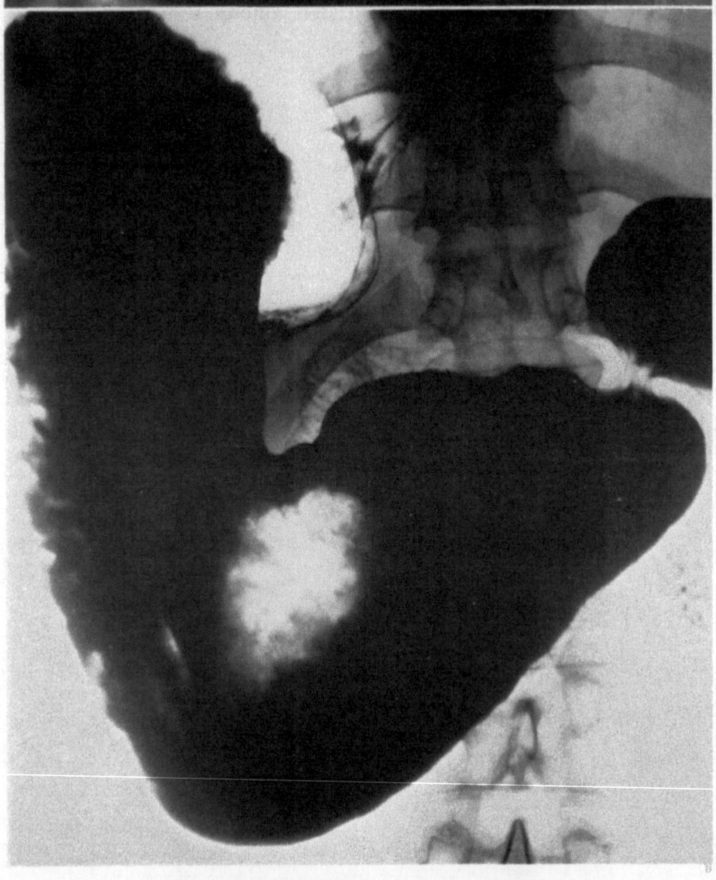

87 b

Fig. 87 a Barium filled stomach in the upright position.

Fig. 87 b Barium filled stomach in the prone position. A large filling defect is noticed near the gastric angle.

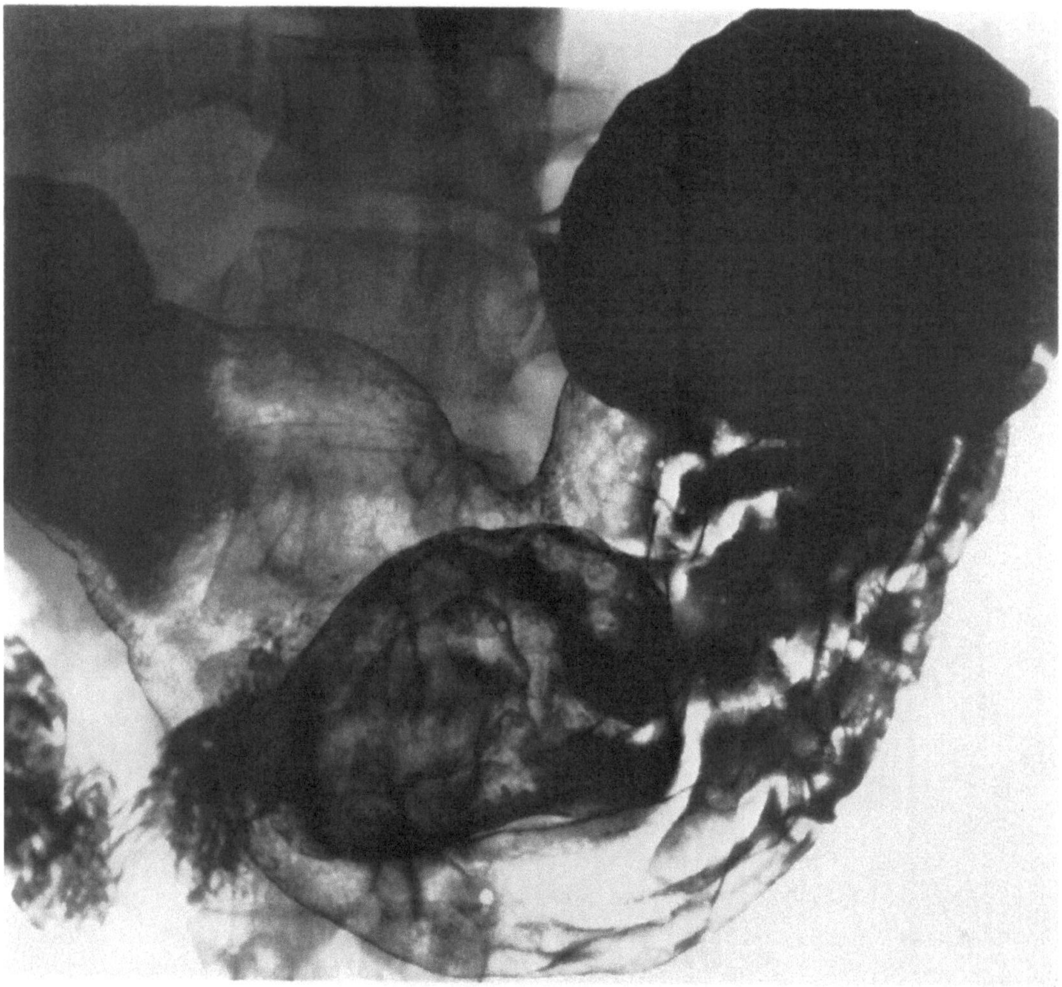

Fig. 87c **Double-contrast study in the supine position.** The whole contour of the sharply bordered tumor is well demonstrated. The tumor may have an uneven surface, judging from the irregular barium flecks on the tumor shadow.

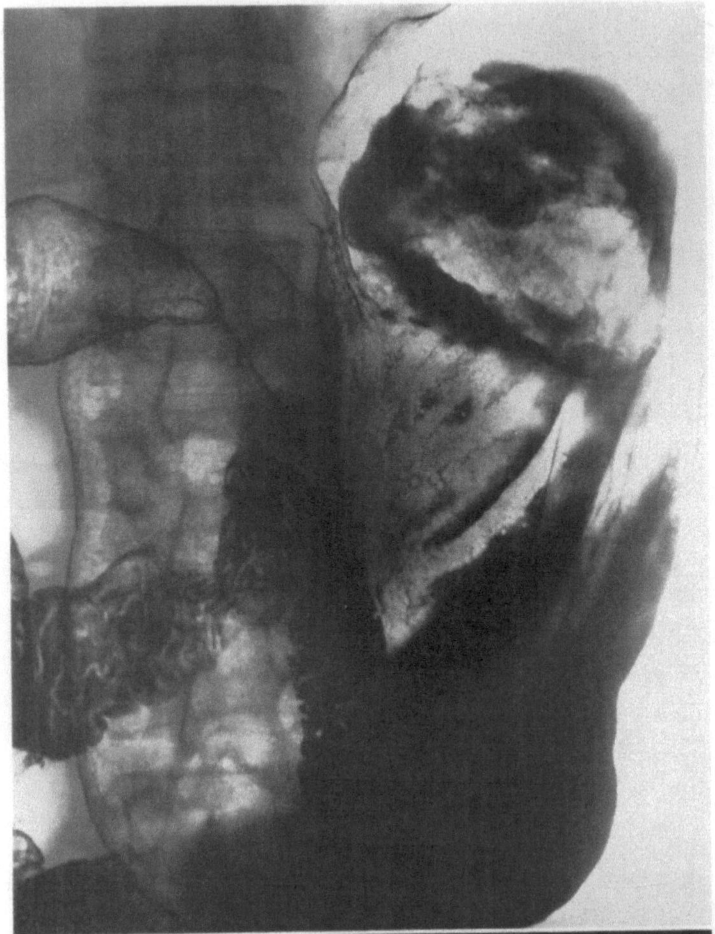

87 d

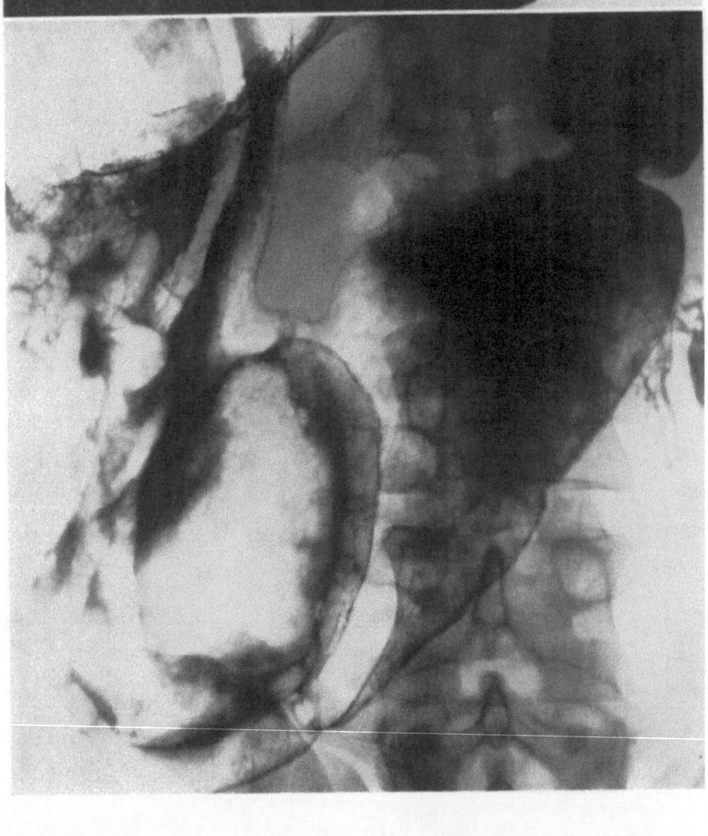

87 e

Fig. 87 d Double-contrast study in the semi-recumbent position. The tumor has been moved to the fornix. Folds converging at the angulus are noticed on the body of the stomach.

Fig. 87 e Double-contrast study in the prone position. A tumor shadow, a profile niche, and a barium fleck adjacent to the niche are found on the anterior wall of the angulus.

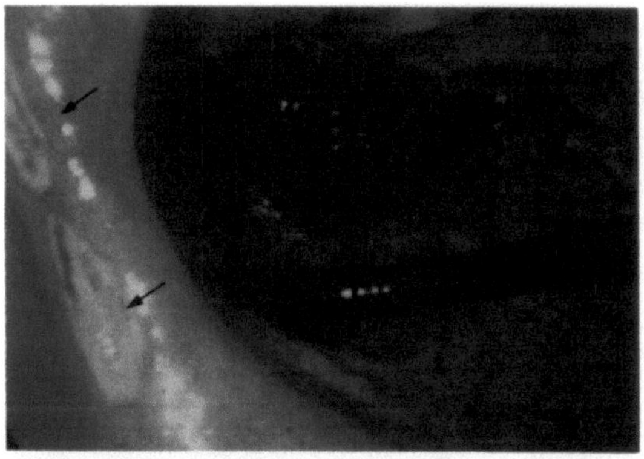

87 f

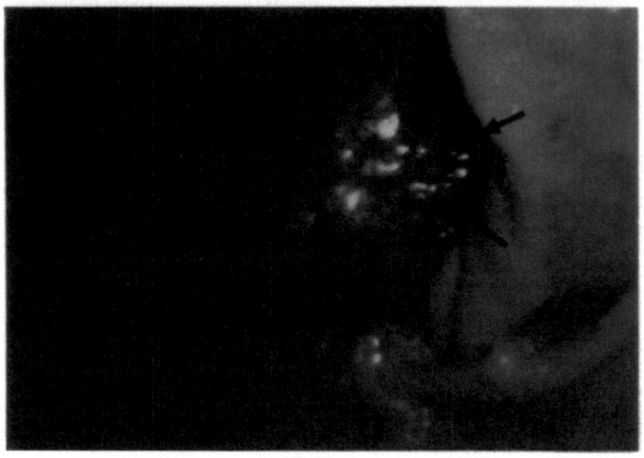

87 g

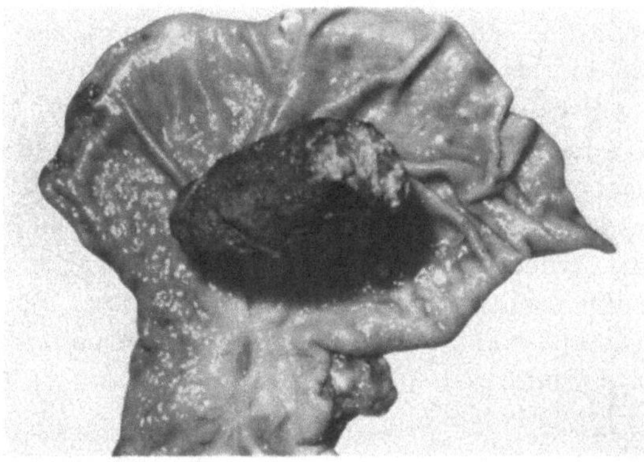

87 h

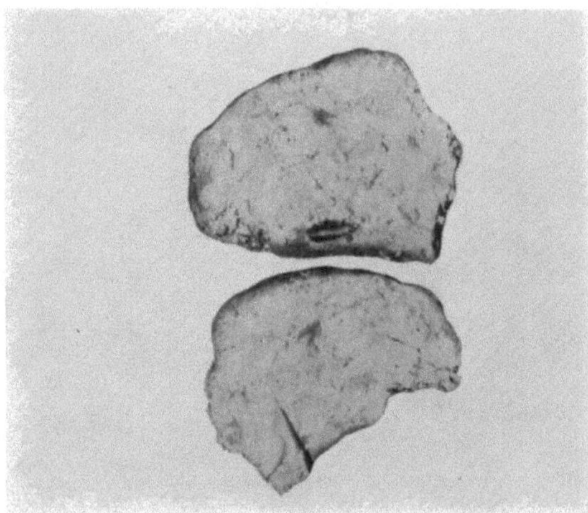

87 i

Fig. 87 f Endoscopic picture. Two spindle-shaped ulcers are seen on the angulus (arrows). The tumor is also seen in a distant view (large arrows).

Fig. 87 g Endoscopic picture. In a close-up view of the tumor, there is a dark-brown, glossy mass (arrows), which proved to be movable by a change of position.

Fig. 87 h Resected specimen. A linear ulcer of the stomach and a bezoar are seen.

Fig. 87 i Cut surface of the bezoar.

Excavated type

A. Typical cases of gastric excavated lesions

Definite and precise diagnoses of almost all types of gastric diseases including gastric cancers necessarily call for histopathological examinations of the gastric tissues. Preoperative examination processes include x-ray and endoscopic examinations which permit macroscopic diagnosis of morphological changes in the object as well as microscopic cytodiagnosis and direct vision gastric biopsy.

In clinical practice based on the above parameters, diagnoses are first made in accordance with the macroscopic peculiarities of lesions that have been detected; however, in those lesions lacking overt peculiarities, diagnoses should be based on the results of cytodiagnoses or gastric biopsies. From this viewpoint, it can be said that the prime objective of conducting x-ray and endoscopic examination is to grasp the macroscopic morphological characteristics of the respective diseases.

1. Excavated types of advanced cancer of the stomach

Borrmann, as shown in Figure 8, classified cancers of the stomach according to macroscopic morphology into four types. In our country, the most widely used macroscopic classification of advanced carcinomas is that of Borrmann. With a yet unclassified type included, advanced cancers of the stomach can be classified into five types. Most of the pathological changes included in this unclassified group show macroscopic changes similar to those in early cancer, which will be explained in the following chapter. Cases we have observed consist of Borrmann type I, 3.3%; II, 32.2%; III, 37.8%; IV, 17.8%; and the unclassified type, 8.9%.

Diagnoses of the excavated type of advanced cancer are made either by x-ray or endoscopic examination of macroscopic findings of the lesions. In the case of small scale pathological changes, particular care is required so that there is no mistaken diagnosis of benign ulcer.

In this chapter, the excavated gastric cancers, Borrmann II (ulcerating carcinoma with elevated margin) and Borrmann III (ulcerating carcinoma with progressive infiltration of the gastric wall) will be demonstrated.

a. Borrmann type II (Noninfiltrative carcinomatous ulcer)

Among the advanced cancers in the stomach, there is a noninfiltrative carcinomatous ulcer, the so-called Borrmann type II cancer. The excavation of this lesion is found on the surface of a localized cancerous protrusion. Macroscopically, the lesion appears like a flower bed with a large ulceration in the center, and the carcinomatous infiltration is usually limited to the surrounding marginal elevation.

The radiological appearance has a typical pattern of an irregularly shaped ulcer with a doughnut-shaped filling defect in the frontal view. In the profile view, it is observed as a "Schattenplus im Schattenminus", or the so-called meniscus sign.

Case 23

c.c.: Dull epigastralgia and emaciation.

57 year-old male.

On x-ray examination, both in mucosal and compression studies, an irregularly shaped ulcer surrounded by a marginal swelling was easily seen on the posterior wall of the antrum. In the barium filled studies in the upright and prone positions (Figs. 88 a, b), a slight irregularity of the gastric wall was noted on the lesser curvature of the lower gastric body, but this finding was undetectable under fluoroscopy. More obvious changes of the gastric wall were seen on the greater curvature of the antrum. In this region, rigidity of the wall and a faint shadow defect were noticeable.

In the double-contrast study in the first oblique position (Fig. 88 c), an irregularly shaped, carcinomatous ulcer surrounded by an oval filling defect was observed on the posterior wall of the antrum. Another lesion of the lower gastric body was seen in this picture as a finding of converging folds with a faint shadow as shown by the arrow. In the compression study with the patient upright (Figs. 88 d, e), the doughnut-shaped tumor was more clearly demonstrated. It did not disappear even under strong compression, leading us to conclude that the protrusion was high and hard.

Protrusions into the stomach can be revealed most effectively by compression studies, and conversely, depressed lesions are most effectively revealed by double-contrast radiography. In the endoscopic picture with a GTF-A (Fig. 88 f), an irregularly shaped ulcer with an uneven floor surrounded by a hard marginal swelling could be seen on the posterior wall of the antrum. Macroscopically (Fig. 88 g), it was a Borrmann type II cancer 3.5×4.0 cm in diameter. Histological examination of the resected specimen (Fig. 88 h) revealed the cancerous infiltration reaching the subserosal layer.

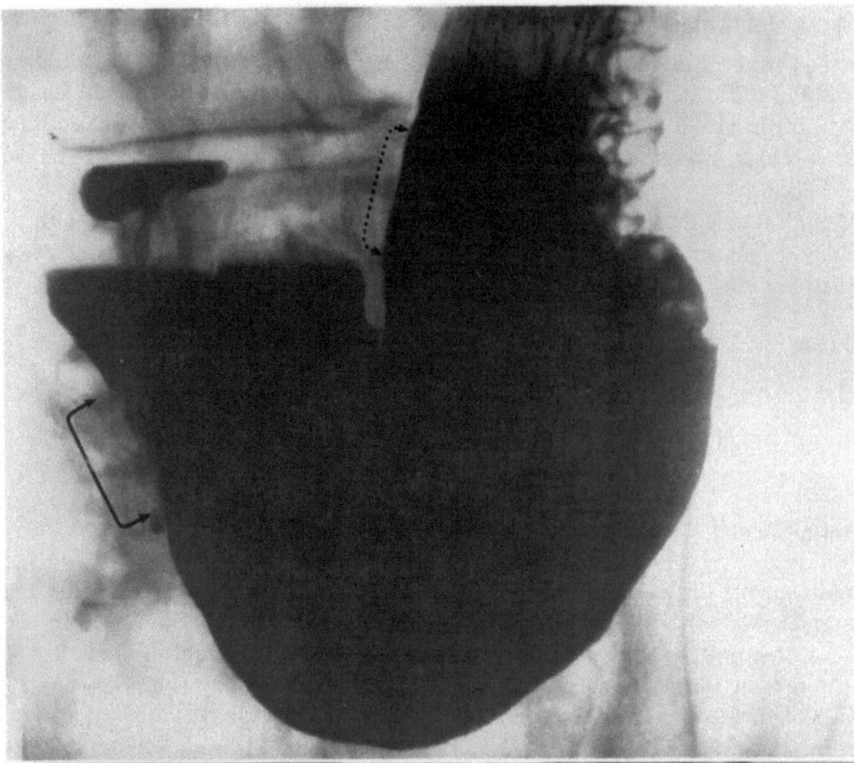

88 a

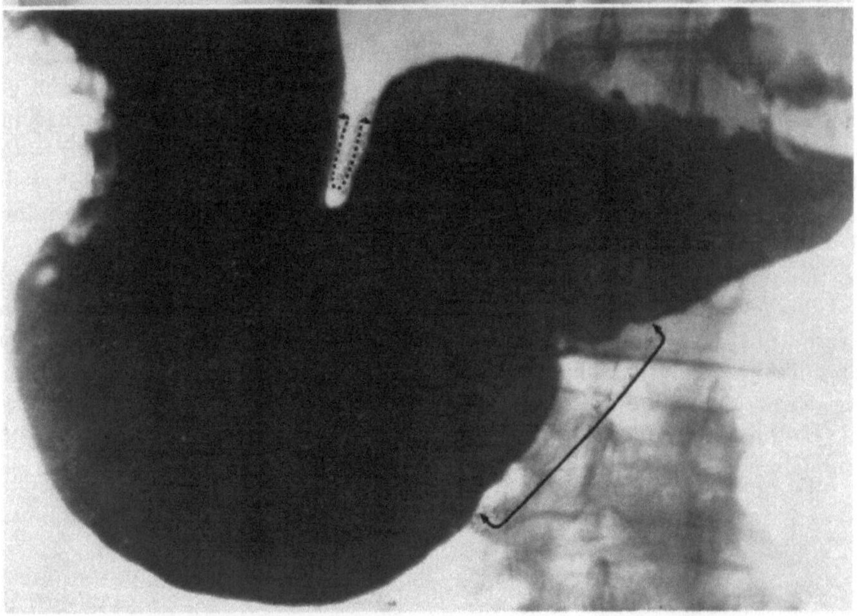

88 b

Fig. 88 a Barium filled study in the upright position. A slight filling defect and rigidity of the wall can be seen on the greater curvature of the antrum. Distensability and irregularity of the lower gastric body were overlooked at the fluoroscopic examination.

Fig. 88 b Barium filled study in the prone position. Findings are more clearly demonstrated in this picture.

88c

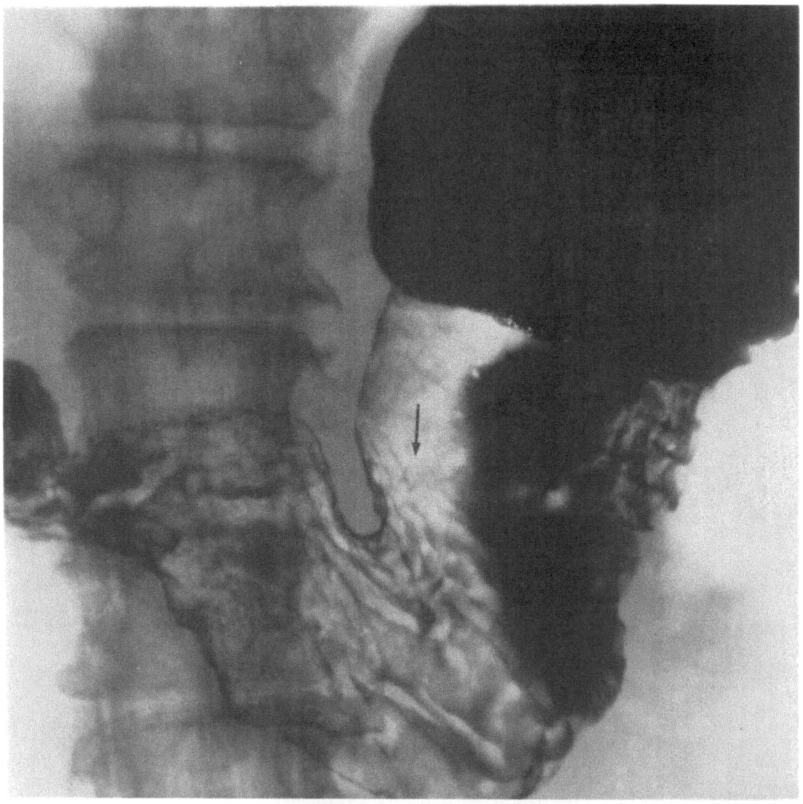

88d

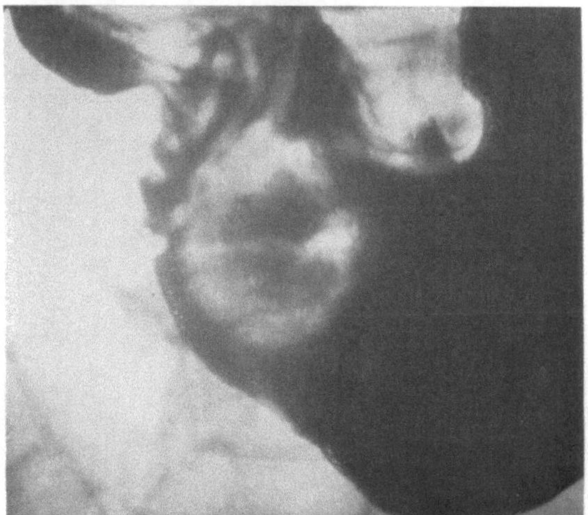

88e

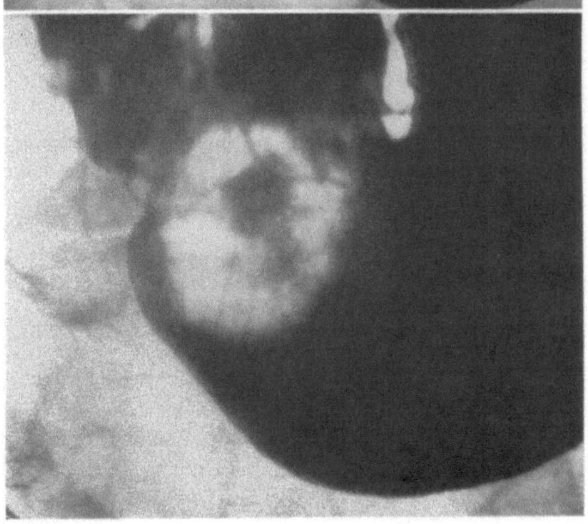

Fig. 88c Double-contrast study in the first oblique position. An amoeboid irregular niche is present on the posterior wall of the antrum. The niche is clearly circumscribed by a rigid marginal protrusion, but the height of the protrusion is difficult to estimate with only this picture. Another lesion of the lower gastric body has apparently left imprints on this picture.

Fig. 88d Compression study with a medium amount of barium.

Fig. 88e Radiograph of the barium filled stomach subjected to full compression. An irregularly outlined defect is clearly demonstrated, but the shape of the central niche is variable. The marginal swelling does not disappear with strong compression.

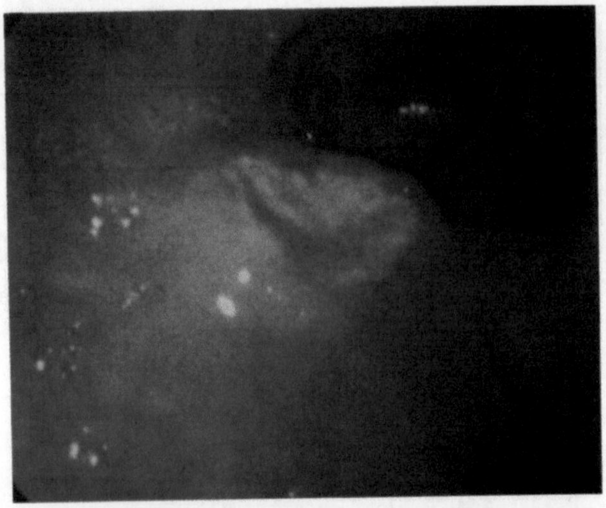

88 f

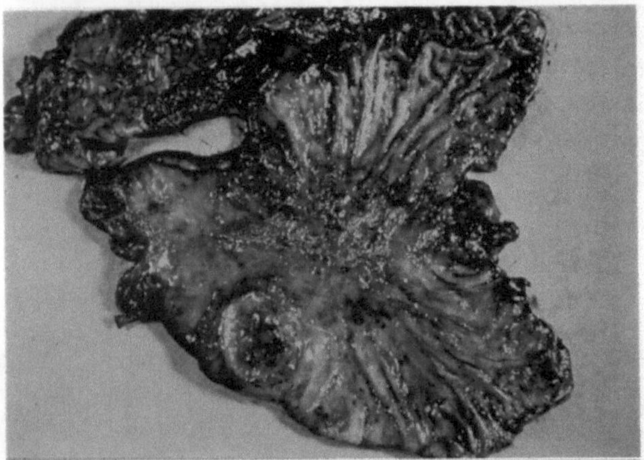

88 g

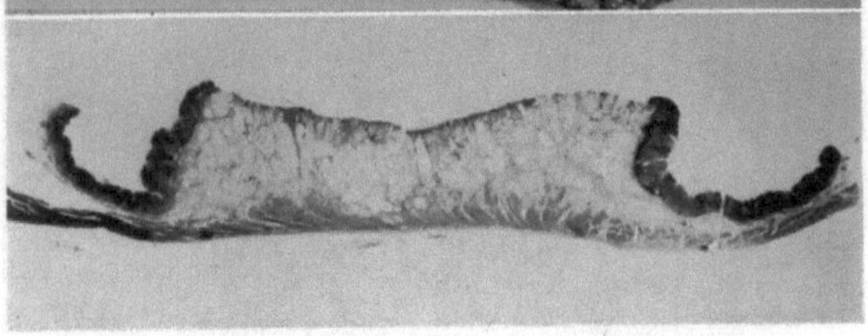

88 h

Fig. 88 f GTF-A picture. An irregularly shaped, white-coated ulcer is surrounded by a marginal swelling which is sharply demarcated from the adjacent mucosa.

Fig. 88 g Resected stomach. A carcinomatous ulcer of the BORRMANN type II and an ulcer-scar at the lesser curvature of the corpus are seen.

Fig. 88 h Histopathological findings. The cancer infiltrated to the subserosal layer, but the horizontal invasion of cancer cells is circumscribed within the marginal swelling.

b. BORRMANN type III (Infiltrating carcinomatous ulcer)

Among the excavated cancers in the stomach, there are the BORRMANN type III cancers, or carcinomatous ulcers with partial infiltrations into adjacent tissues. Macroscopically, the lesions are large, irregular ulcerations surrounded by marginal elevations, but are not circumscribed and partly broken down by cancerous infiltrations. Radiologically, they can be seen as irregular niches with partly circumscribed protrusions and with evidences of marginal infiltrations. Gastrofiberscopy is often useful to confirm the characteristics of these lesions.

Case 24

c.c.: Epigastric distress for several years.

39 year-old female.

In the examination of the mucosal relief with a small amount of barium (Fig. 89 a), sudden interrupted folds were revealed on the lesser curvature of the lower gastric body. In the compression study with a relatively small amount of barium (Fig. 89 b), an irregularly shaped, flat ulcer and surrounding translucency were seen. With fluoroscopy, this shallow niche was not clearly revealed.

A double-contrast study with a small amount of air and barium is shown in Figure 89 c. In this picture, an irregularly shaped, shallow depression with converging folds can be seen on the posterior wall at the angle. In this radiograph, only the shape of the lesion could be demonstrated in comparison with the radiograph of the barium filled stomach subjected to full compression taken with the double-contrast method shown in Figure 89 f. However, in our investigation, few amount double-contrast studies were valuable for routine x-ray examinations, especially to discover the depressed lesions. With the barium filled studies in the upright and prone positions (Figs. 89 d and e), a niche was revealed on the depressed rigid wall (niche en castre) on the lesser curvature of the lower gastric body.

In the double-contrast study with the patient supine (Fig. 89 f), a sharply demarcated, markedly irregular, shallow ulcer was clearly demonstrated on the posterior wall of the lower gastric body. On the greater curvature side, the ulcer margin was surrounded by a rigid mucosal protrusion, and other portions of the marginal swelling were broken down. In addition to these findings, the markedly rigid wall of the lesser curvature, indicated that the lesion was apparently an advanced cancer of the BORRMANN type III.

The gross picture of the surgical specimen is shown in Figure 89 g. An irregularly shaped shallow ulcer was revealed on the posterior wall surrounded by a marginal protrusion on the greater curvature side and a marginal infiltration on the lesser curvature side. Histopathologically, it was established as an adenocarcinoma tubulare mucocellulare with invasion to the subserosa.

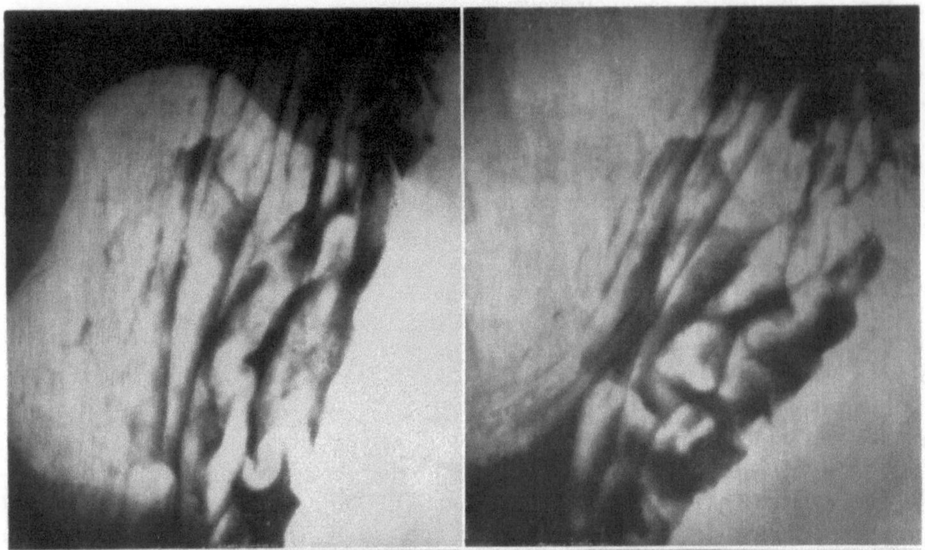

89 a/89 b

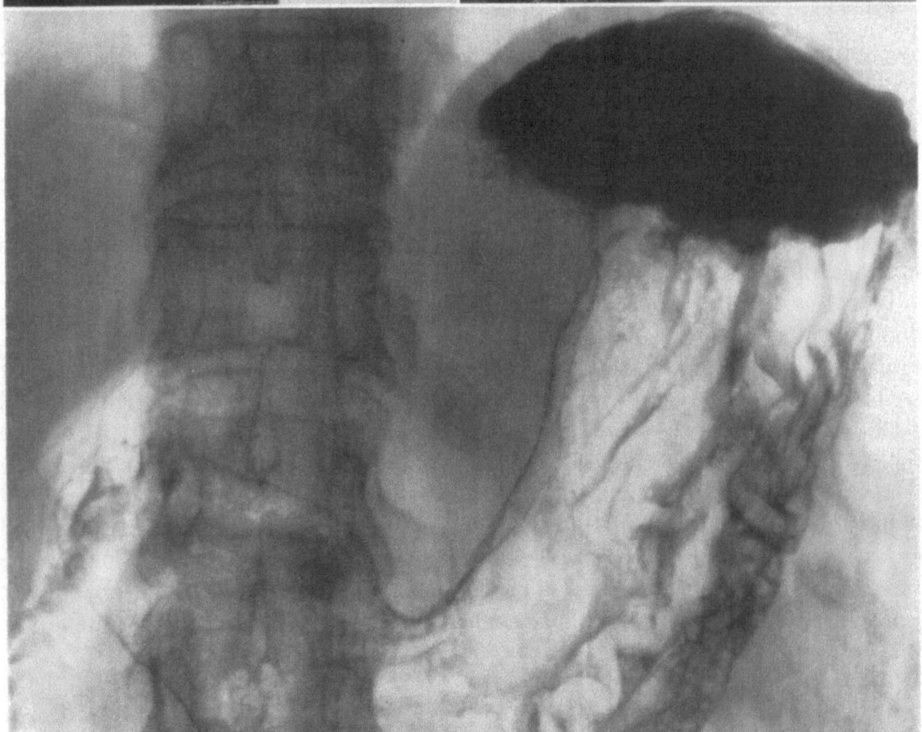

89 c

Fig. 89a Mucosal study. Mucosal convergence and partly interrupted folds are seen.

Fig. 89b Compression study. An irregular, shallow ulceration is surrounded by convergent and interrupted folds.

Fig. 89c Double-contrast study. Use of this technique makes it easy to demonstrate shallow, depressed lesions.

89 d

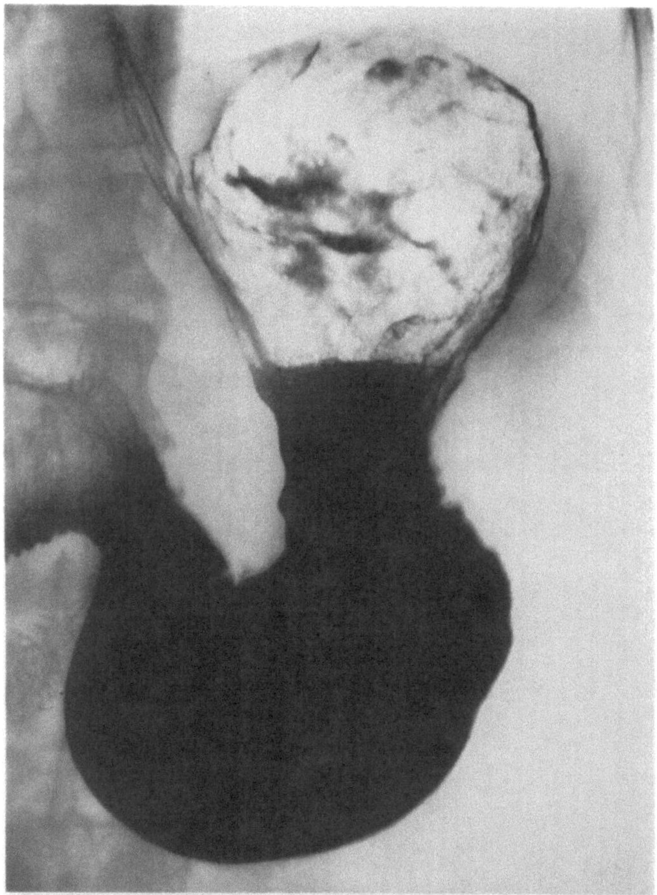

89 e

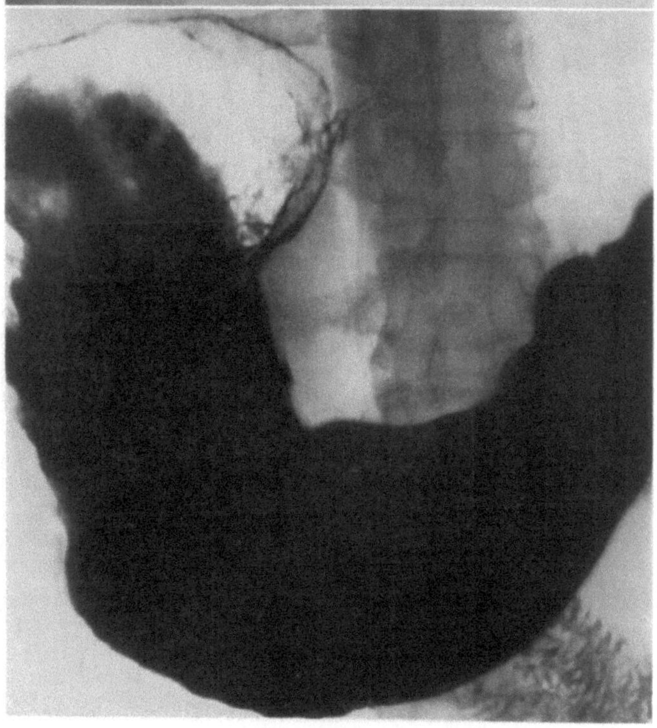

Fig. 89 d Barium filled study in the upright position. A "niche en castre" is clearly demonstrated on the lesser curvature of the body. Rigidity and indentation of the gastric wall indicates the carcinomatous infiltration of this lesion.

Fig. 89 e Barium filled study with the patient prone.

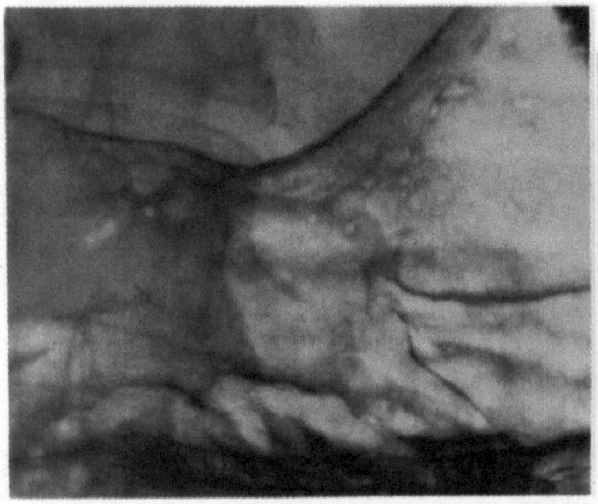

89 f

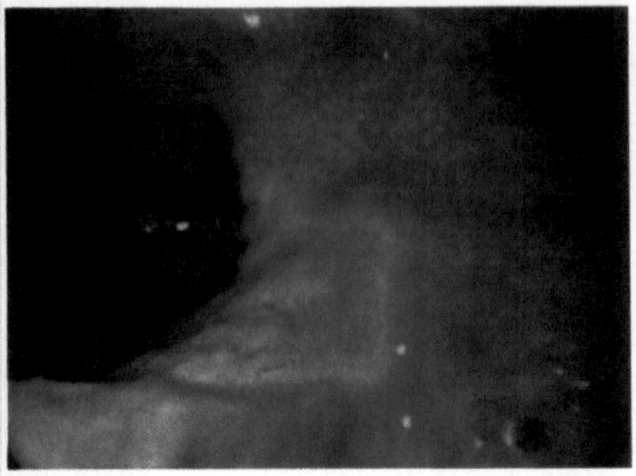

89 g

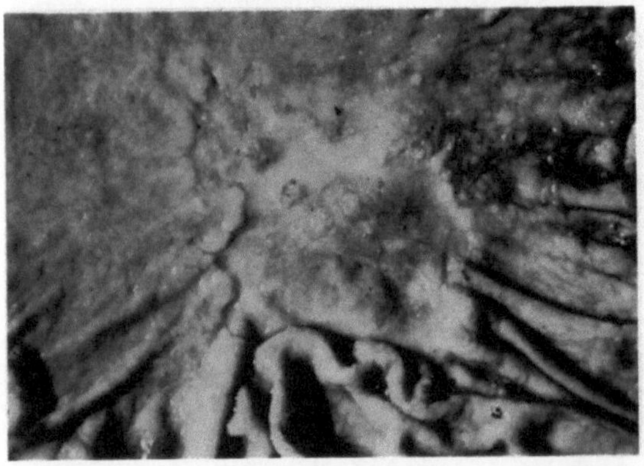

89 h

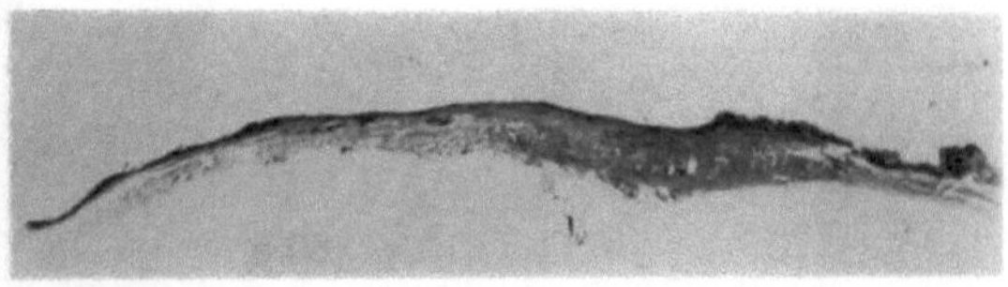

89 i

Fig. 89 f Double-contrast study in the supine position. In this picture, the details are very clearly demonstrated.

Fig. 89 g Endoscopic picture five days before operation (GTF-A). On the lesser curvature of the angulus, a sharply demarcated, shallow ulceration is observed and the surrounding mucosa is markedly elevated and rigid. Some converging folds are nodularly interrupted at its elevated margin on the posterior side. On the other side, the surrounding mucosa is patchily discolored. This lesion is easily diagnosed endoscopically as an infiltrating carcinomatous depression.

Fig. 89 h Resected stomach. An irregularly shaped, carcinomatous depression with infiltration is noticed. In general, depressed lesions of the stomach can be most clearly demonstrated on double-contrast radiographs.

Fig. 89 i Histopathological findings. Histologically, the lesion is revealed as an adenocarcinoma tubulare mucocellulare which has infiltrated to the subserosal layer.

2. Excavated types of early gastric cancer

The macroscopic classification of early cancer is shown in Figure 9 as follows: 1) protuberant early cancer, 2) superficial early cancer, and 3) excavated early cancer. They have further classified superficial early cancer into superficial elevated type (IIa), superficial flat type (IIb) and superficial depressed type (IIc). This means the basic classification includes the five types of I, IIa, IIb, IIc and III. Thus, excavated types of early gastric cancer are type IIc and type III. The difference between the two is that the depression of the former is limited to the mucosa. Practically speaking, however, there are mixed types of IIa+IIc, IIc+III, or III+IIc, and the authors feel that a simple classification in compliance with the major types of the disease would be much more helpful in making a diagnosis. In our studies, lesions of type I were observed in 5% of the cases, IIa in 19%, IIb in 1%, IIc (incl. IIc+III) in 65%, and type III (incl. III+IIc) in 10%.

Though early cancer of the excavated type belongs to IIc and III, the incidence of these types of cancer is much more frequent than the rest. Figure 91 indicates the results of routine x-ray examinations of early cancer of the types IIc and III. In type IIc, a number of lessions have been confirmed by means of double-contrast radiography. In type III, it is possible to find lessions in almost all cases, yet benign ulcers are likely to be misdiagnosed as cancer in these cases.

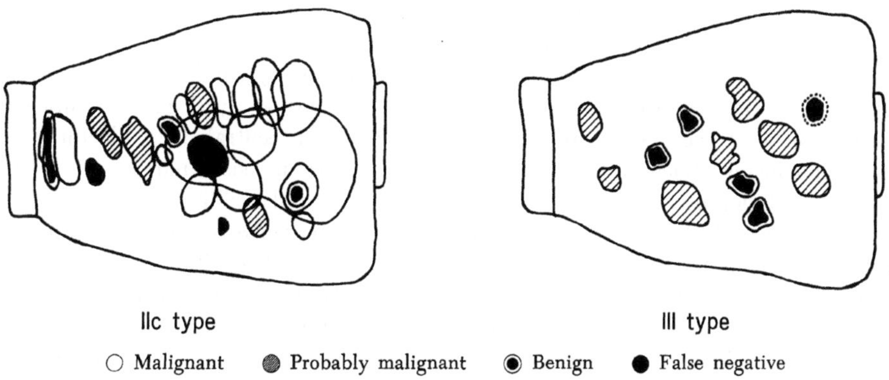

Fig. 91 Routine x-ray diagnosis of excavated early gastric cancer.

a. Type IIc (Superficial depressed type) early gastric cancer

The type IIc early gastric cancer has been defined as a cancerous erosion in which the depression is limited to the mucosa and the cancerous invasion is only in the mucosa or submucosal layer, without infiltration to the muscular layer proper. The IIc+III type early gastric cancer is included in this category.

In our investigations, the macroscopic characteristics of the lesions are observed to be as follows:

1. The floor of the shallow depression shows reddish discoloring, villous depression with a granular appearance.
2. The contour of the depressions is irregular and sharply demarcated. In some cases the depression has a double contour.
3. The surrounding mucosa shows interruption and flattenning of the mucosal folds. Marginal hyperemia or hemorrage are valuable for a differential diagnosis.

Case 25

c.c.: Epigastric pain and heart-burn for two months.

37 year-old female.

In the barium filled studies in the upright position (Fig. 91 a) and prone position (Fig. 91 b), the irregular widening of the gastric angle was impressive. In this region, rigidity of the wall and faint saw-tooth irregularities could be seen. These findings indicated the existence of a large lesion, rather than multiple lesions. The double-contrast study (Fig. 91 c) showed an irregular, shallow niche at the angle. An oval, faint fleck with a central deep ulceration was associated with convincing mucosal thickening and partly with mucosal narrowing. Occasionally, superficial mucosal depression appears demonstrated as granular filling defects in the double-contrast studies (Fig. 91 d). A barium fleck with rugal convergence is commonly found whenever mucosal studies with a small amount of barium are performed (Fig. 91 e). These findings were convincing evidences that the lesion was a typical IIc+III type early cancer.

Gastrofiberscopic findings (Fig. 91 f) revealed an ulceration which was coated by a dirty-whitish, thin exudate in its central region. An irregular IIc depression with an uneven, patchy reddened floor was noted surrounding the ulceration. In these pictures, a shallow, irregular depression surrounded by flattened mucosal folds around the marginal area was found. This finding is reported to be "the typical pattern of double contour". The gross specimen (Fig. 91 g) was almost identical to the pre-operative radiograph and endoscopic picture. The sharply demarcated depression was recognized as a IIc+III type early cancer and the cancerous infiltration was limited to the submucosal layer.

91a

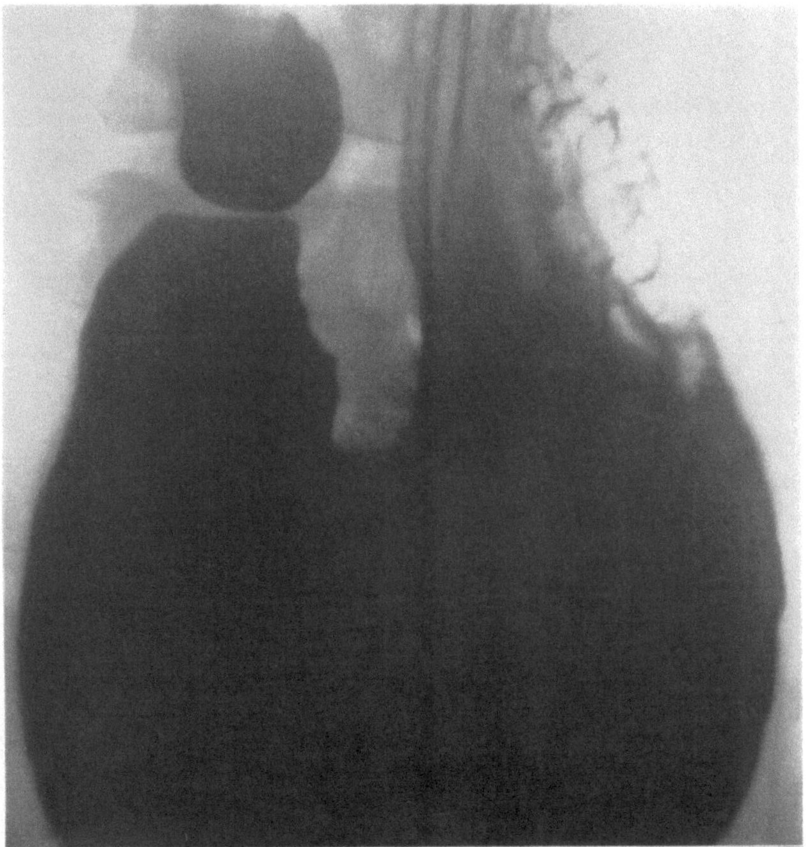

91b

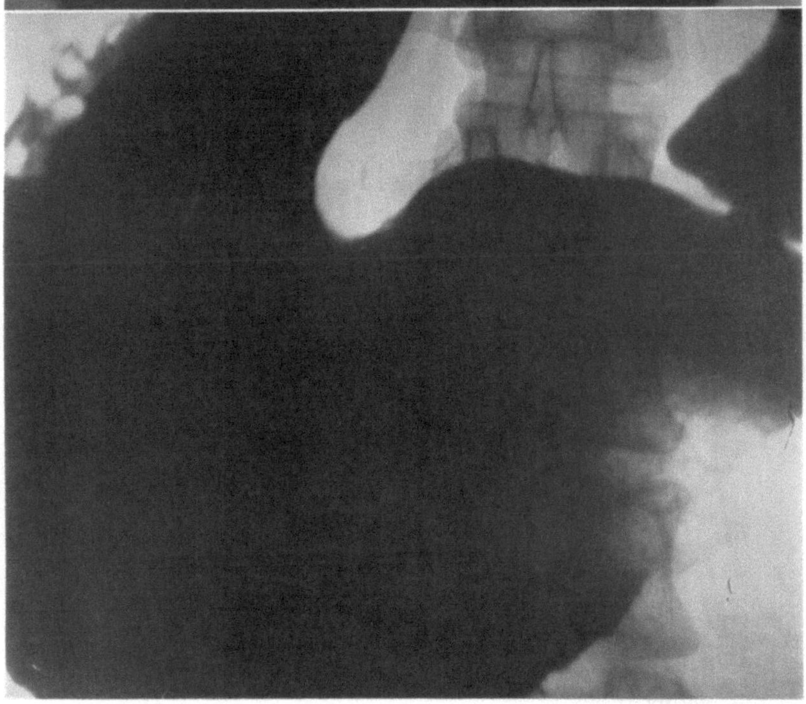

Fig. 91a Barium filled stomach in the upright position.

Fig. 91b Barium filled stomach in the prone position. The lesser curvature of the angular region is widened and rigid. This marginal line consists of the floor of the lesion.

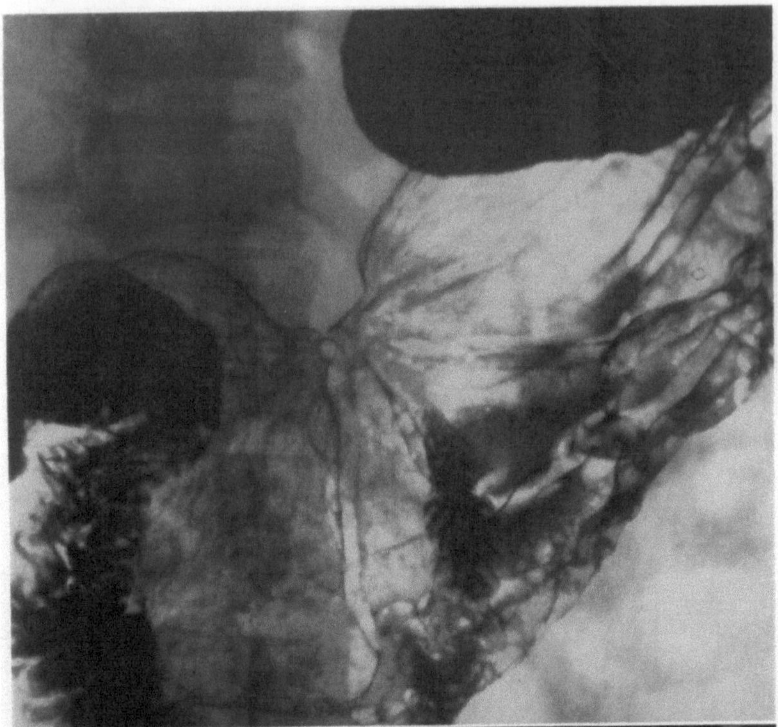

91c

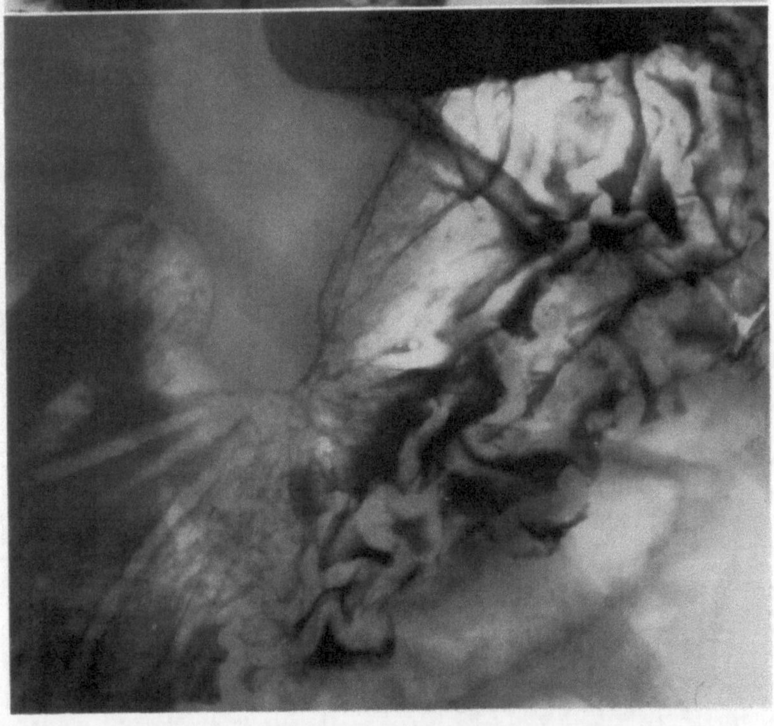

91d

Fig. 91c Double-contrast study. A sharply demarcated, shallow depression is observed inside the marginally deformed wall. Typical findings of a type IIc (or IIc+III) early cancer are demonstrated in this picture.

Fig. 91d Double-contrast study in the left oblique position. In this picture, the lesion appears to be a granular mucosal protrusion and was diagnosed mistakenly as a filling defect. The border of the cancerous erosion is not clear, but irregularly shaped, globular granules show the characteristics of this lesion.

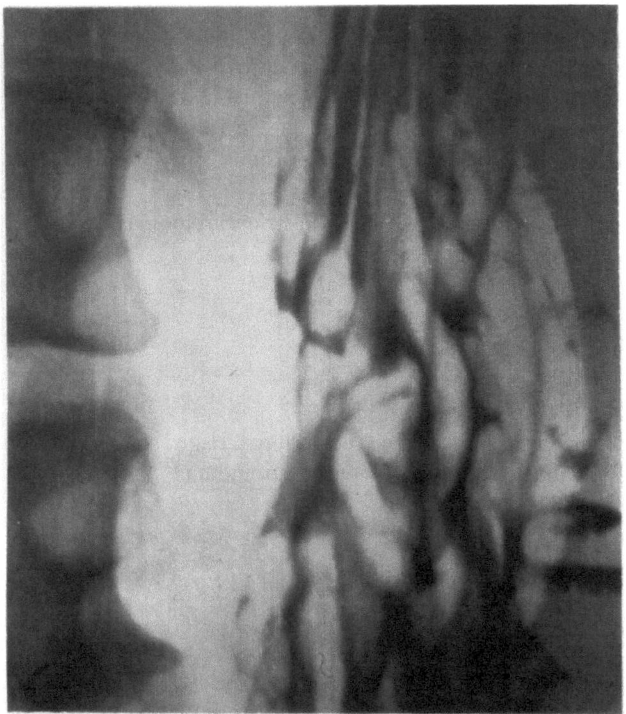

91e

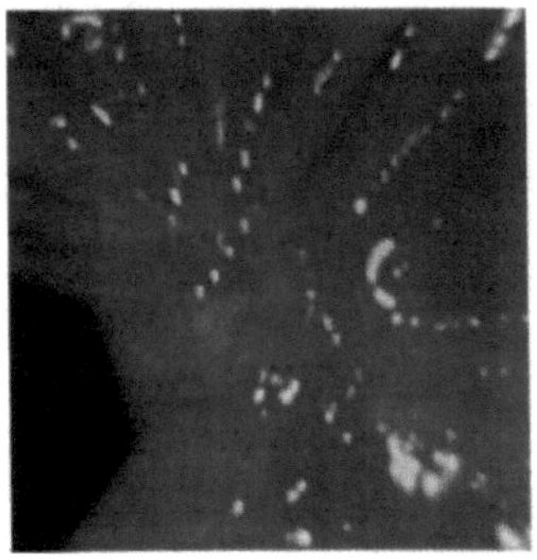

91f

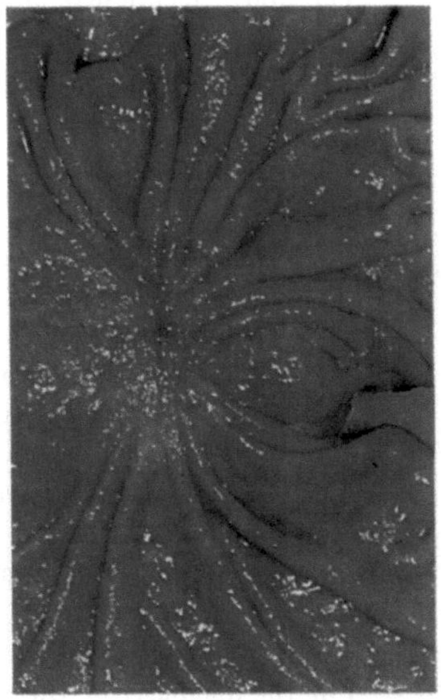

91g

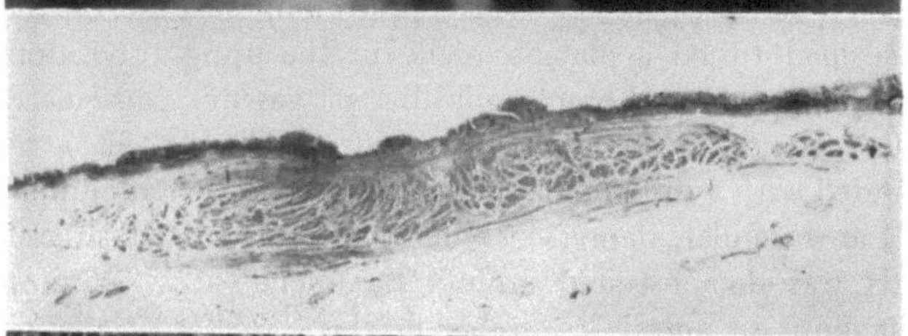

91h

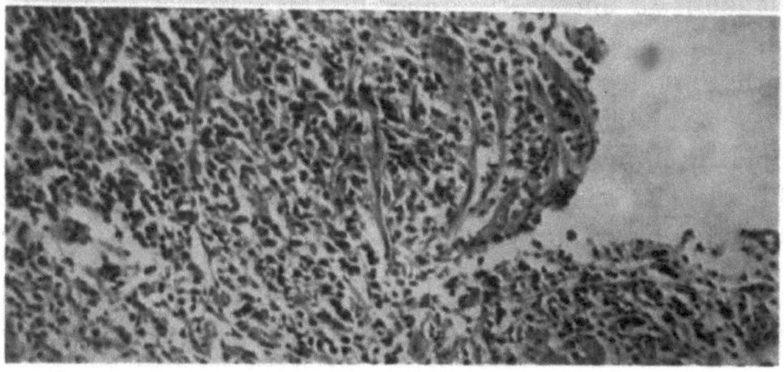

91i

Fig. 91e **Mucosal study.** An irregular, shallow depression and interruption of mucosal folds are observed.

Fig. 91f **Endoscopic picture.** A dirty-whitish-coated ulcer surrounded by the reddened, villous erosion is visible. These are the typical features of a IIc+III type early cancer.

Fig. 91g **Resected stomach.** The gross specimen shows a type IIc early cancer with an unmarked III lesion.

Figs. 91h and g **Histopathological findings.** Histologically, the cancerous infiltration has partially invaded the submucosal layer at the central region of the ulceration.

b. Type III (Excavated type) early gastric cancer

The difference between a type IIc and a type III is that the depression of the former is limited within the mucosa while the excavation of the latter into the gastric wall is prominent. It is almost impossible to diagnose accurately this type of early cancer using the present techniques of roentgenology and gastrofiberscopy. Practically, however, the so-called lesions of the type III early cancer are recognizable as small areas of cancerous erosions surrounding peptic ulcers.

Presently, it is useful to differentiate the excavated type early gastric carcinomas from the benign peptic ulcers according to the following characteristics:

1) Marginal protuberance of the crater
2) Demarcated excavation
3) Irregularly shaped ulcer
4) Gigantic ulcer
5) Rigidity of the converging folds

The above mentioned findings are suspicious of this type of lesion. High acid values in gastric analysis are occassionally encountered with this type of early carcinoma.

Case 26

c.c.: Discomfort in the epigastrium for three months.

47 year-old male.

The barium filled studies (Figs. 92 a, b) indicated an abnormal, protruding shadow on the lesser curvature of the antrum, which seemed to be a plateau niche in the upright position, and a slightly rigid concavity in the prone position. Fluoroscopically, it was not particularly difficult to discover these niches in this region. In the double-contrast study (Fig. 92 c), an irregularly shaped ulceration was demonstrated with a distal mucosal elevation. In the radiographs from the compression study (Figs. 92 d, e), an irregular, depressed niche was clearly demonstrated. Abrupt interruption of the mucosal folds was demonstrated around the niche. The compression study was most effective for the diagnosis of antral lesions as in this case, especially on the lesser or greater curvature.

For the diagnosis of this case, the authors preferred x-ray findings to endoscopy even though, the preoperative differential diagnosis was very difficult, *i.e.*, advanced cancer, type IIc early cancer or type III early cancer. Endoscopically, it was not possible to confirm whether the lesion was malignant or benign (Fig. 92f). The surgical specimen revealed a relatively shallow type III early cancer (Fig. 92 g), and the cancerous invasion was limited to the submucosal layer histologically (Fig. 92 h).

92a

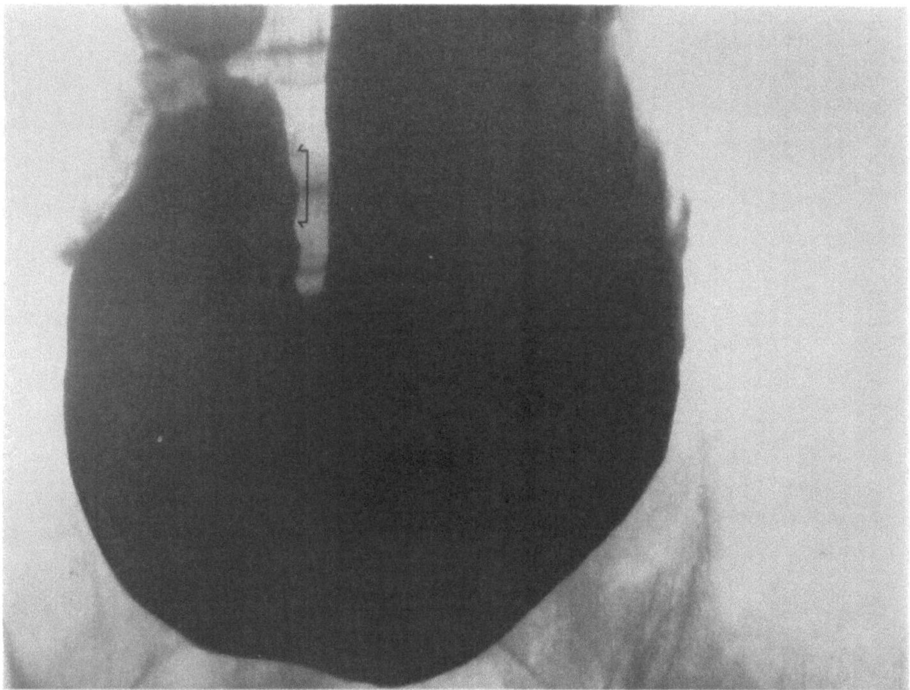

92b

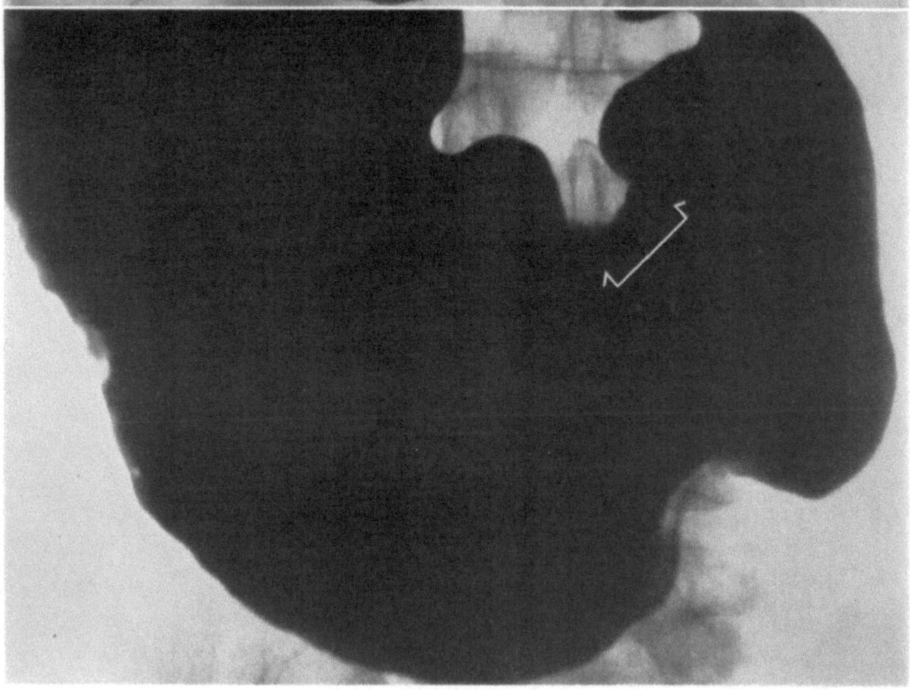

Fig. 92a Barium filled stomach in the upright position. Irregularity of the antrum is observed.

Fig. 92b Barium filled stomach in the prone position. Marginal concavity and rigidity of the wall are noticed.

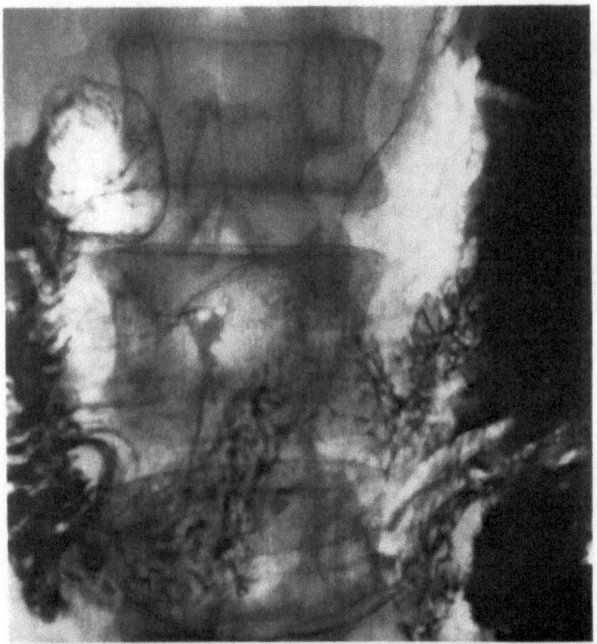

92c

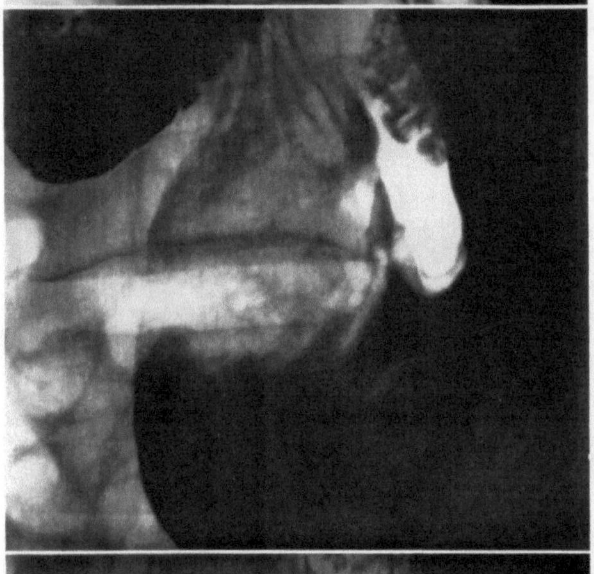

92d

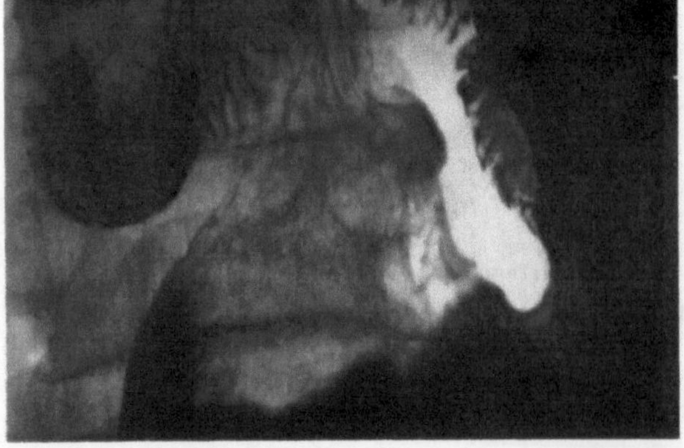

92e

Fig. 92c Double-contrast study. A relatively small niche is demonstrated. The form of the niche is sharply demarcated and irregular.

Figs. 92d and e Compression study. The depressed niche is surrounded by a faint, mucosal protrusion and interruptions of the mucosal folds are seen.

92f
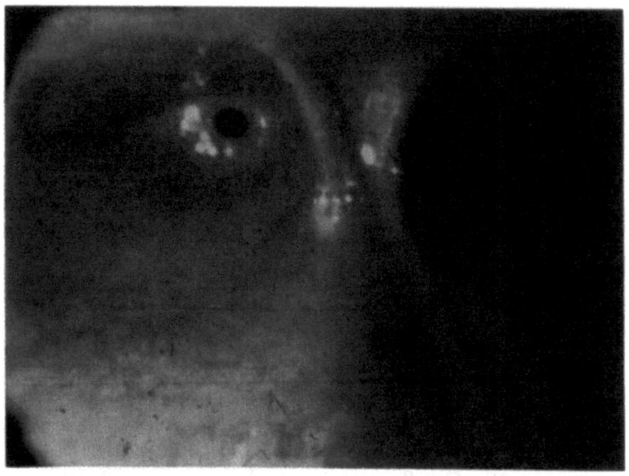

92g
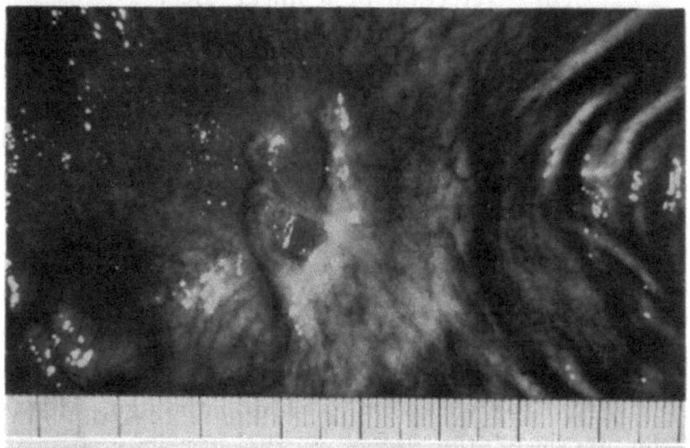

92h
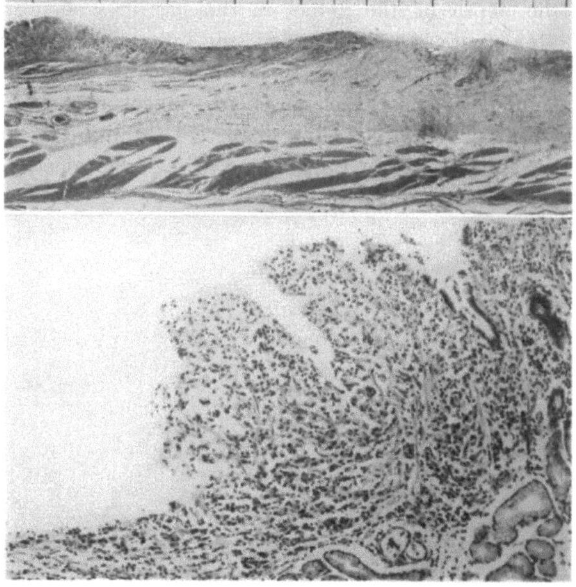

Fig. 92f Endoscopic picture. An irregularly shaped, shallow ulcer is seen on the lesser curvature of the antrum.

Fig. 92g Resected stomach. An irregularly shaped ulceration and its surrounding mucosal elevation are present.

Fig. 92h Histopathological findings. The lesion is revealed as an adenocarcinoma tubulare mucocellulare histologically.

3. Gastric ulcer

A gastric ulcer is defined as a circumscribed substance defect of the gastric wall that involves not only the mucosa but also the muscularis mucosa. A benign ulcer usually has a sharp, clean-cut border and is surrounded by an inflamed mucosa. The floor is clean and covered by a thin, whitish coat. A benign ulcer crater appears roentgenologically in profile as a penetrating niche or, in the frontal view, as a sharply outlined and circumscribed barium fleck surrounded by a halo or a ring-like collar of inflamed submucosa. The contour and surrounding mucosa of the ulcer are usually smooth and clean.

Gastrofiberscopy is of great value in diagnosing gastric ulcers, especially flat ulcers in the final stages of healing. The practical importance of the diagnostic problems of gastric ulcers are as follows:

1) Accurate diagnosis of an acute or chronic ulcer
2) Confirmation of the protractability of a peptic ulcer
3) Detection of a linear ulcer
4) Differentiation between benign and malignant ulcers

In differential diagnosis of benign and malignant ulcers, all the evidences available with the use of radiologic and gastrofiberscopic examinations are needed. There are some malignant ulcers which simulate benign ulcers, causing diagnostic difficulties. The shape and depth of the crater, mucosal protrusion around the crater, and surrounding mucosal folds are valuable for differentiation.

In contrast peptic ulcers, cancerous ulcers are defects produced on the surface of the protuberant membrane. Consequently, peptic ulcers have secondary walls produced by inflammatory swelling or autoplasticity on the margins of the ulcers, and thus the craters or the walls of the ulcers are flat and the surrounding membrane is soft.

From the viewpoint of histopathology, MURAKAMI has classified peptic ulcers according to the depth of the defect in the gastric wall. This classification has been widely adopted as MURAKAMI's Ul classification not only in clinical medicine but also in the field of pathology. Preveously stated (Fig. 10), Ul-I indicates a defect of the mucous membrane which is not deep enough to reach the muscularis mucosae and is called an erosion. Ul-II is an ulcer reaching the submucosal layer which pierces through the muscularis mucosae. Ul-III is an ulcer reaching the muscular layer proper, and Ul-IV is an ulcer reaching the serosa after completely penetrating the muscular layer proper.

a. Acute ulcer

It is still difficult to differentiate between an acute ulcer proper and an exacerbated chronic ulcer. Histopathologically, in an acute ulcer the border may be flat, but is often elevated and surrounded by mucosal edema without radiating folds. An acute ulcer is characterized by the absence of granulation and fibrous tissue.

Case 27

c. c.: Hematemesis and melena after steroid therapy for nephrosis.

52 year-old male.

The first x-ray examination before steroid therapy (Figs. 93 a, b) revealed no evidence of abnormality in the stomach. This was true of both the barium filled study and the double-contrast study (Fig. 93 c). Retrospectively, the only area of mucosal unevenness was detected on the posterior wall of the antrum. It is shown by the arrow on the double-contrast study.

After seven days of hematemesis, the patient received x-ray and endoscopic examinations. The x-ray films from the second examination are shown in Figures 93 d–g. Barium filled studies in the upright and prone positions exhibited an angular, gigantic niche and a small niche on the lesser curvature of the antrum (Figs. 93 d, e). In the compression study (Fig. 93 d), the angular ulcer is clearly demonstrated as an oval-shaped and smoothly outlined niche. The double-contrast study (Fig. 93 e) demonstrated both the angular and antral ulcer niches. The angular ulcer was smoothly rounded without converging folds and the mucosal surface around the ulcer was smooth and markedly edematous. These findings indicated an acute gastric ulcer. On the contrary, the antral small niche was surrounded by converging folds. This case was diagnosed as an acute angular ulcer and an acute exacerbated ulcer of the antrum induced by steroid administration.

The next day, the patient underwent endoscopic examination. Endoscopic examination revealed two ulcers on the lesser curvature of the gastric angle and the antrum (Figs. 93 f, h). Macroscopically, a grayish, hemorrhagic ulcer was demonstrated at the angle, but the surrounding mucosa was smooth and rather edematous (Fig. 93 g). Another lesion, a white-coated, round, well-defined ulcer with converging folds was demonstrated in the antrum. Histopathologically, the oval ulcer at the angle was revealed to be an acute ulcer and the pyloric lesion as a chronic ulcer. It is most important to differentiate between an acute giant ulcer and a type III early cancer.

A similar endoscopic picture of III+IIc type early cancer is shown in Figure 93 i. In this picture, an angular hemorrhagic ulcer having patchy discoloration and a depression indicated a small area of cancerous erosion. Note the difference between the two endoscopic findings.

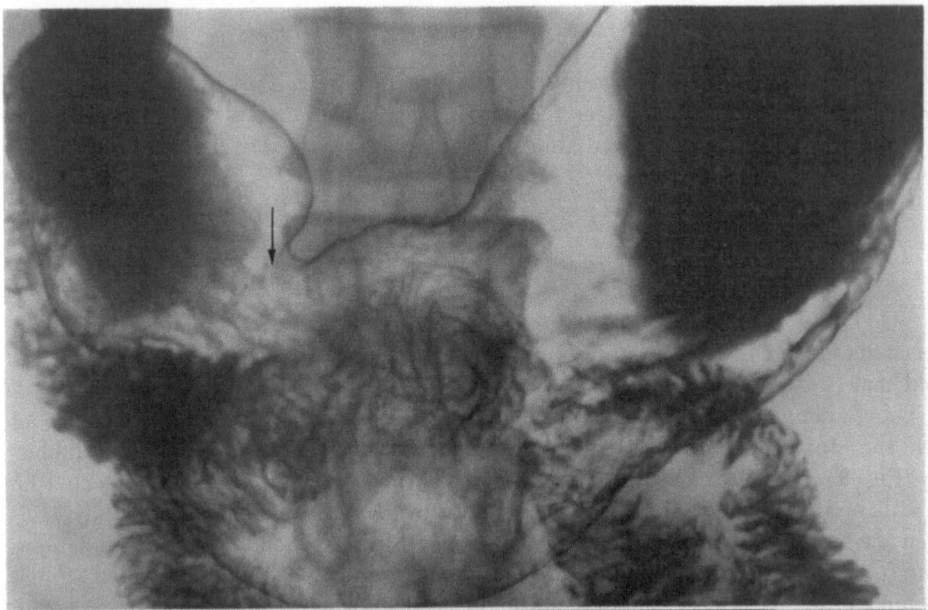

93a

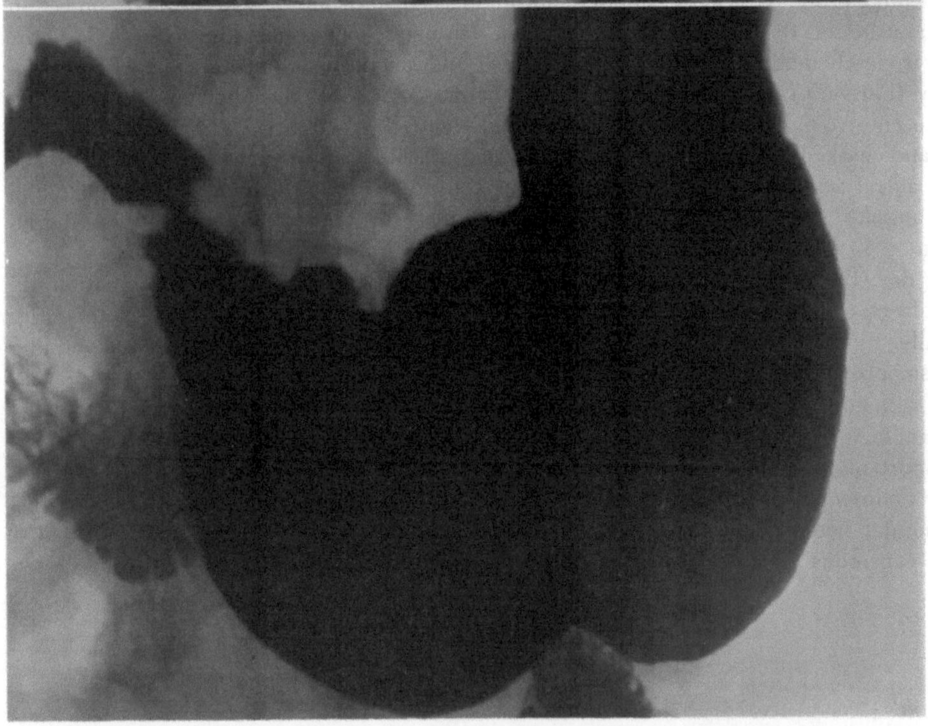

93b

Fig. 93a Double-contrast study before steroid therapy. Mucosal uneveness and fine mucosal convergency are shown by the arrow.

Fig. 93b Barium filled stomach in the upright position after steroid therapy. Multiple ulcer niches are clearly demonstrated on the lesser curvature.

93c

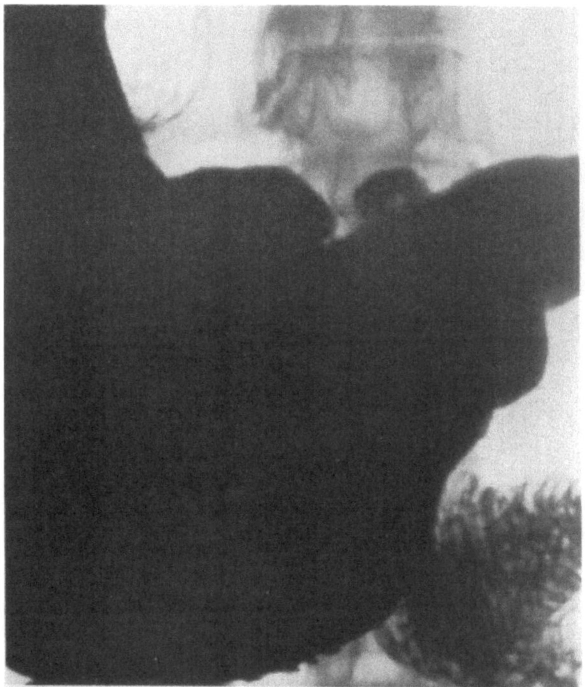

93d

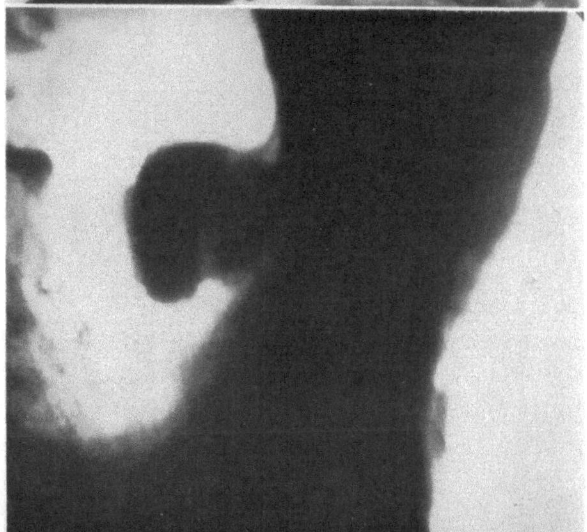

93e

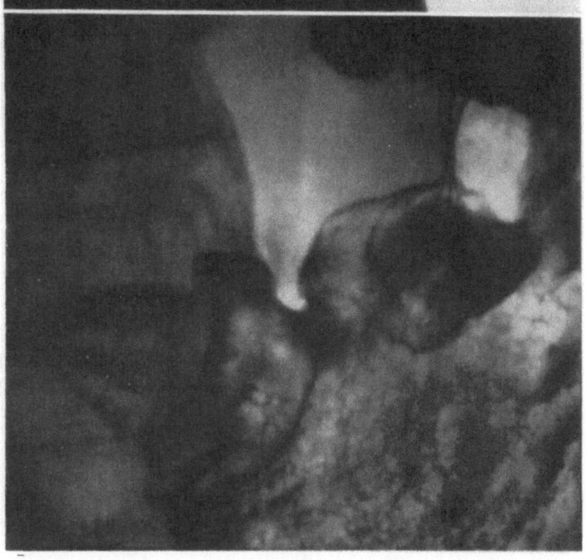

Fig. 93c Barium filled stomach in the prone position.

Fig. 93d Compression study. A clearly defined niche is demonstrated on the lesser curvature of the gastric angle.

Fig. 93e Double-contrast study. The angular ulcer is demonstrated by frontal view and the antral one shown in profile.

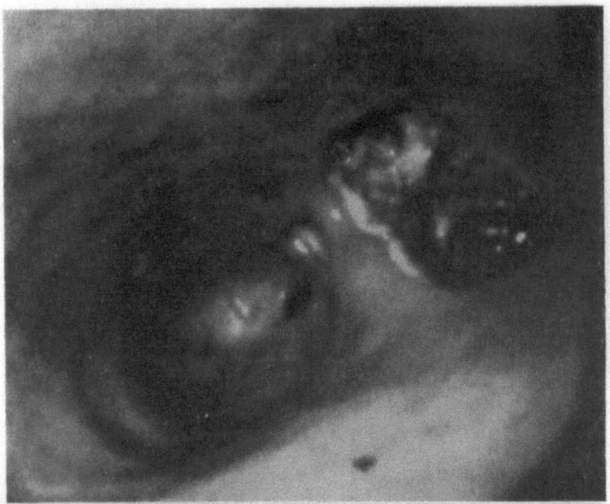

93f

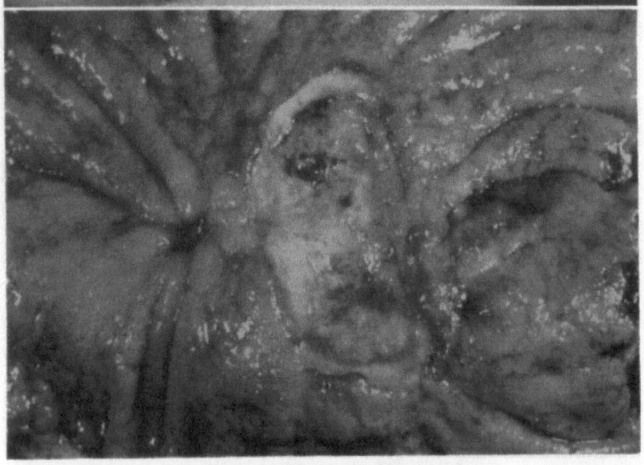

93g

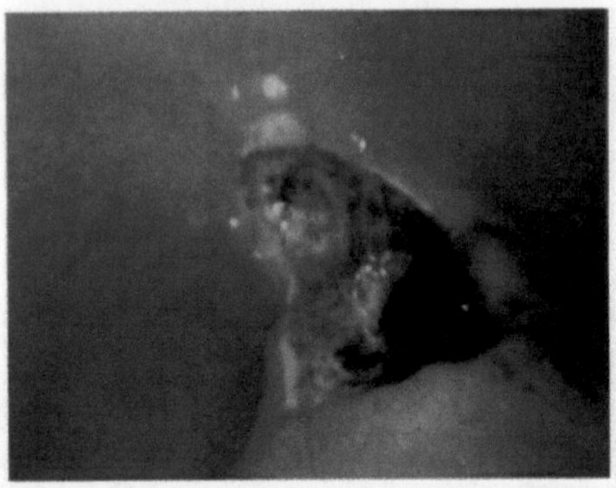

93h

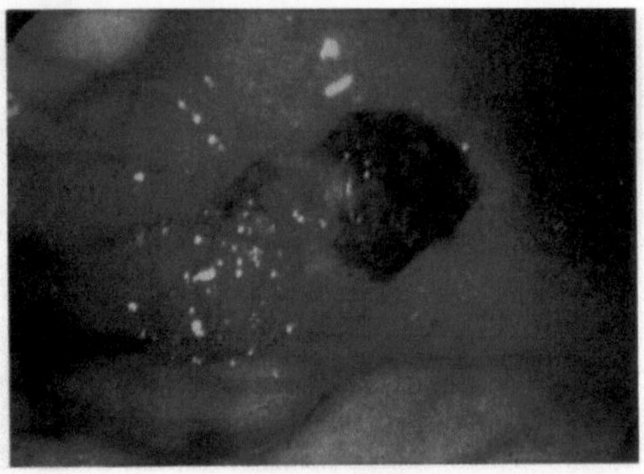

93i

Fig. 93f Endoscopic picture.

Fig. 93g Resected stomach.

Fig. 93h Endoscopic picture of acute ulcer.

Fig. 93i Endoscopic picture of a III+IIc type early cancer.
Compare the differences of these endoscopical findings.

b. Chronic gastric ulcer

Almost all peptic ulcers are characterized by their clinical courses of remission and exacerbation, therefore, most ulcers are chronic ulcers in various stages. Usually convergence of mucosal folds and marginal mucosal protuberances without edema represent chronic gastric ulcers.

Radiologically, SHIRAKABE has pointed out that suspicious findings for protractability of gastric ulcer are as follows:

1) A sharply demarcated ulcer crater with an uneven floor
2) A marked convergence of the mucosal folds and an interruption without surrounding edema of the gastric wall.

Endoscopically, we point out similar problems: multiple ulcers in contact with one another crossing the longitudinal axis of the stomach, a nodular thickening of the ulcer margin, and a cleancut border of the ulcer-coat with marked convergence.

1) Flat non-penetrating ulcer

Case 28

c. c.: Hunger pains in the epigastrium and a loss of appetite.

69 year-old male.

A small niche was demonstrated on the lesser curvature of the antrum in the radiograph of the barium filled stomach (Fig. 94 a).

The double-contrast study revealed frontal view of the niche. Although the shape of the niche seemed to be slightly varied in these three radiographs (Figs. 94 b, c, d), this ulceration was oval and the surrounding mucosal findings proved that it was shallow. A spreading barium fleck with granular appearance was observed on the oral side of the niche.

When these findings are observed, one must be careful to differentiate scarring ulcers from the III+IIc type early cancer. Endoscopic findings proved that it was a benign ulcer in the healing stage (Figs. 94 e, f).

The characteristic features of benign ulcers in the healing stage are as follows:

1) In the radiographs of the double-contrast study, the granular appearance surrounding the niche is similar to the normal gastric areas.

2) The border of the niche is not sharp, and the shape of the niche is easily changeable with photographic conditions.

3) Endoscopically, concavities surrounding the ulcer coat appear to be homogeneously reddened and gradually spreading.

The gross specimen demonstrated that this lesion was a shallow, oval ulceration with slight mucosal convergency (Fig. 94 g). Histologically, it was revealed as a chronic gastric ulcer which should have been classified under Ul-III.

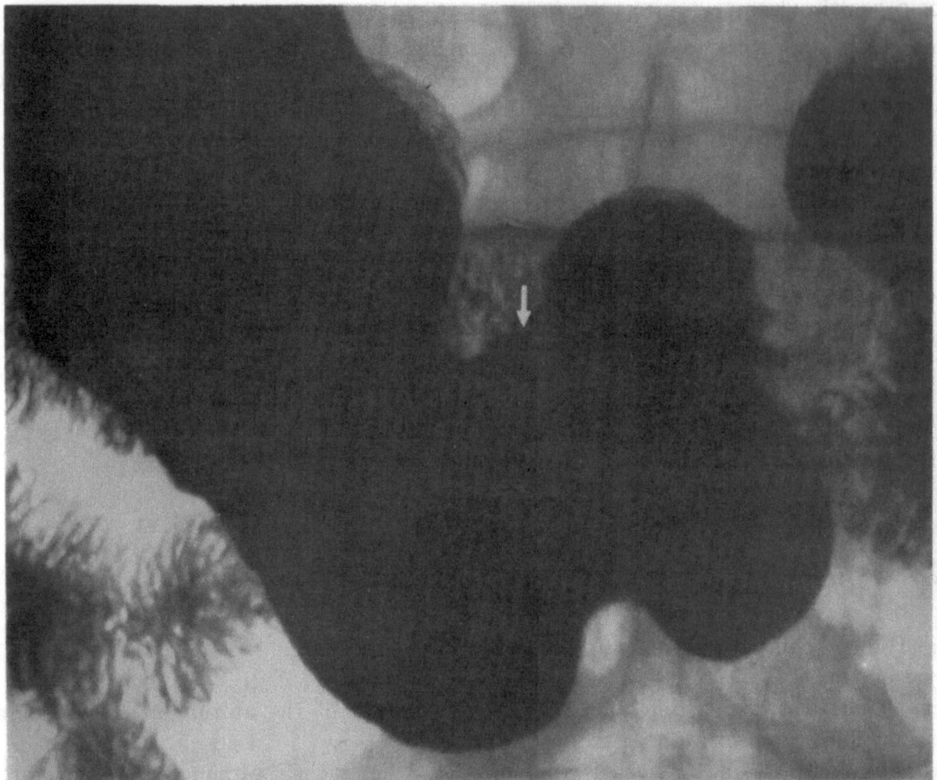

94 a

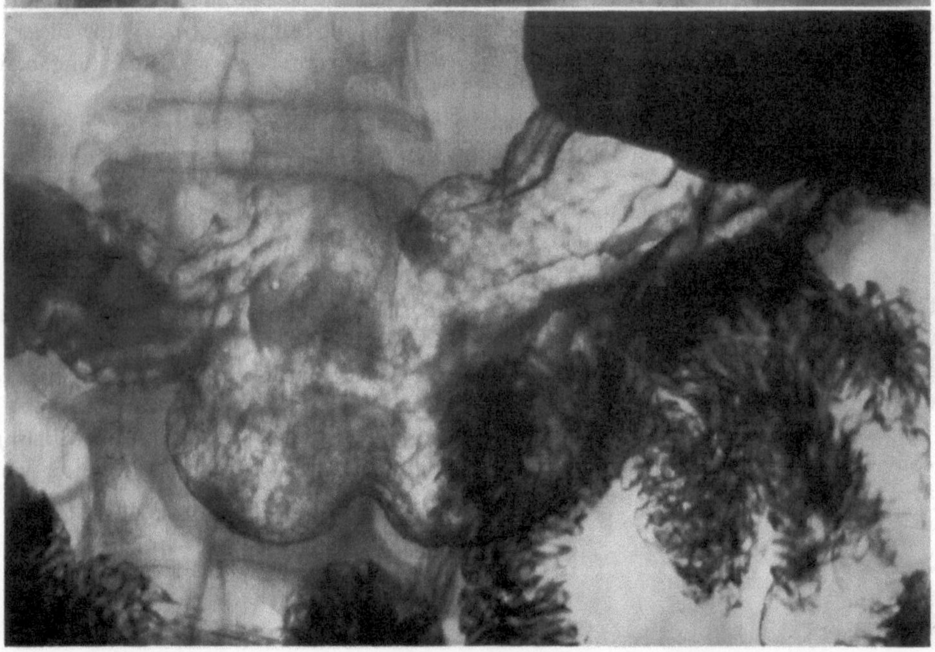

94 b

Fig. 94 a Barium filled stomach in the prone position.

Fig. 94 b Double-contrast study. Round ulcer is seen at the gastric angle.

94 c

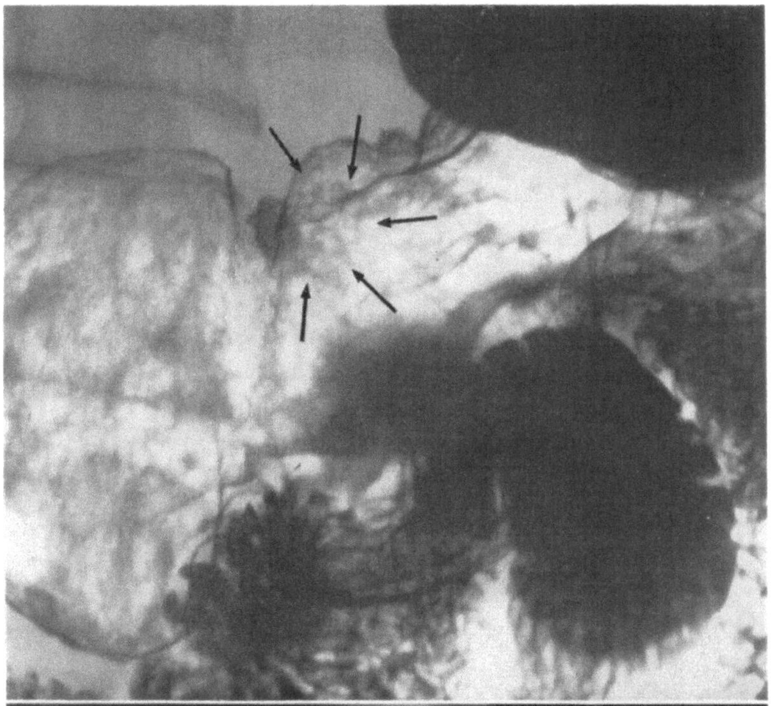

94 d

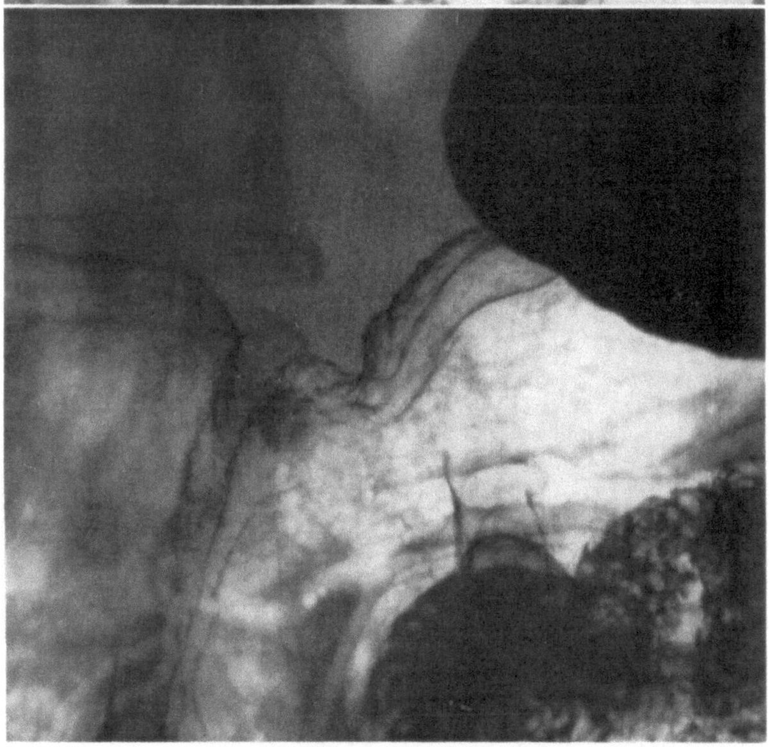

Fig. 94 c and d Double-contrast studies. The shape of the niche differs variously in these pictures. A faint granular shadow on the oral half of the niche (arrow) is noticed. It usually means the presence of a focal gastritis around the chronic gastric ulcer.

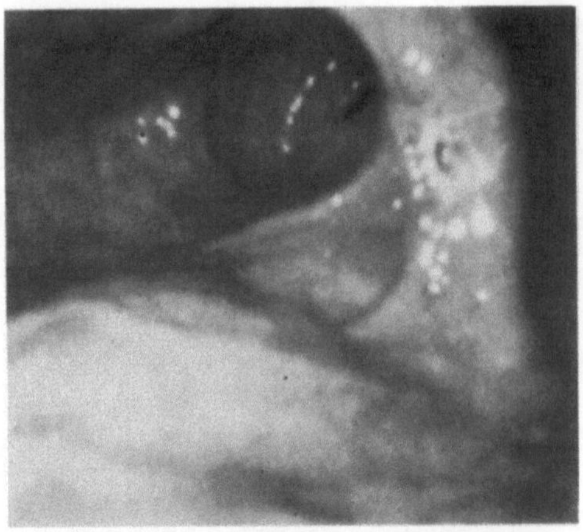

94e

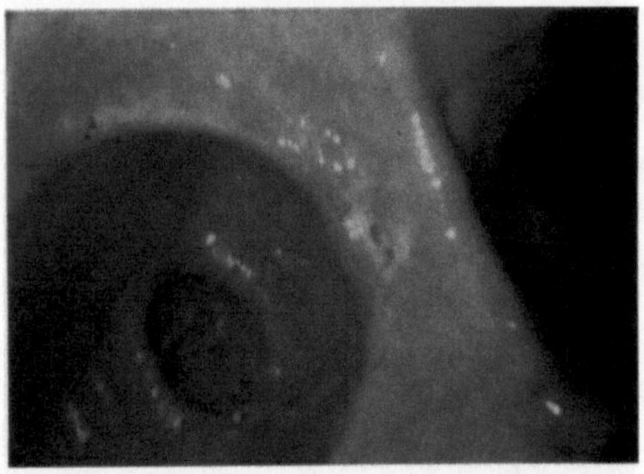

94f

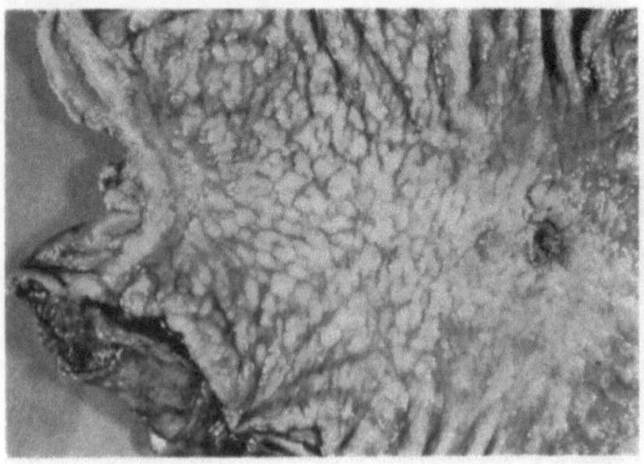

94g

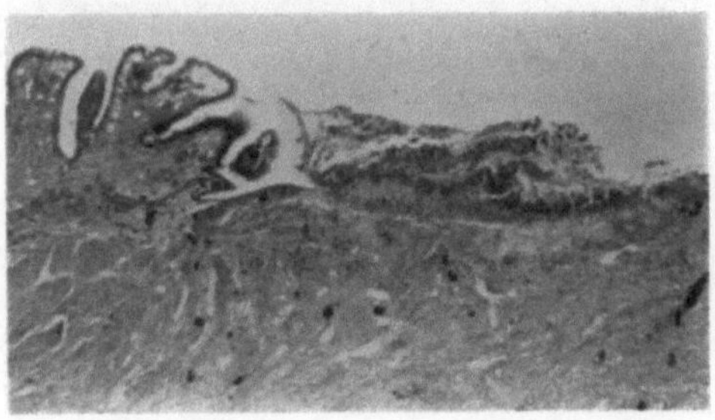

94h

Figs. 94e and f Endoscopic pictures. An irregularly shaped, shallow ulcer surrounded by a red halo is seen. Gastric biopsy proved it to be benign.

Fig. 94g Resected stomach. Macroscopically, the surrounding mucosa of the round ulcer shows uneveness similar to a type IIc early cancer.

Fig. 94h Histopathological findings. This lesion was revealed as a benign ulcer penetrating to the muscular layer proper (Ul-III).

2) Deep penetrating ulcer

Bases of gastric ulcers generally consist of granulation and fibrous tissues; in some, however, the base consists of a capsule of the pancreas and/or another organ neighboring the stomach. These conditions are recognized as chronic, covered perforations and frequently called "penetrating ulcers".

Case 29

c.c.: Epigastric pain.

52 year-old male.

One year ago he was admitted to another clinic for a gastric ulcer.

The barium filled study revealed a large niche surrounding a slight concavity of the gastric angle and showed moderate shortening of the lesser curvature (Figs. 95 a, b). This finding indicated that the lesion was not a round ulcer, but probably a linear ulcer. In the double-contrast study (Fig. 95 c), an irregular niche connected with a linear ulcer was demonstrated on the posterior wall of the gastric angle. This was easily diagnosed as a deep ulceration.

Mucosal folds were markedly convergent and interrupted at the edge of the niche both in the double-contrast and compression studies (Figs. 95 c, d). In the compression study, the ulcer floor looked granular and uneven. The clearly bordered niche indicated it to be a deep ulceration, whose floor was changed by the adjacent organs or adherent to them. Therefore, this lesion could be diagnosed as a penetrating ulcer. The photograph taken by GTF-A (Fig. 95 e) revealed a deep niche at the angle, surrounded by a linear-shaped, reddened, concave mucosa. This could easily be diagnosed as a deep ulceration, not a penetrating ulcer.

This lesion could be diagnosed endoscopically as a short, linear ulcer with an irregular, deep ulceration. Careful attention must be paid to the endoscopic differential diagnosis between depressions of the type II c early cancer and ulcer scars. The gross specimen (Fig. 95 f) showed the lesion to be a linear ulcer whose central circular region was adherent to the omentum major.

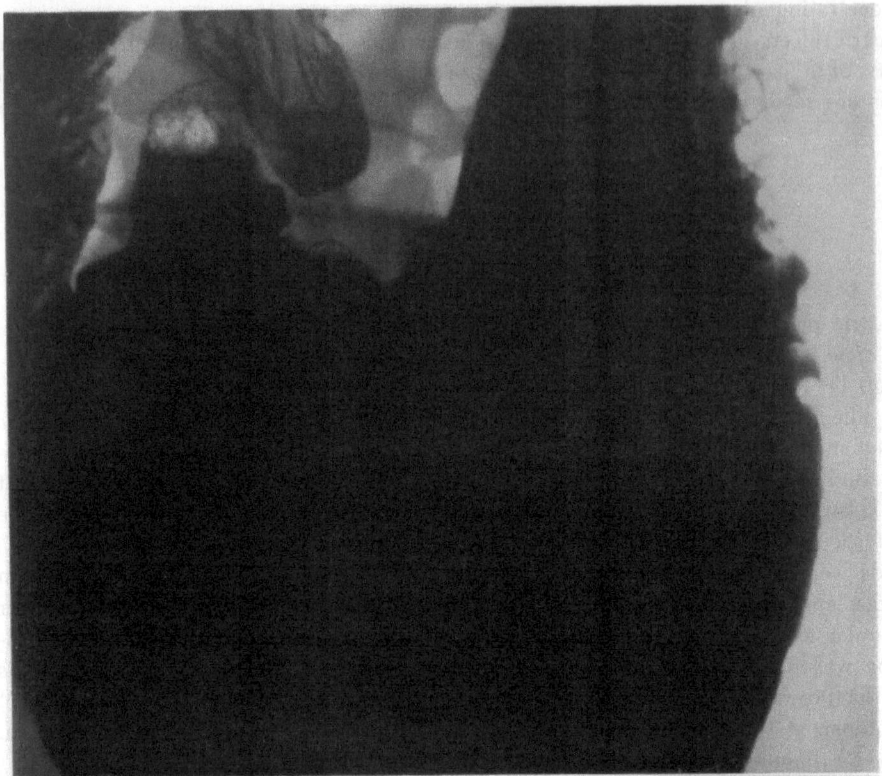

95 a

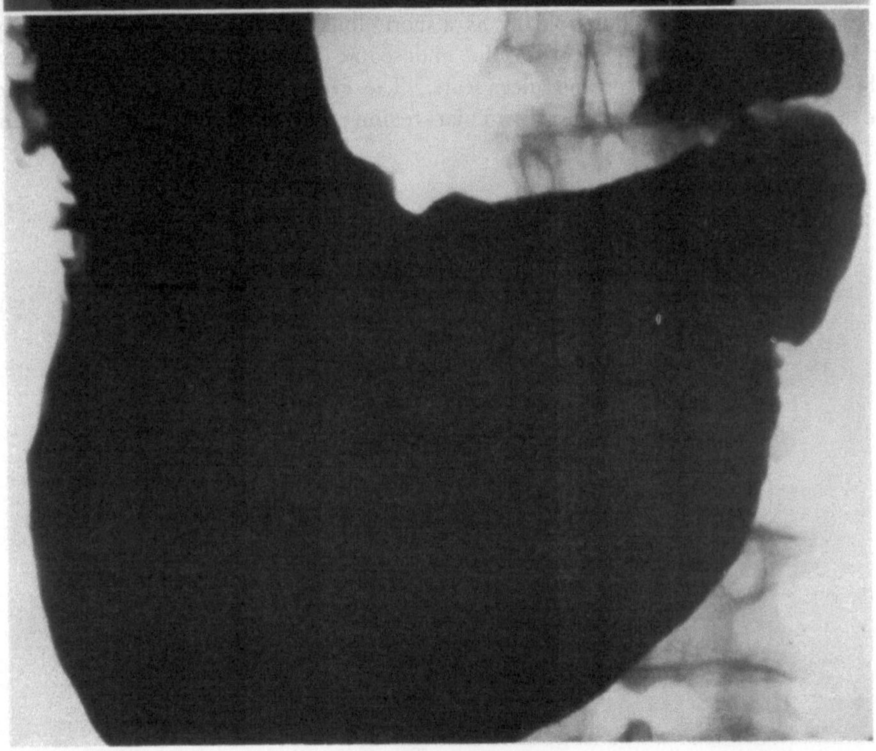

95 b

Figs. 95 a and b Barium filled studies in the upright and prone positions. The angular niche is fairly well demonstrated. Shortening of the lesser curvature and a stenotic pylorus are demonstrated.

95 c

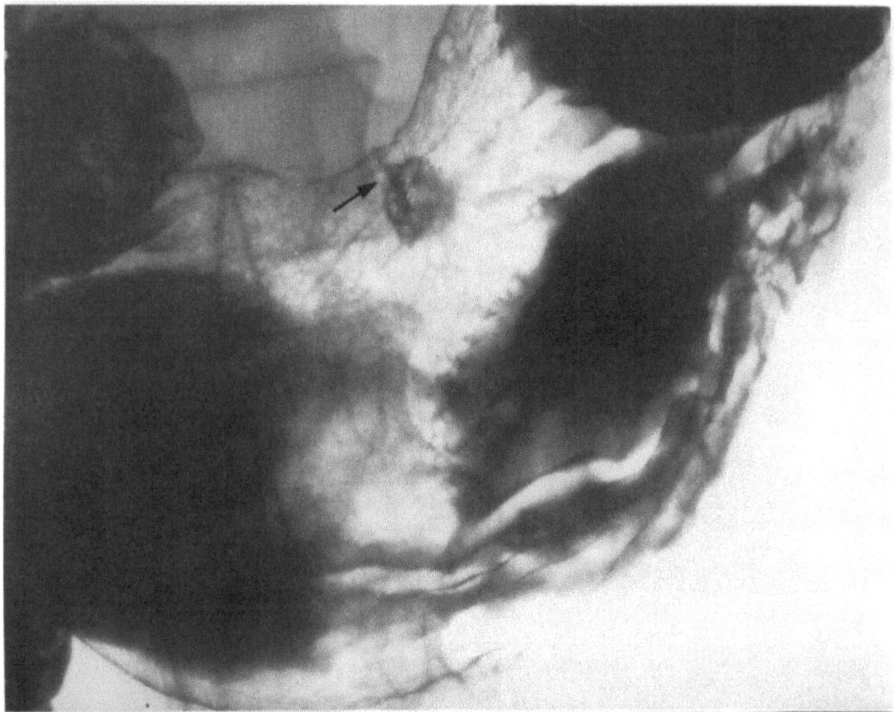

95 d

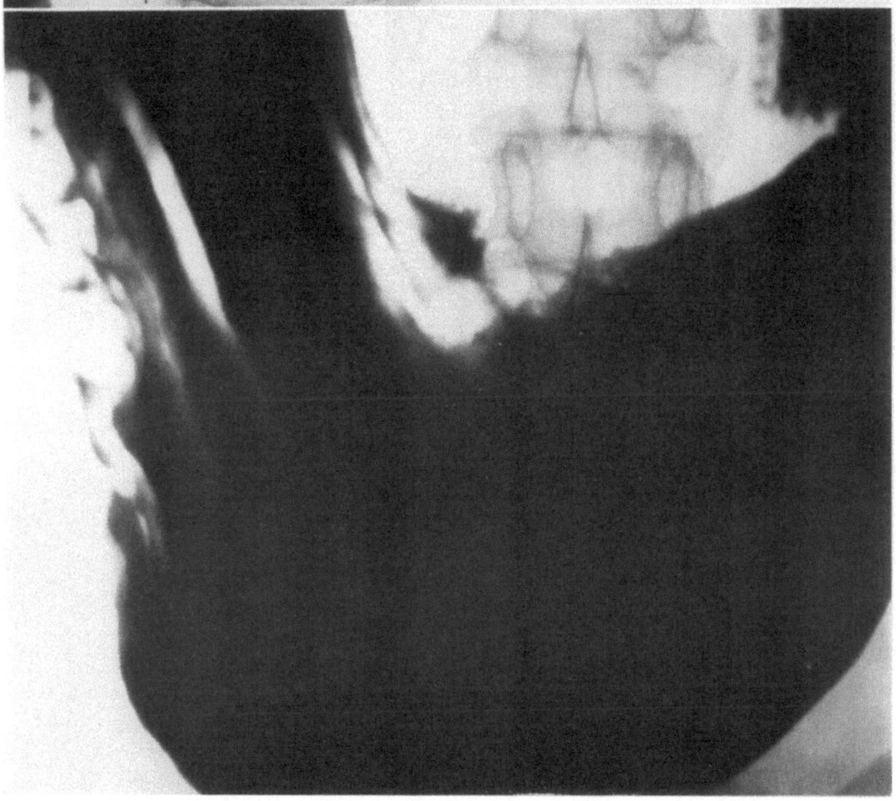

Fig. 95 c Double-contrast study. A linear niche (arrow) from the round niche to the lesser curvature is observed on the gastric angle.

Fig. 95 d Compression study in the prone position. The irregular, uneven floor of the niche indicates penetration.

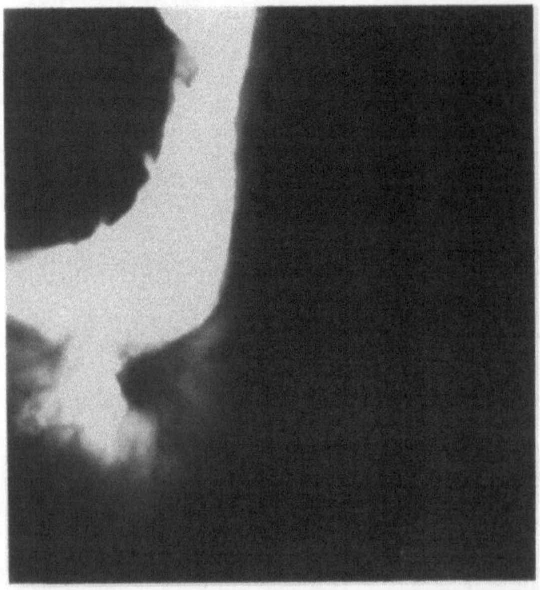

95e

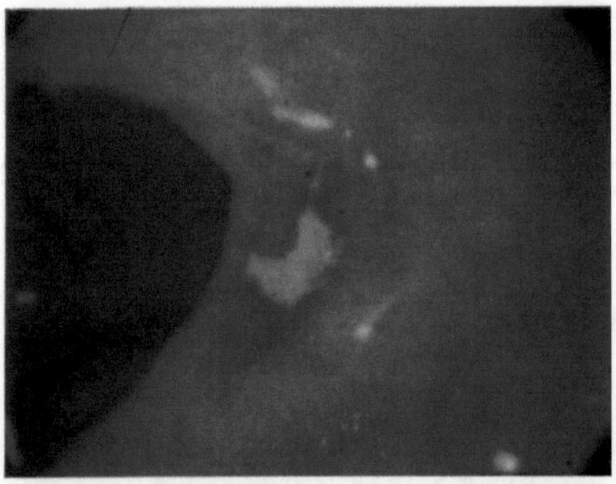

95f

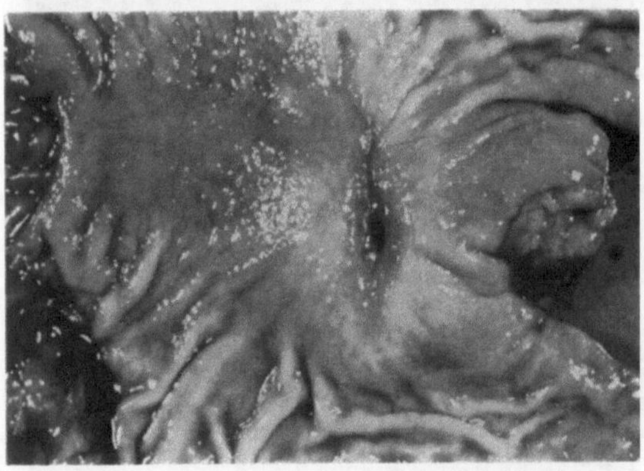

95g

Fig. 95e Compression study in the upright position.

Fig. 95f Endoscopic picture. A deep ulcer with associated linear reddening is seen.

Fig. 95g Resected stomach. A short linear ulcer-scar connecting with a round ulcer is seen. The central part of the ulcer was adherent to the omentum major. Histopathologically, the ulceration reached the serosal layer (Ul-IV).

3) Multiple gastric ulcer

For an accurate diagnosis of multiple lesions in the stomach, it must be emphasized that careful attention should be paid to the entire stomach, not only to the region in which conspicuous lesions are found. SHIRAKABE and KUMAKURA have reported that multiple gastric ulcers show deformities of the gastric wall radiologically. Their main characteristics are as follows:

1) Hourglass deformity or indentation on the greater curvature of the body
2) Accessory pocket-like distension of the lesser curvature of the body
3) Straightening of the lesser curvature
4) Widening of the gastric angle
5) Shortening of the distance from the gastric angle to the pyloric ring.

These criteria are useful in diagnosing multiple ulcers and gastrofiberscopy has great value in confirming multiple lesions.

Case 30

c. c.: Nausea, vomitting, and epigastric pain.

49 year-old male.

The barium filled stomach in the prone position (Fig. 96 a) fortunately showed the lesion with compression of the abdominal wall. In this radiograph, multiple niches were recognized, one on the gastric angle and the other on the lesser curvature of the antrum. Note the angular smooth widening and shortening of the distance from the gastric angle to the pyloric ring.

In the double-contrast studies (Figs. 96 b, c), kissing ulcers on the angle and the other niche on the pyloric side of the lesser curvature were demonstrated. Multifocal convergence of mucosal folds were seen in this picture. Widening of the gastric angle and pyloric dislocation with a bulbar deformity were also demonstrated in this picture. The compression study of the duodenal cap revealed a round ulcer with convergence of the duodenal mucosal folds (Fig. 96 e). The compression study of the antrum (Fig. 96 d) revealed a shallow ulcer with markedly converging folds, but it was more difficult to demonstrate lesions separately because these ulcers were located close to each other.

Generally speaking, when we find one niche, it is important to pay careful attention to the possible discovery of multiple deformities such as those mentioned above. Supplementally, endoscopy is highly effective in diagnosing multiple lesions. A gross inspection of the surgical specimen (Fig. 96 f) revealed multiple gastroduodenal ulcers including ulcer scars.

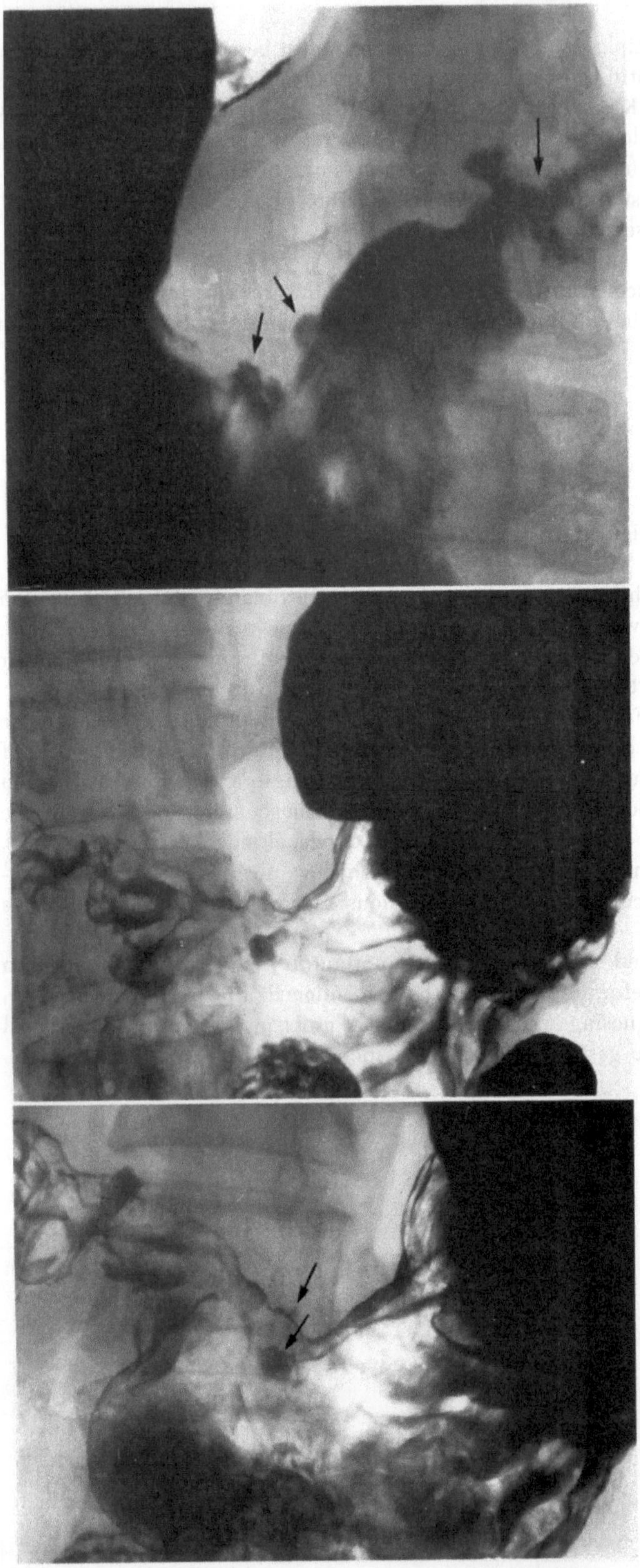

Fig. 96 a Radiograph of the barium filled stomach in the prone position. Angular and antral multiple niches and a bulbar deformation are demonstrated.

Fig. 96 b Double-contrast study.

Fig. 96 c Double-contrast study (fist oblique position). There are two niches on the gastric angle. One is circular in shape while the other is seen on the lesser curvature.

96 d

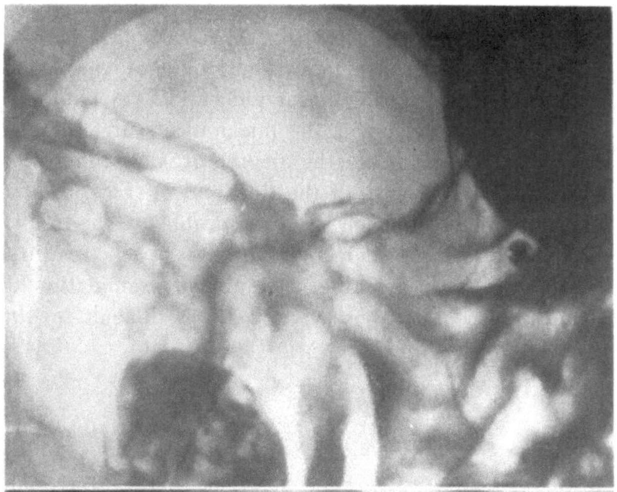

96 e

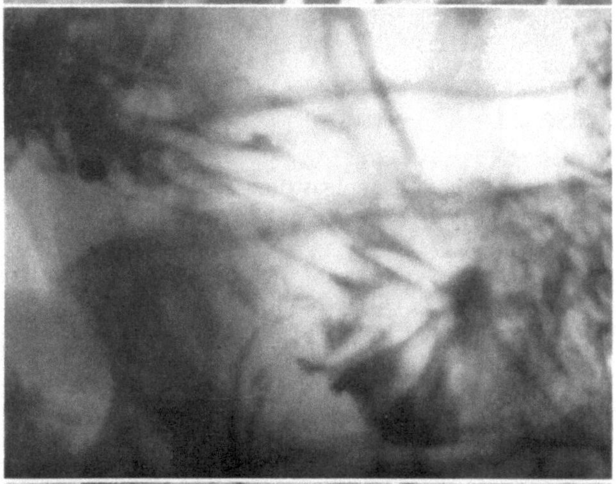

96 f

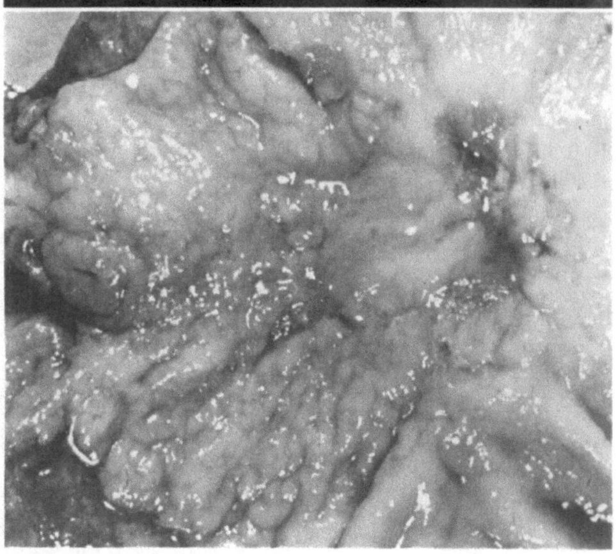

Fig. 96 d Compression study of the pyloric region. It is difficult to differentiate this mucosal convergency with a shallow depression on the lesser curvature of the antrum from a type IIc early cancer.

Fig. 96 e Compression study of the duodenal cap. A duodenal ulcer with markedly converging folds is seen.

Fig. 96 f Resected stomach.

4) Linear ulcer

It has been established that MURAKAMI first recognized that linear ulcers in the stomach are represented by a conspicuous shortening of the lesser curvature, and that SHIRAKABE first succeeded in demonstrating linear niches in x-ray photographs by using the double-contrast method.

Ordinarily the longer the linear ulcers are, the shorter the distance between the ulcer and the pylorus. Therefore, the degree of shortening of the lesser curvature and gastric deformity is varied by the length of the linear ulcer (Figs. 97 a, b). Cases in which marked shortening and deformity of the stomach are recognizable are the results of long linear ulcers, while cases in which there are only mild shortenings of the lesser curvature are due to the presence of shorter linear ulcers. Generally speaking, a combined examination by x-ray and gastrofiberscopy has increased diagnostic accuracy, however, it still is difficult to obtain direct findings of linear ulcers endoscopically.

Case 31

c. c.: Dull pain in the epigastrium for several years.

48 year-old male.

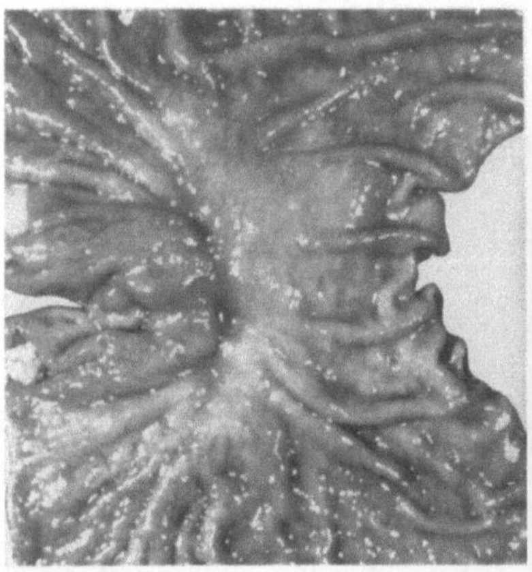

97 a

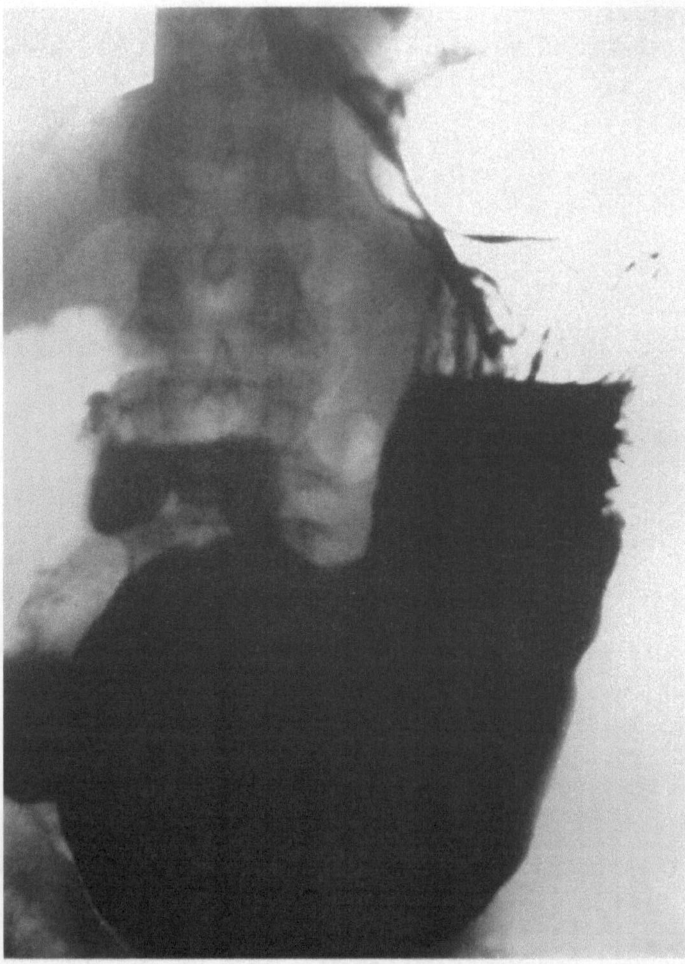

97 b

Fig. 97 a Resected stomach. A long linear ulcer is observed.

Fig. 97 b Barium filled stomach in the upright position. Marked shortening of the lesser curvature is demonstrated.

Case 32

c.c.: A sensation of fullness in the epigastrium and epigastrial pain for several months.
61 year-old male.

A small fingertip-sized niche was noticed at the gastric angle in the radiographs of the barium filled stomach (Figs. 98 a, b). A mild shortening of the lesser curvature and a marked indentation on the greater curvature of the antrum were also observed in both pictures. Therefore, the lesion was suspected of not being a simple ulcer, but a part of a linear ulcer or multiple ulcers.

The double-contrast studies (Figs. 98 d, e) showing a linear ulcer of the gastric angle and a barium filled niche were only a part of this linear ulcer. It should be mentioned that the appearance of the niche was variable depending on the amount of insufflated air. In this case, the mucosal (Fig. 98 c) and compression studies (Fig. 98 f) did not demonstrate this linear ulcer adequately.

The endoscopic picture (Fig. 98 g) showed a bamboo-leaf-shaped, long ulcer which extended over the posterior and anterior wall on the lesser curvature of the angular region. The linear ulcer was relatively broad and moderate in length and endoscopically easily diagnosed as a linear ulcer. In general, endoscopic diagnoses of linear ulcers are rather difficult. Linearshaped mucosal reddening and an echelon-shaped deformity at the angle often indicate the existence of linear ulcers.

The surgical specimen (Fig. 98 h) revealed a linear ulcer of the gastric angle measuring 3.5 cm in length.

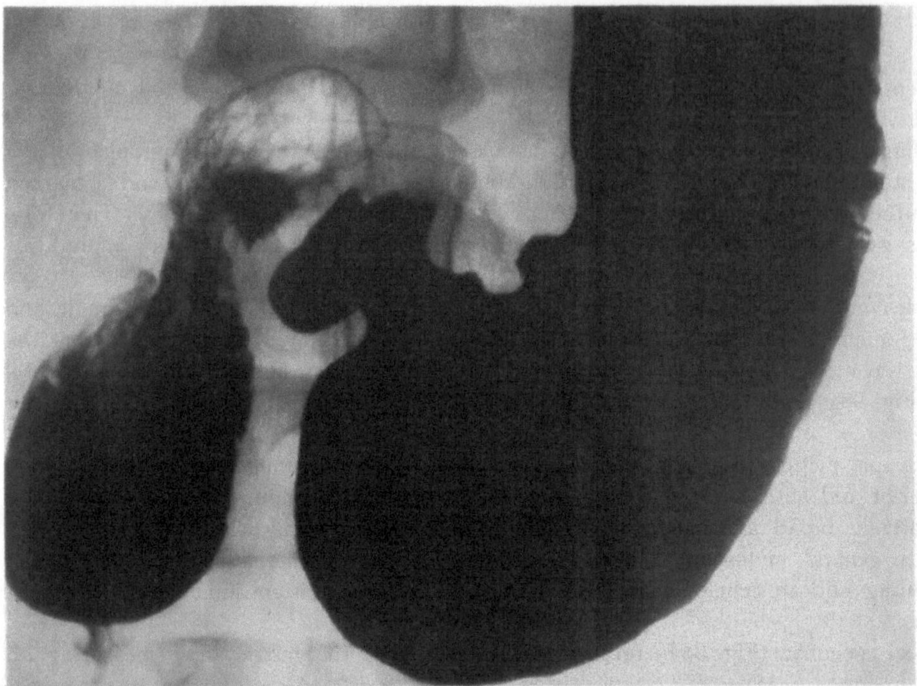

98 a

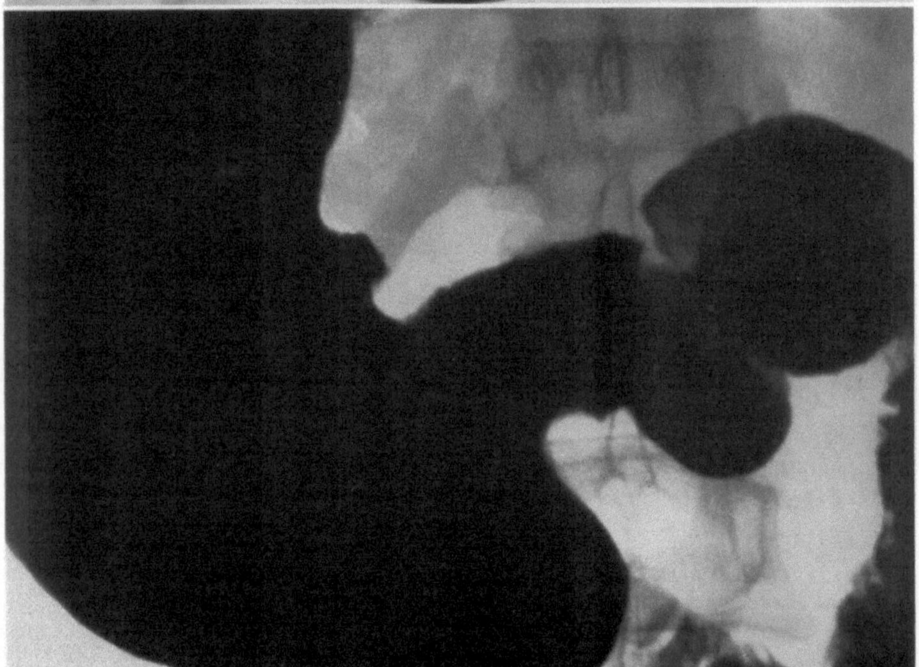

98 b

Figs. 98 a and b Barium filled stomachs in the upright and prone positions. Note the angular niche on the depressed wall due to an edematous swelling. A slight shortening of the lesser curvature and a marked indentation on the greater curvature on the antrum are seen.

98 c

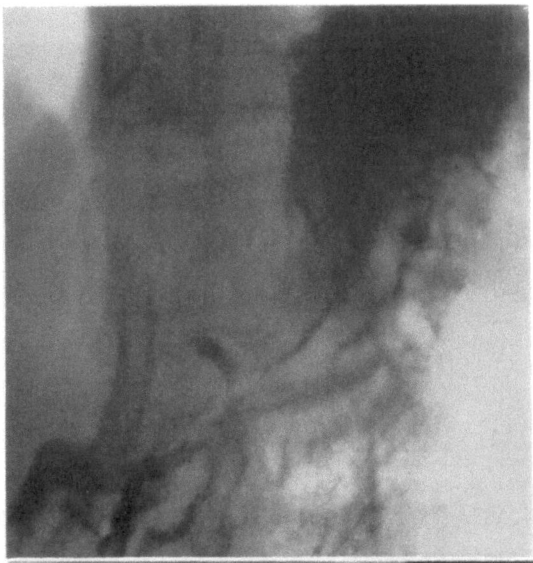

98 d

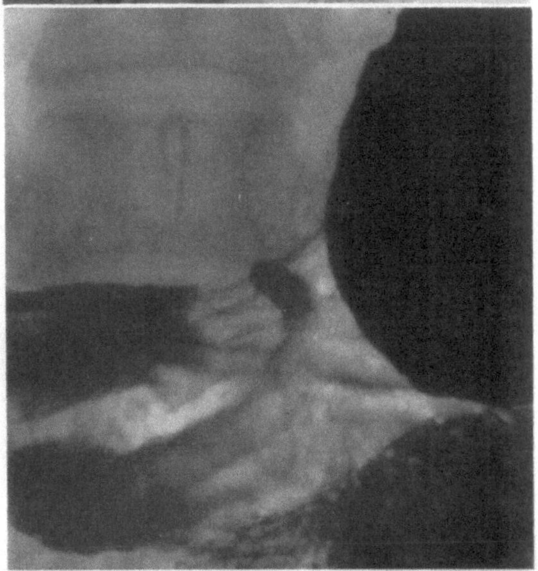

98 e

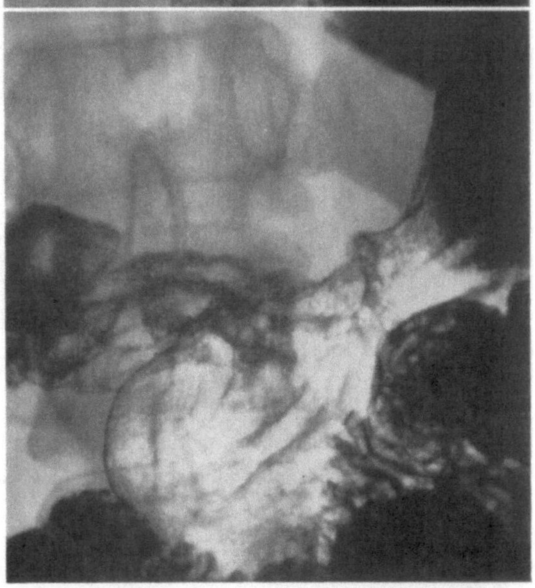

Fig. 98 c Mucosal study. A deep niche at the gastric angle with a marked convergence of the mucosal folds is clearly observable.

Fig. 98 d Double-contrast study in the supine position. A linear ulcer is clearly demonstrated.

Fig. 98 e Double-contrast study in the first oblique, supine position.

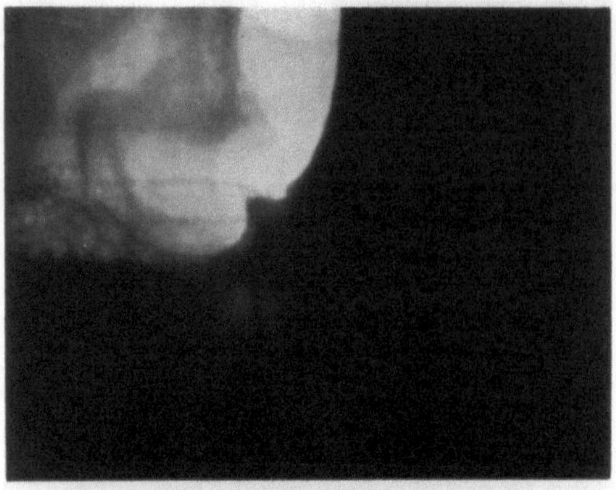

98 f

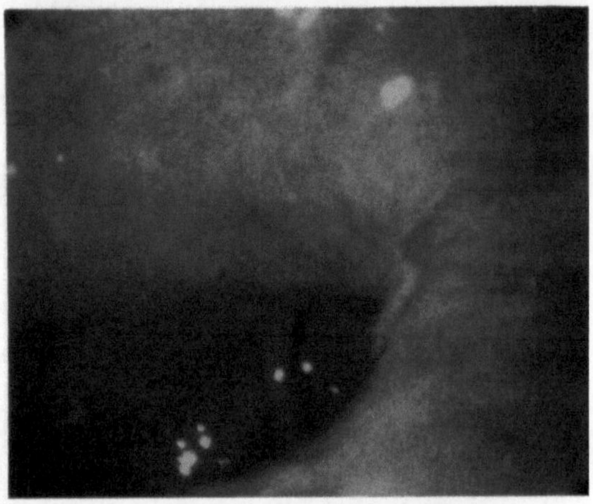

98 g

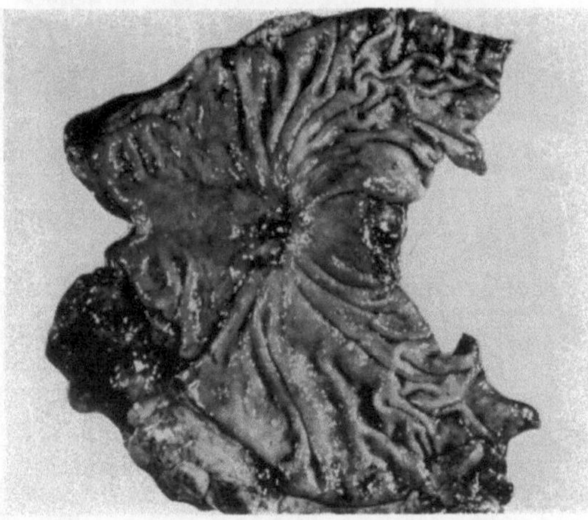

98 h

Fig. 98 f Compression study.

Fig. 98 g Endoscopic picture. A linear ulcer is clearly demonstrated.

Fig. 98 h Resected stomach. Relatively short linear ulcers are seen at the gastric angle.

c. Ulcer scar (Scarring ulcer)

When the healing tendency of gastric ulcers is dominant, a thin layer of mucosal cells grows across the defect (^{2}Ul), gradually transforming into a columnar regenerating epithelium, although the scarring area is slightly depressed compared with the surrounding normal mucosa (^{3}Ul), and finally becomes normal mucosa (^{4}Ul) as the ulcer heals.

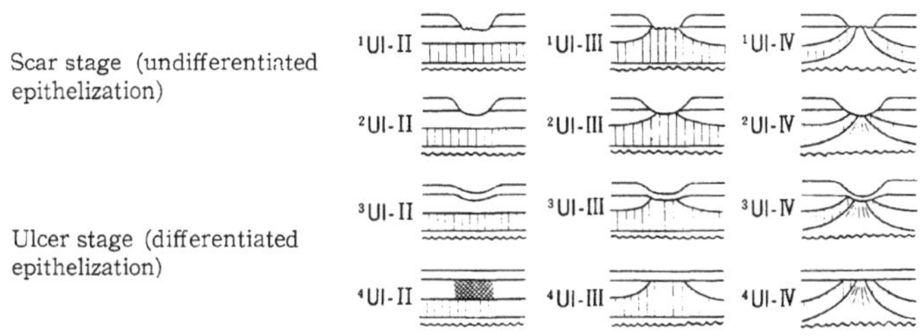

If the discovered ulcer is acute and if it heals promptly, there may be almost no scarring, so an undetectable ulcer scar may be present macroscopically.

Macroscopic characteristics of ulcer scars are classified according to the radiating folds, abnormal granulation or uneveness of the floor, and endoscopic discoloration.

Case 33

c.c.: Epigastric fullness and eructation.

46 year-old female.

The barium filled stomach in the upright position revealed a marked deformity of the entire stomach. Incisura formation on the greater curvature of the lower gastric body and an irregularity of the gastric wall on the confronting lesser curvature were most impressive (Fig. 99 a).

With serial double-contrast studies, these lesions were clearly demonstrated. In the double-contrast study with a small amount of barium and air (Fig. 99 c), only one or two lesions could be demonstrated with difficulty. Medium or full amounts of air in the double-contrast studies (Figs. 99 b, d) revealed the details of this lesion. On the greater curvature side in these pictures, three lesions with converging folds could be distinguished and recognized as multiple ulcer scars. Another lesion with a fine mucosal convergence was demonstrated on the lesser curvature, and the coverging folds with a reticular mucosal surface indicated the mechanism of the narrowing of the gastric lumen.

A serial double-contrast examination is an indispensable method for the determination of gastric ulcer scars roentgenologically. But, on the other hand, a supplemental endoscopic examination is desirable. The photograph by GTF-A (Fig. 99 e) showed a reddish, discolored depression with converging folds on the posterior wall. On the floor of this depression, there was no ulcer coating and no marked uneveness. These endoscopic findings were diagnosed as ulcer scars. It is essential to know the differences in endoscopic features of ulcer scars and the type IIc early cancer. The histological findings of the resected specimen (Fig. 99 f) demonstrated a long linear ulcer-scar with multiple ulcer scars on both the anterior and posterior walls (Fig. 99 g).

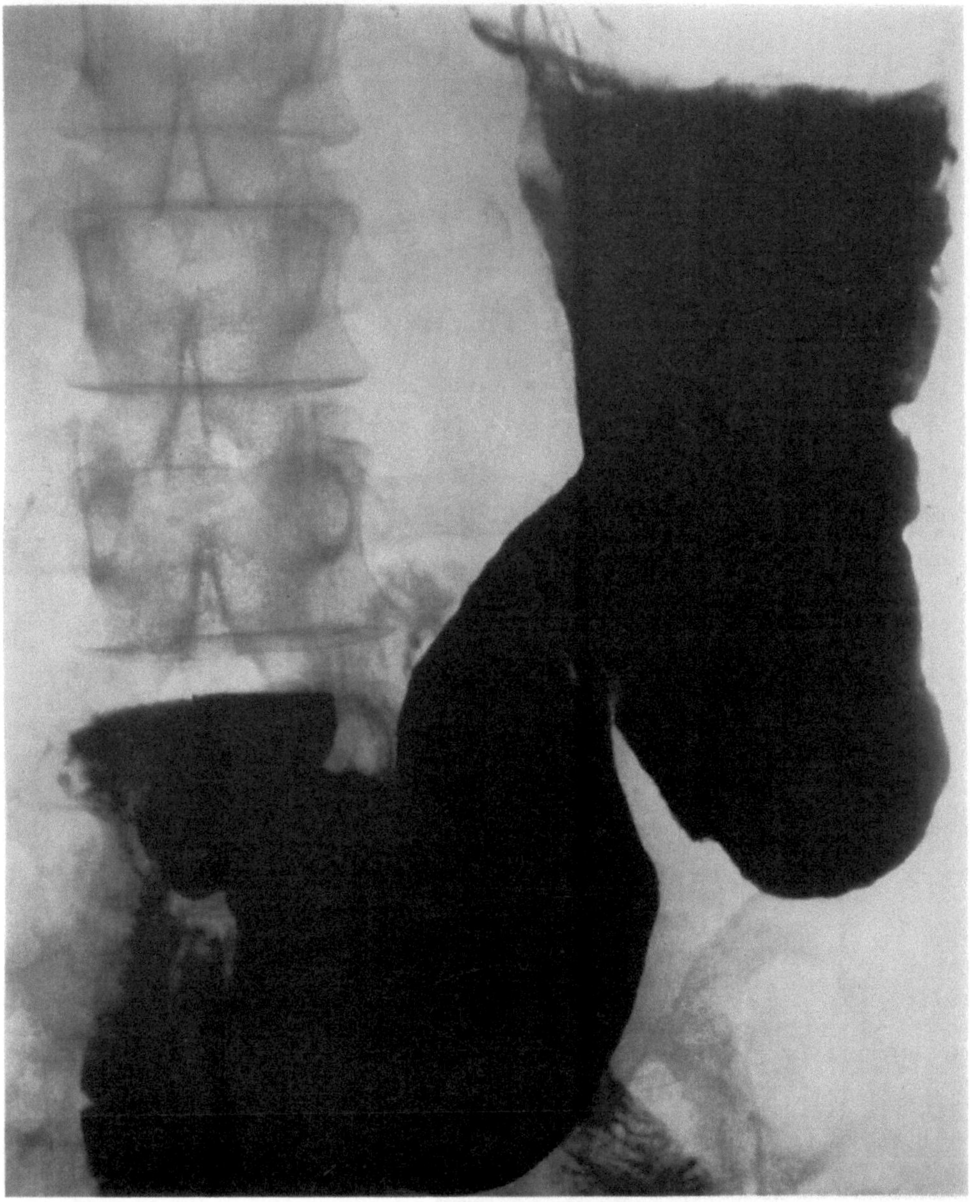

Fig. 99 a Barium filled stomach in the upright position. A typical hour-glass stomach is demonstrated.

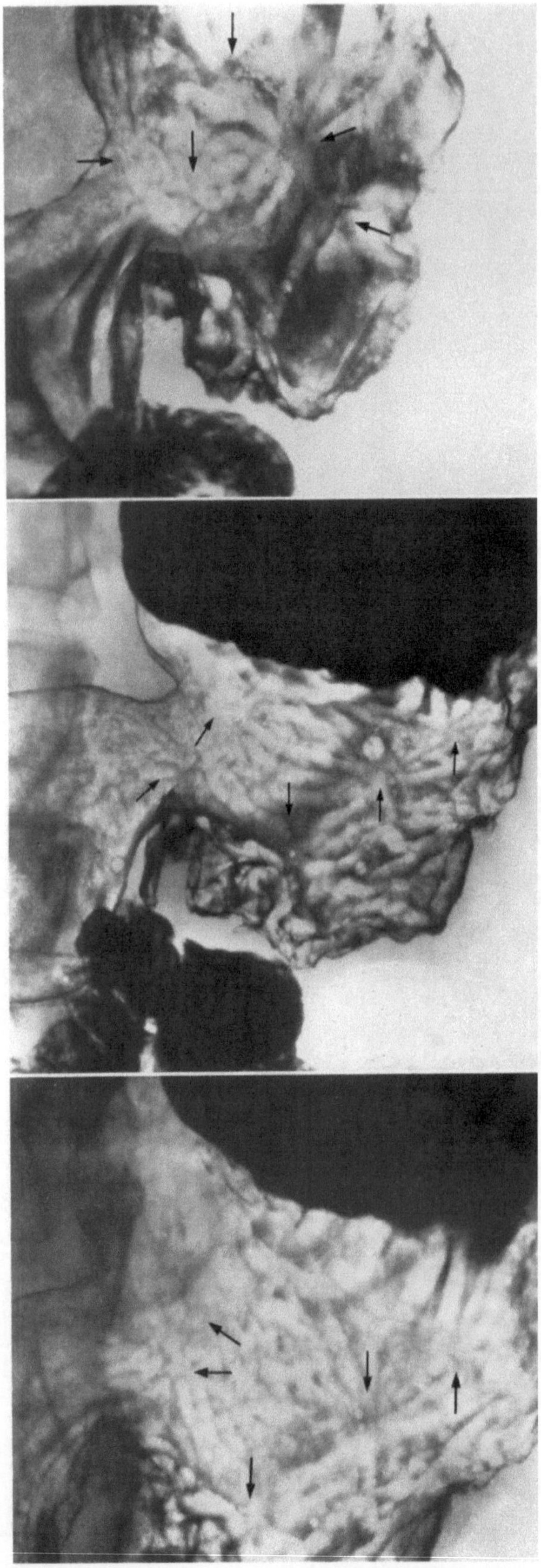

99b

99c

99d

Figs. 99b, c, and d Serial double-contrast studies. Multiple ulcer scars with radiating folds are clearly seen.

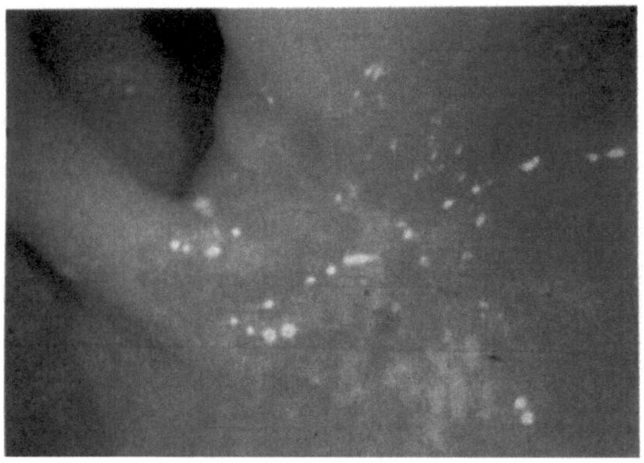

99e

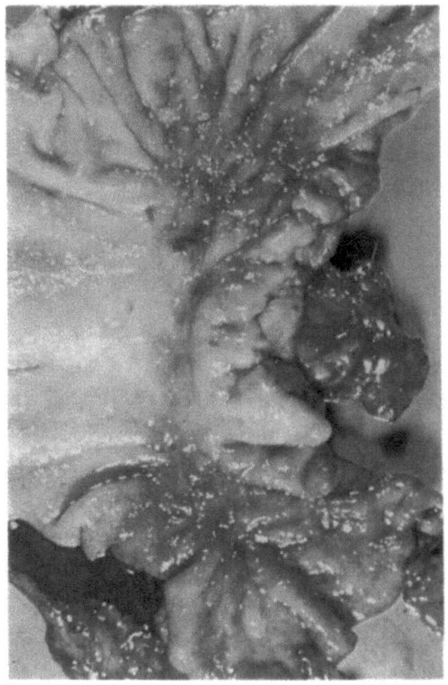

99f

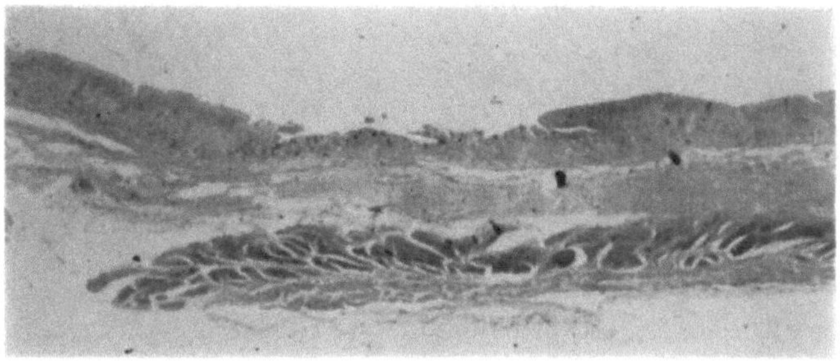

99g

Fig. 99e Endoscopic picture.

Fig. 99f Resected stomach.

Fig. 99g Histopathological findings. Histologically, the lesion was diagnosed as a partially lineally shaped ulcer scar.

4. Erosion of the stomach

Erosions are defined as defects of the gastric wall which are limited only to the mucosal layer histopathologically. The recent development of endoscopic examination of the stomach enables the diagnosis of minor gastric erosions. It is known that there are two types of gastric erosion, the so-called punctiform and varioliform (WALK). The authors divided the gastric erosions into two main groups:

1) Flat erosion: This type of gastric erosion is a simple, defective lesion of the mucosal layer.
2) Erosive gastritis: A defect of the mucosal layer surrounded by edematous (immature type) or fibrous (mature type) mucosal elevations.

The layer of the gastric membrane is 1–2 mm thick. There is a very shallow erosion which may not be detected by x-ray or macroscopic examinations.

Erosions which may easily be detected by means of x-ray or macroscopic examinations are:

1) erosions which are large and relatively deep
2) erosions with protuberant surrounding membranes
3) erosions with flash or discoloration

Consequently, it can be said that erosions which may be clinically diagnosed are very limited. It must be remembered that it is difficult in some cases to differentiate erosions from flat peptic ulcers or cancerous erosions.

a. Flat erosion

It is very likely that flat-surfaced erosions exist independently in most cases. Macroscopically or on x-ray film, they appear similar to the superficial excavated type of early cancer.

Case 34

c.c.: Distress in the epigastrium for two months.

62 year-old female.

This lesion escaped fluoroscopy, although it left imprints on the radiograph. The barium-filled stomach in the prone position (Fig. 100 a) revealed no evidence of abnormalities on either the lesser curvature or the greater curvature of the stomach contour. The double-contrast study in the first oblique position (Fig. 100 b), with no interference from the spinal shadow, revealed two portions with faint barium flecks. A granular, uneven surface of the surrounding mucosa was also noted. These findings were suspected roentgenologically to be erosions or shallow ulcers. The endoscopic finding (Fig. 100 c) showed reddened and slightly whitish discoloration in the central area above the angular region. The lesion was recognized as a flat erosion endoscopically, but it was difficult to differentiate this lesion from a small lesion of the type IIc early cancer. Malignancy was not demonstrated on gastric biospy, but gastrectomy was performed at the request of the patient. The gross specimen exhibited flat erosions which were very difficult to detect macroscopically (Fig. 100 d). Histologically, this lesion proved to be benign erosions (Fig. 100 e).

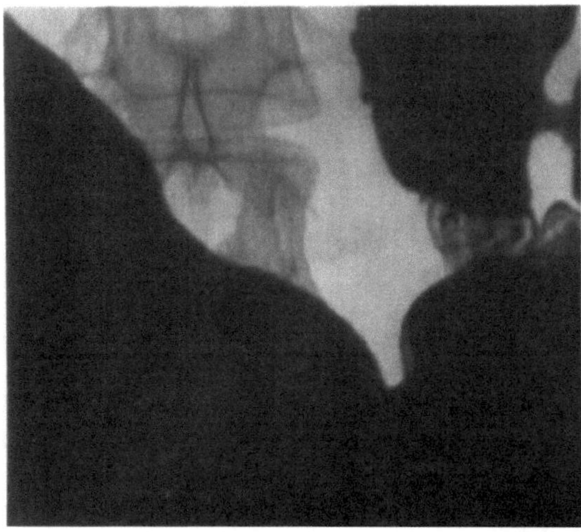

100 a

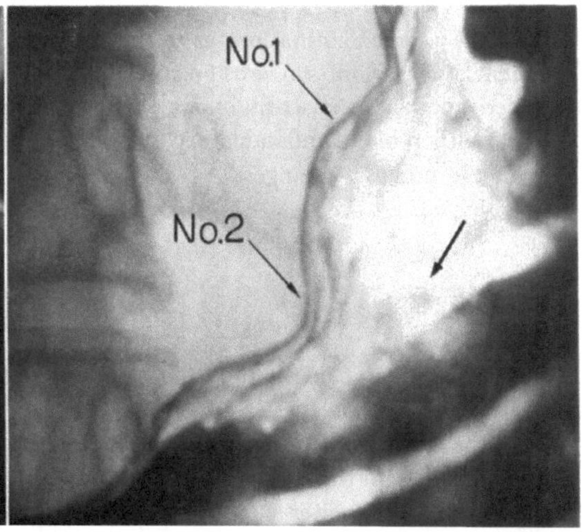

100 b

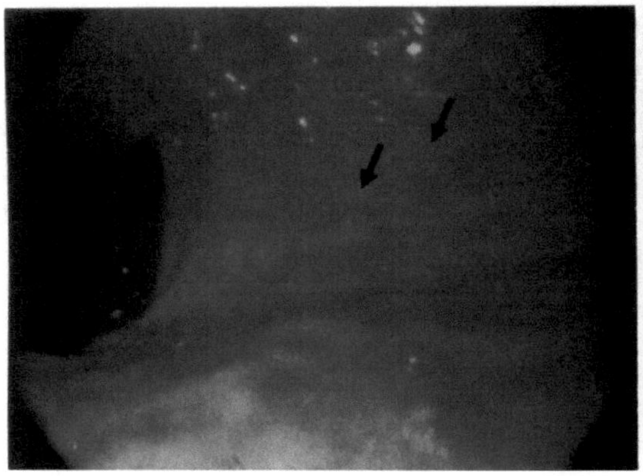

100 c

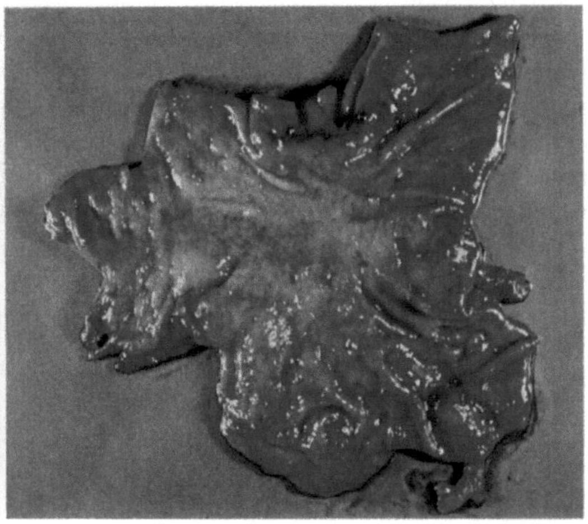

100 d

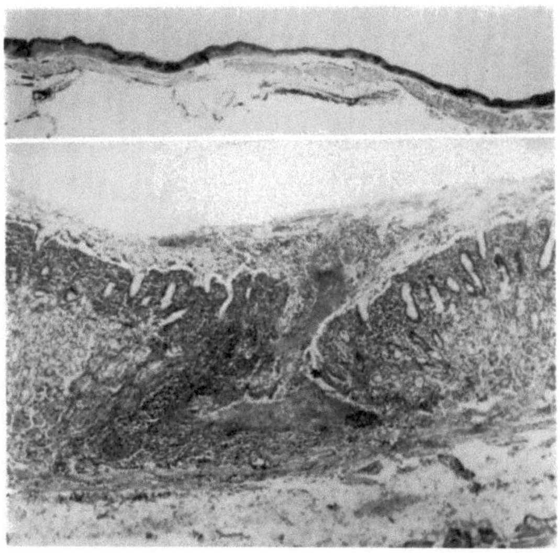

100 e

Fig. 100 a Barium filled stomach in the prone position. The barium filled stomach shows no abnormal contour.

Fig. 100 b Double-contrast study. In the disignated (arrow) region, reticular barium flecks are seen.

Fig. 100 c Endoscopic picture. Multiple reddened and discolored areas can be seen.

Fig. 100 d Resected stomach. Flat, hemorrhagic erosions are scattered from the antrum to the lower body.

Fig. 100 e Histopathological findings. Histologically, this lesion proved to be a flat-type erosion on the atrophic mucosa.

b. Erosive gastritis

In the x-ray examination, as in the microscopic examination of red blood cells in the urinary sediment, the varioliform erosion appears in the form of a filling defect with a central dot. It is called an erosive gastritis or a dellengastritis. A protuberance on the surrounding membrane consists either of an inflammatory swelling or hyperplasia of the foveolar epithelium with some irreversible mucosal changes.

Case 35

c.c.: Hunger pain in the epigastrium for a month.

31 year-old female.

In the barium filled stomach, there were no abnormalities except for a hyperspastic condition in the antrum. In the double-contrast study (Fig. 101 a), several varioliform erosions were demonstrated from the greater curvature to the lesser curvature in the prepyloric region. One of them was relatively large on the side of the lesser curvature, and the other was located just on the lesser curvature. Therefore, a part of this lesion was demonstrated as a marginal protrusion in the lateral view.

The endoscopic finding revealed multiple, arranged, localized mucosal swellings, and erosions which were located at the top of these protrusions (Fig. 101 b). This type of erosion is endoscopically called a varioliform or " erosive " gastritis. In the resected stomach, there were many erosions scattered on the surface of the antral region. The histological finding (Fig. 101 c) revealed an erosion, which reached into 2/3 of the depth of the mucosal layer and was surrounded by protrusions of the neighboring mucosa. A marginal protrusion of the erosion was recognized as a hyperplastic change of the foveolar epithelium. On the x-ray film, this protrusion was demonstrated as faint filling defects. There were many difficult problems regarding the pathogenetic correlation of this gastric erosion with other gastric diseases.

101 a

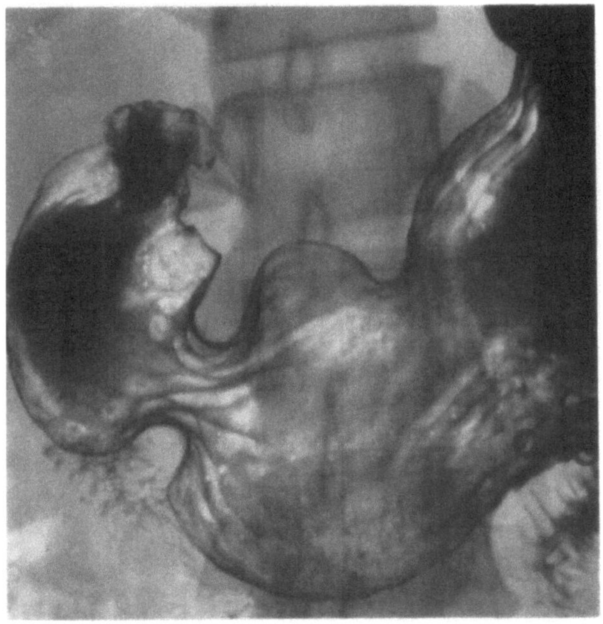

101 b

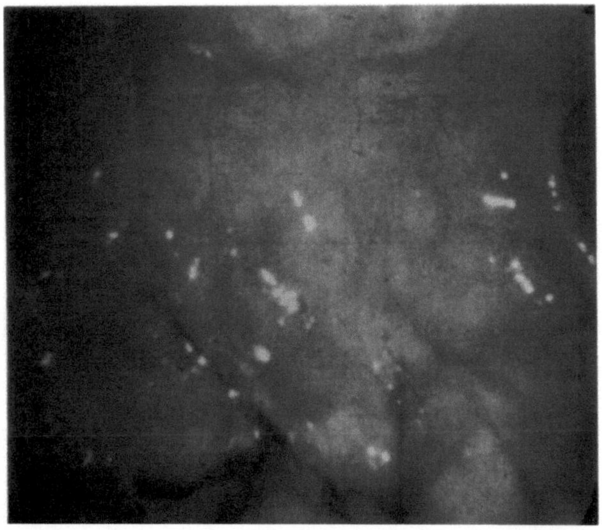

101 c

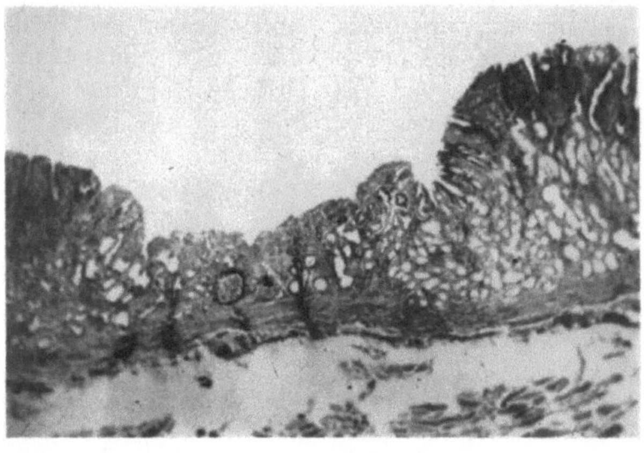

Fig. 101 a Double-contrast study. A small filling defect with a central dot is seen.
Fig. 101 b Endoscopic picture. Varioliform erosions are seen.
Fig. 101 c Histopathological findings.

From our experience, we have found that an erosion is first produced in the form of a flat-surfaced erosion, changes into a varioliform erosion because of a delay in treatment, and then further develops into gastric polyps (Fig. 102).

The dotted line in Figure 102 denotes cases suspected of cancerous change during the course of treatment.

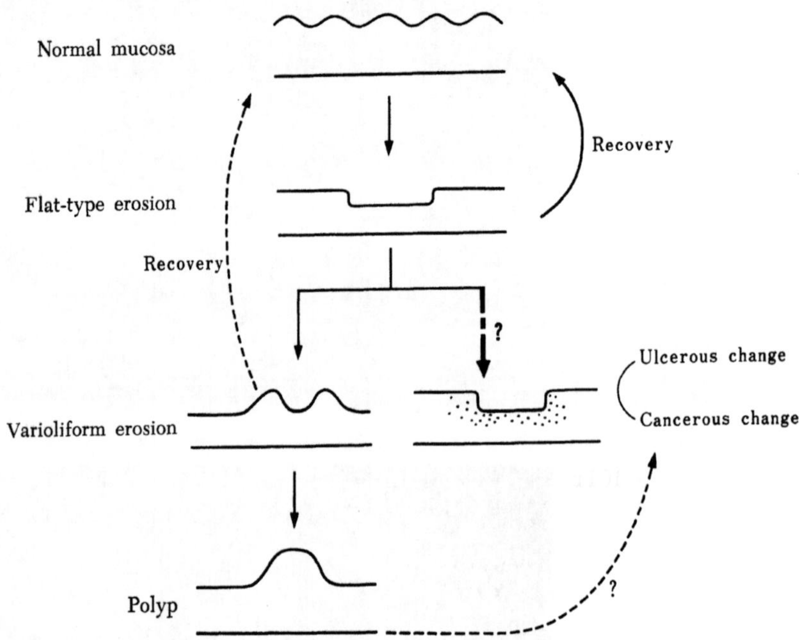

Fig. 102 Fate of erosion.

B. Indistinguishable cases

We have discussed how to make differential diagnoses of typical depressed lesions of the stomach. However, actual cases which cannot always be differentiated easily according to their proper type are frequently encountered. The reasons for this difficulty are considered chiefly as: small lesions; flat, unrestricted depressions without cicatricial deformities; and the location of the lesion. There are few problems in obtaining correct diagnoses, so a habit must be formed of reading x-ray and gastrofiberscopic evidence in accordance with the basics of x-ray and endoscopic examinations.

1. Small size type IIc early gastric cancer

Case 36

c.c.: Dull pain in the epigastrium.

32 year-old female.

In the first x-ray examination, only the scarring ulcer of the gastric angle was detected, and a small IIc of the greater curvature was overlooked. Figures 103 a and b show the x-ray photographs of the first examination. No particular alteration was noted except a slightly uneven surface of the gastric angle.

Three months after the first examination, the patient received an x-ray and endoscopic re-examination due to the lack of relief from her complaints. The second x-ray examination (Figs. 103 e–i) was successful in demonstrating the lesion on the greater curvature of the lower gastric body though this was accomplished with difficulty. In the double-contrast study in the supine position (Fig. 103 c), converging mucosal folds were revealed on the greater curvature. There seemed to be a lesion on the anterior wall. The double-air-contrast studies in the prone position (Figs. 103 d, e) clearly demonstrated a small IIc type early carcinoma on the greater curvature of the lower gastric body.

However, it was more clearly revealed in the compression studies (Figs. 103 f, g) as an irregularly shaped, superficial depression surrounded by interrupted folds and a granular mucosal protuberance. This lesion was easily diagnosed with this compressed picture as a small IIc type early carcinoma. Accordingly, it must be emphasized that compression studies should be used in combination with mucosal studies or double-contrast examinations to make correct diagnoses of lesions which are localized on the greater curvature, especially with minimal lesions.

On an endoscopic examination (Fig. 103 h), an irregularly shaped, superficial depression was demonstrated, and a fiberscopic biopsy revealed an adenocarcinoma mucocellulare (Fig. 103 c). A histopathological examination of the resected stomach (Fig. 103 j) revealed a small type II c early gastric carcinoma.

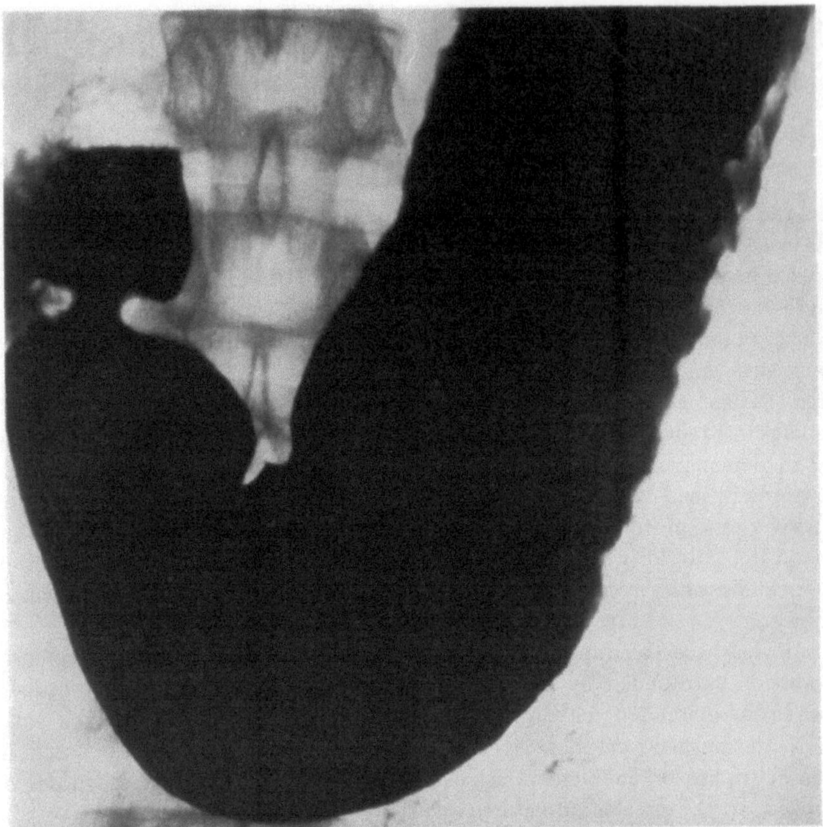

103a

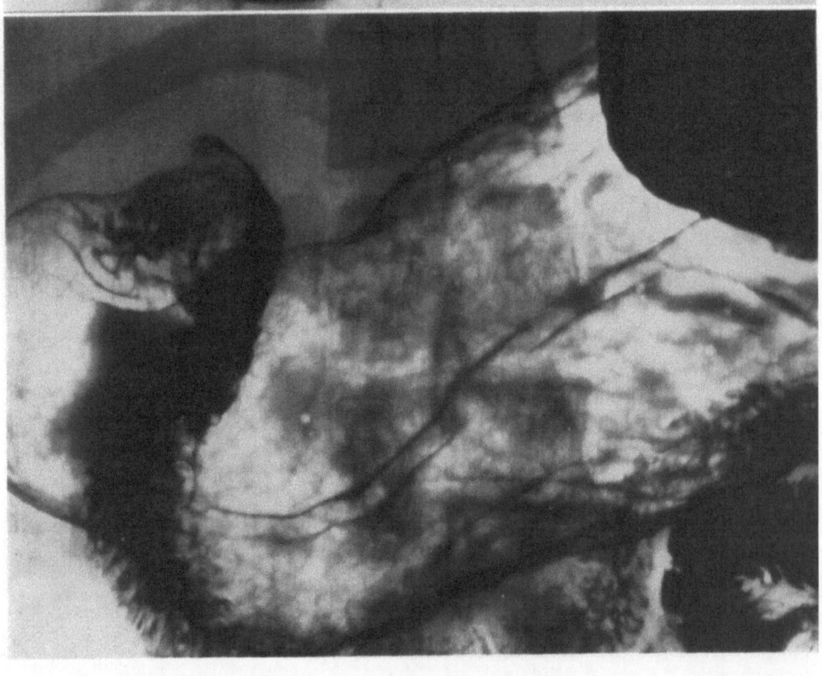

103b

Fig. 103a Barium filled stomach in the upright position. No particular changes are evident.

Fig. 103b Double-contrast study in the supine position. A localized mucosal uneveness on the gastric angle is seen and diagnosed as a scarring ulcer; however, a type IIc early cancer is overlooked on the greater curvature.

103c

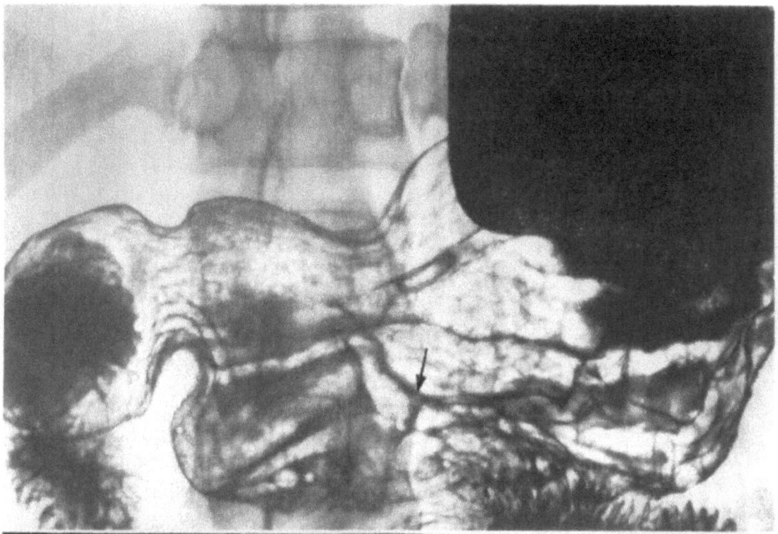

103d

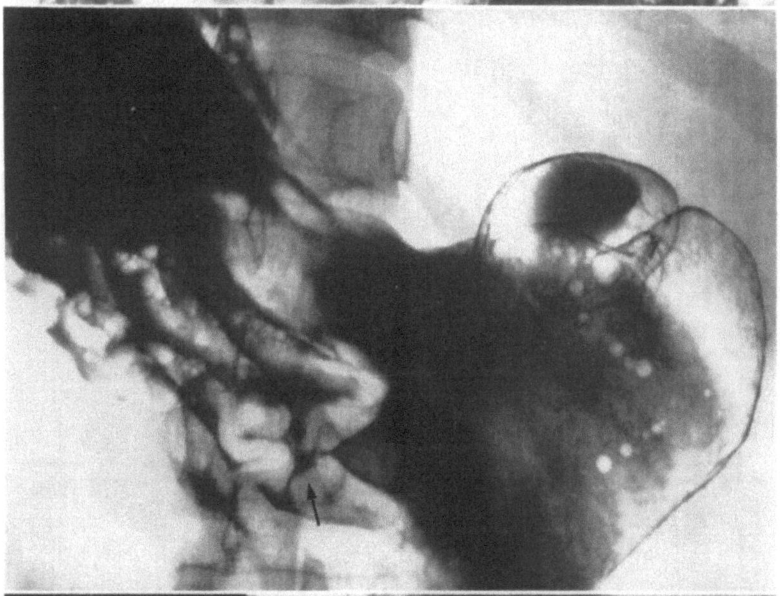

103e

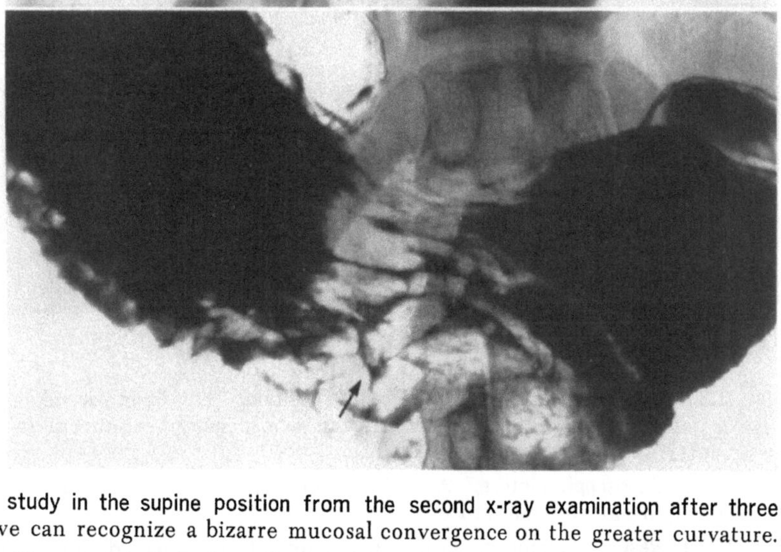

Fig. 103c Double-contrast study in the supine position from the second x-ray examination after three months. In this picture, we can recognize a bizarre mucosal convergence on the greater curvature.

Figs. 103d and e Prone double-contrast study from the second x-ray examination. A small, superficial depression with interrupted, thickened mucosal folds is revealed on the greater curvature. The contour of the depression is not clearly demonstrated.

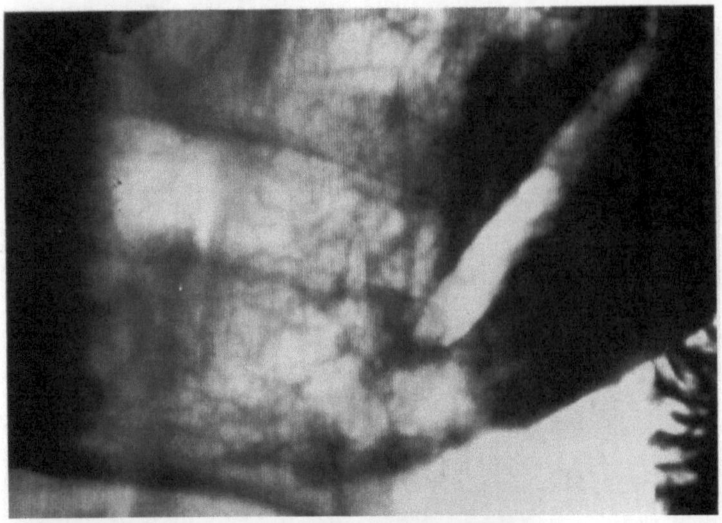

103 f

103 g

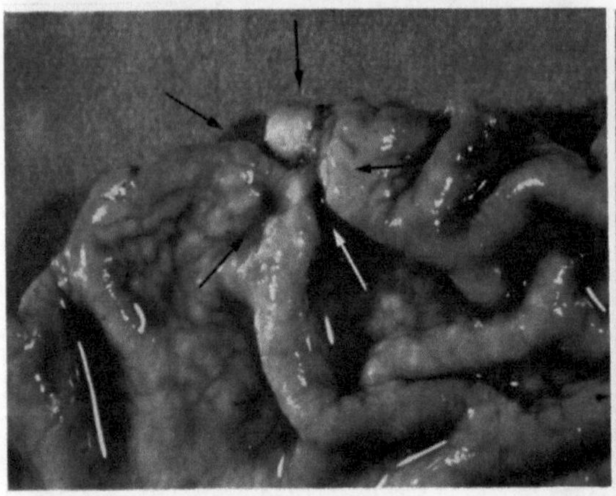

103 h

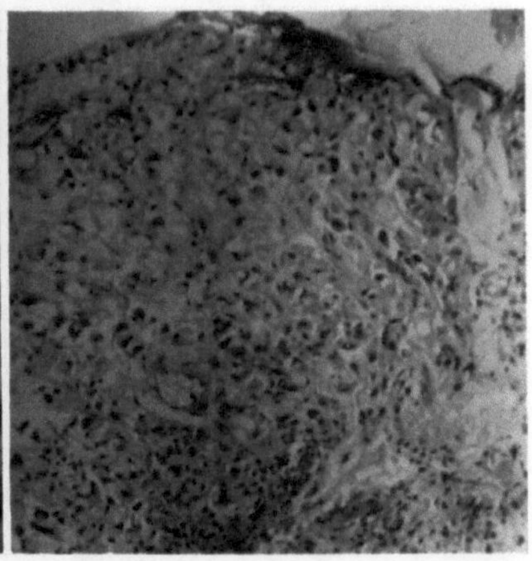

103 i

Fig. 103 f Compression study in the upright position. This picture taken under slight compression reveals an amoeba-like, shallow depression whose marginal mucosa is granular and elevated due to an interruption of the mucosal folds.

Fig. 103 g Endoscopic picture. A typical cancerous erosion with surrounding mucosal protuberance is seen on the greater curvature of the angle.

Fig. 103 h Resected stomach. Gross inspection of the resected stomach revealed a flat, sharply demarcated lesion measuring 0.7×0.8 cm in size (arrows). Histologically, it is an adenocarcinoma tubulare mucocellulare and invasion is limited to the mucosal layer.

Fig. 103 i Biopsic histology. Adenocarcinoma tubulare mucocellulare.

2. Indistinctly bordered, very shallow type IIc early carcinoma (IIb-like lesion)

Even in cases of the superficially excavated type (IIc), some are difficult to diagnose because of a blurred excavated border. In such cases, it is necessary to look for abnormal granular findings on the membrane and a moderate change in the mucosal folds. On the other hand, most cases of type IIc with blurred border are mucosal carcinomas. It is not easy to diagnose the depth of type IIc cancerous invasions.

The authors feel that the sharpness of the border and the protuberance of the mucosa in the excavated type IIc are helpful in the diagnosis of cancerous invasions. To be more exact, type IIc with blurred borders, lacking mucosal protuberances is cancers of the membrane in most instances. On the other hand, lesions with clear borders and diffuse protuberances surrounding the lesion are deep enough to reach the lower layer of the membrane (Table 3).

Table 3 Relationship between cancerous invasion and marginal protrusion in the IIc type gastric cancer

Invading stage		Type A protrusion	Type B protrusion
M	16	87.5 (%)	12.5 (%)
SM	18	28 〃	72 〃
PM↓	13	30 〃	70 〃

Relationship between cancerous invasion and sharpness of excavated border in the IIc type gastric cancer

Sharpness of the excavated border	M	SM	PM↓
indistinctly bordered	2	1	0
partly, distinctly bordered	7	5	2
distinctly bordered	7	12	11

Type A (rugal protrusion type)

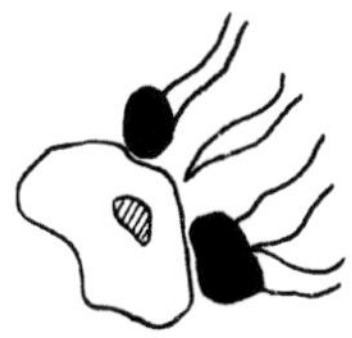

Type B (diffuse protrusion)

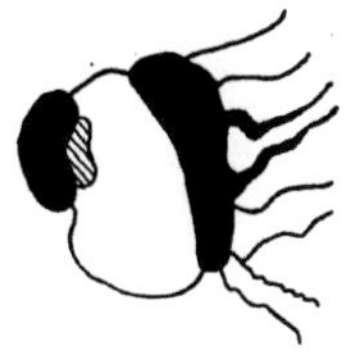

Case 37

c.c.: loss of appetite.

44 year-old female.

On the first routine x-ray examination, there were no particular abnormalities except a slight irregularity on the lesser curvature of the corpus (Fig. 104 a). The double-contrast study in the first x-ray examination taken by a beginner (Fig. 104 b) also demonstrated a slight distensibility of the lesser curvature, although the mucosal surface of the gastric wall was not observable. The patient underwent an endoscopic examination in which a gastrocamera with a fiberscope was used.

Photographs taken with the GTF-A (Figs. 104 c, d and e) demonstrated a wide-spreading lesion on the lesser curvature of the gastric corpus. The lesion was endoscopically recognizable chiefly as a discolored area with a bleeding spot in the central region, slightly depressed in part, but not sharply demarcated. Due to these endoscopic findings, the lesion was suspected as being a IIc type early cancer. However, it was difficult to differentiate this lesion from benign lesions.

The results of a supplemental second x-ray examination are shown in Figures 104 f, g and h. The double-air-contrast study in the supine and first oblique positions revealed a coarse, reticular-surfaced, depressed lesion surrounded by numerous radiating folds on the posterior wall of the corpus. The lesion measured 7.0×4.0 cm in size. In the compression studies (Figs. 104 i, j), two flat ulcerations could be seen in the uneven, reticular area. The lesion was diagnosed radiologically as a widespread, slightly depressed type of a IIc early carcinoma and was confirmed by a biopsy examination as an adenocarcinoma tubulare (Fig. 104 k). Macroscopically (Fig. 104 l), there were two, flat ulcerations and their surrounding mucosal surface was uneven and slightly depressed.

According to the histopathological examination, the lesion proved to be a mucosal adenocarcinoma, and it spread widely as shown by the arrow (Figs. 104 m, n). Correct diagnoses require the use of biopsy techniques or cytological examination.

104a

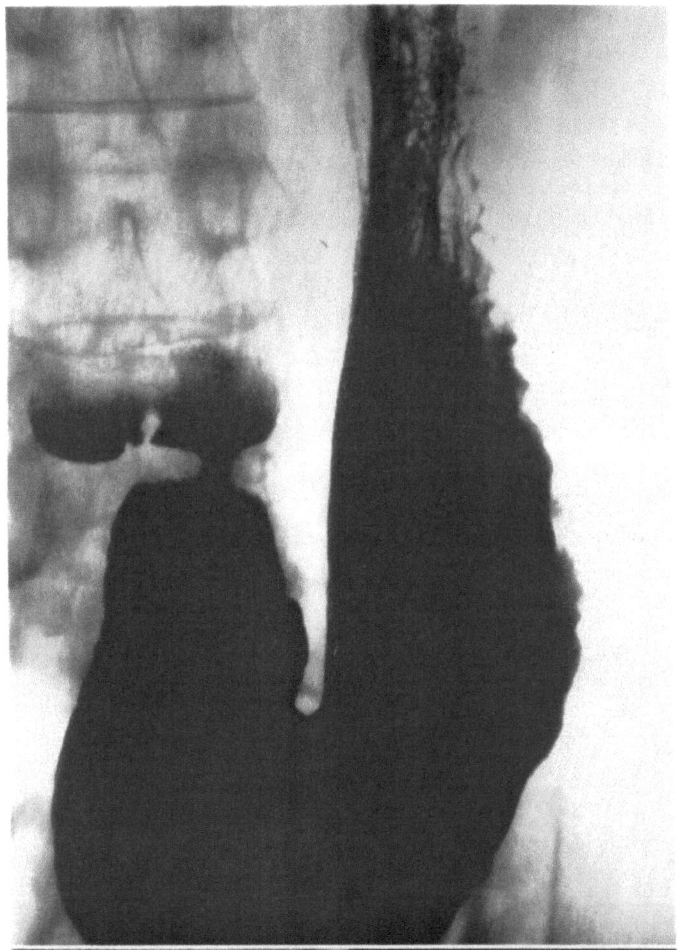

104b

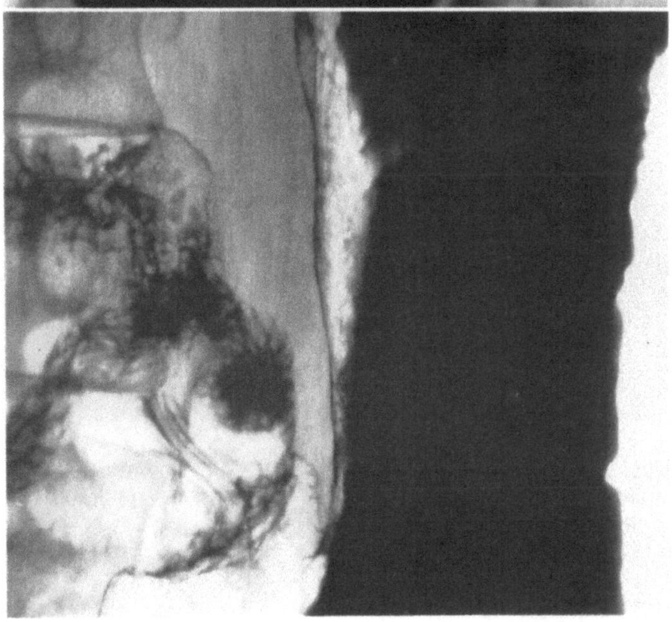

Fig. 104a Barium filled stomach from the first routine examination. One can only detect a slight irregularity of the gastric wall on the lesser curvature.

Fig. 104b Poor double-contrast picture taken by an inexperienced examiner. The irregularity of the lesser curvature and the abnormal mucosal folds of the gastric corpus should not be misread.

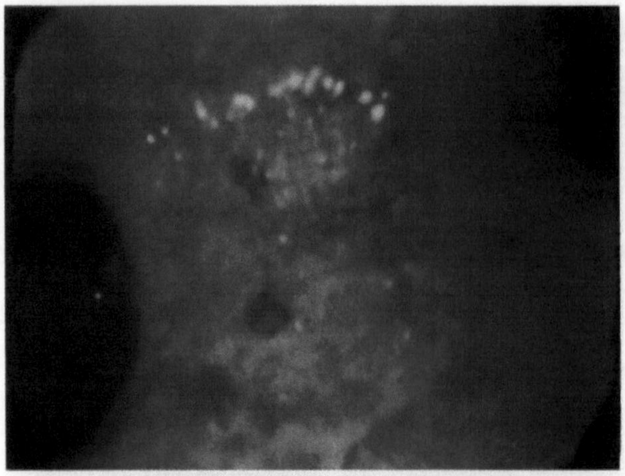

104c

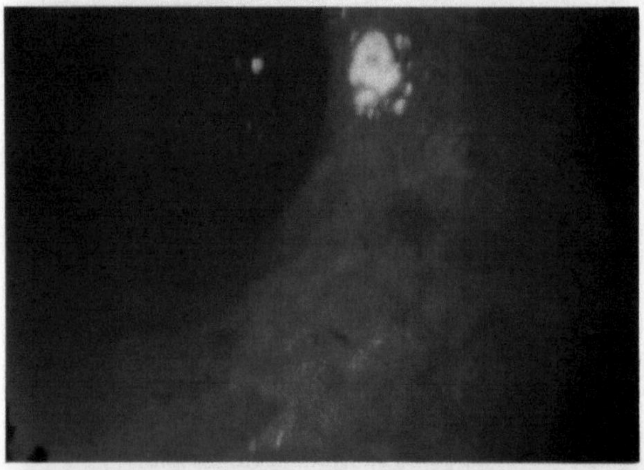

104d

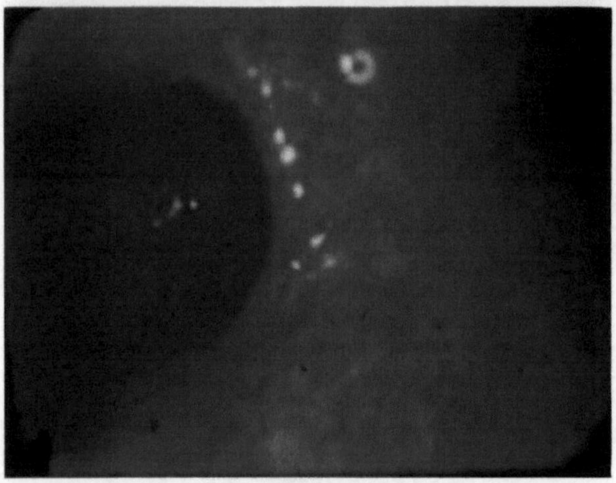

104e

Figs. 104c, d and e Endoscopic pictures. Sharply demarcated, mucosal discoloration is clearly revealed on the posterior wall. Several bleeding spots and a thin, foamy, mucous coat are demonstrated in the broad, discolored area.

104 f

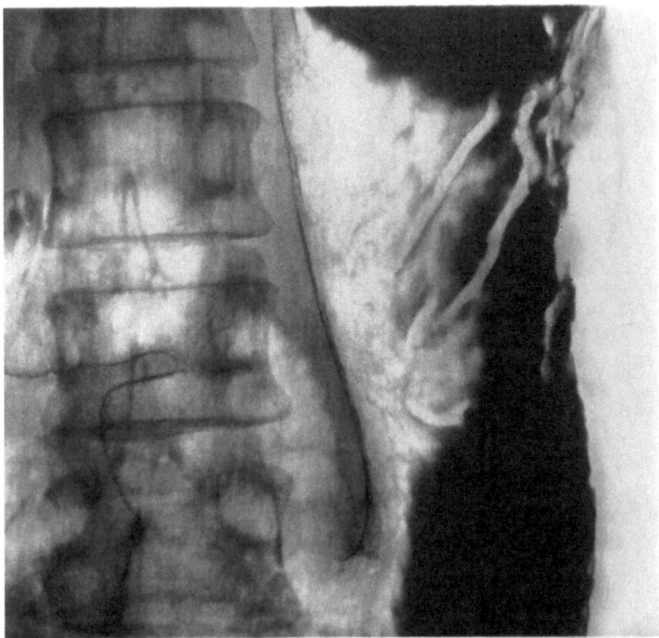

104 g

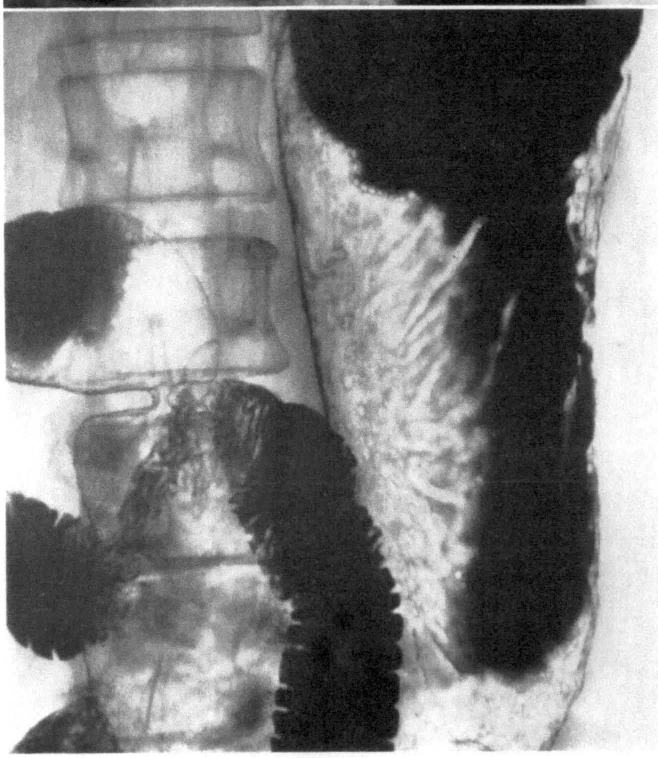

Figs. 104 f and g Double-contrast studies from the second x-ray examination. A slightly depressed lesion surrounded by numerous radiating folds are clearly demonstrated, but a differential diagnosis of this lesion is difficult.

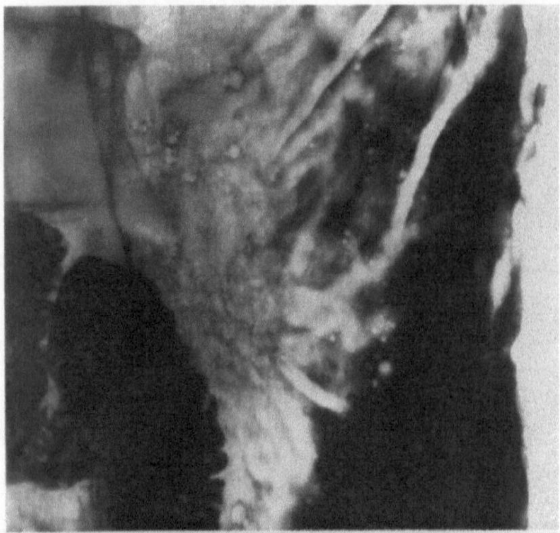

104h

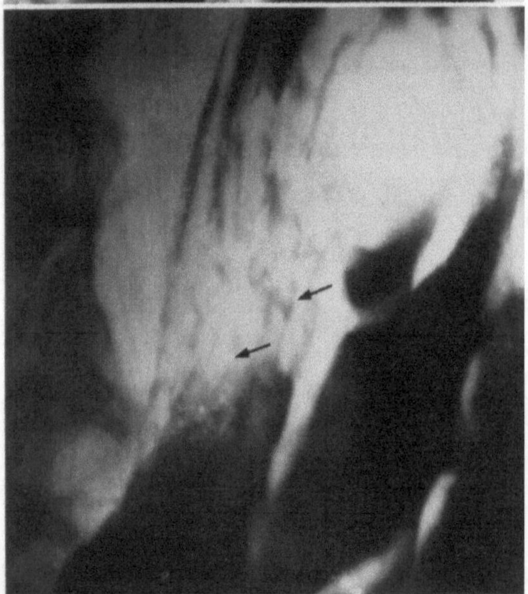

104i

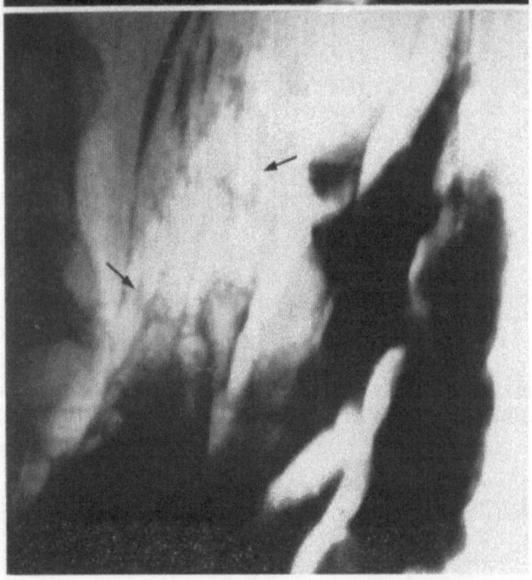

104j

Fig. 104h Double-contrast study from the second x-ray examination. A slightly depressed lesion surrounded by numerous radiating folds is clearly demonstrated.

Figs. 104i and j Compression studies. There are two ulcerations in the lesion.

104k

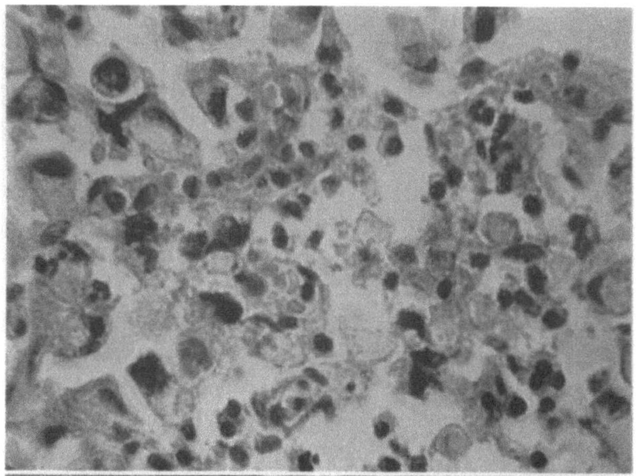

104l

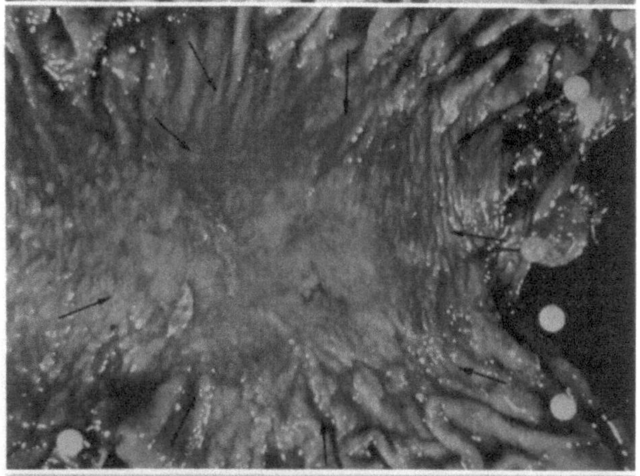

104m

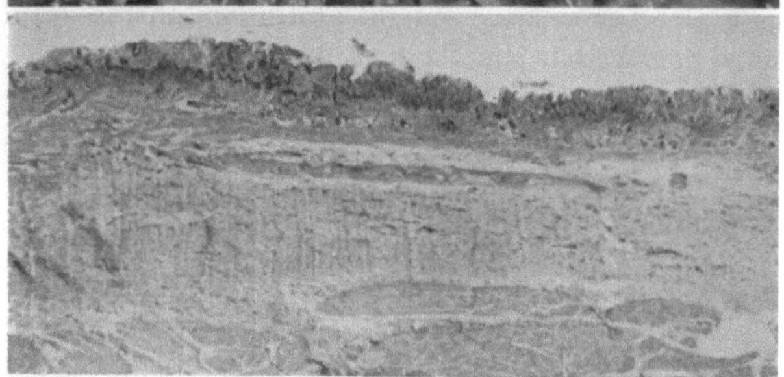

104n

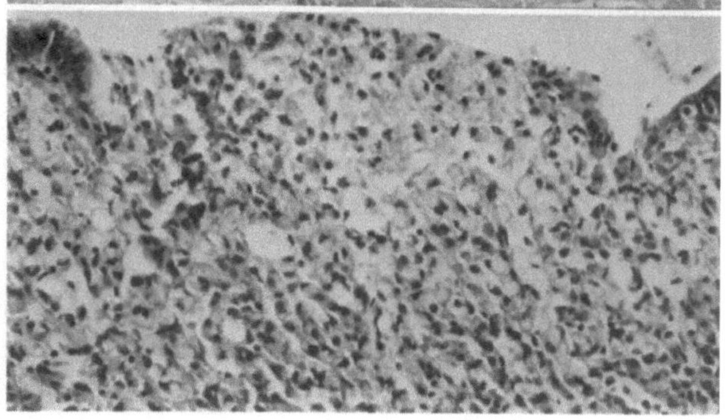

Fig. 104k Biopsy specimen. A biobsy study shows it to be an adenocarcinoma tubulare.

Fig. 104l Resected stomach. There are several flat ulcerations in the broad, shallow depression. The spreading of the cancerous infiltration on the mucosa is shown by arrows.

Figs. 104m, n Histopathological findings. Histologically, the lesion is revealed to be an adenocarcinoma tubulare and is limited to the mucosal layer.

3. Benign or malignant ulcer

As previously described with regard to the diagnosis of benign and malignant ulcers, there are a number of cases which are difficult to diagnose differentially. Despite progress in the techniques of x-ray and endoscopy, the following excavated types are still difficult to diagnose precisely. 1) Pure type III early cancer: This is the excavated type of early cancer without an excavation or a protuberance, which is formed by benign ulcers with cancerous changes in the surrounding membrane. Consequently, the diagnosis of such cases can only be made by means of a cytodiagnosis or gastric biopsy. Most of the cases classified as type III are the type referred to as "a small area of cancerous erosion surrounding a peptic ulcer." Particular care must be exercised in diagnosing small cancerous erosions. 2) Cases of malignant cycle (described previously). 3) Type IIc early cancer localized in one area of a linear ulcer. 4) Ulcer observed in a relatively early scirrhus carcinoma.

It is not always easy to differentiate the proper nature of benign and malignant ulcers, especially in cases of a scirrhus carcinoma of the gastric wall. On the other hand, it is known that ulcers of the greater curvature are frequently malignant. Actually, diagnostic difficulties arise with ulcerations which simulate ulcer niches.

Case 38

c.c.: Epigastric pain and emaciation.

28 year-old female.

The barium filled stomach (Fig. 105 a) demonstrated a peanut-sized niche on the greater curvature of the upper gastric body. This niche looked like a benign ulcer, but slight concavity was demonstrated around the gastric wall. In the compression studies (Figs. 105 b, c), both in the supine and upright positions, a marginal concavity was clearly revealed, and it was diagnosed as a niche en castre. A rigid protrusion on the greater curvature and interrupted, rigid folds were demonstrated in these pictures.

The endoscopic finding (Fig. 105 d) showed an irregularly shaped ulcer on the greater curvature of the corpus. The adjacent reddening and interruption of the mucosal folds were suspicious of malignancy, but the biopsy findings were benign. However, this niche disappeared within a month, so we could not make the correct diagnosis of a malignant ulcer. Four months later, epigastralgia and emaciation became severe, and the patient received a second x-ray examination. The lesion was radiologically diagnosed as a scirrhous carcinoma of the gastric body (Fig. 105 e). Soon there after, the patient died, and the histopathological examination revealed a scirrhous carcinoma (Fig. 105 f).

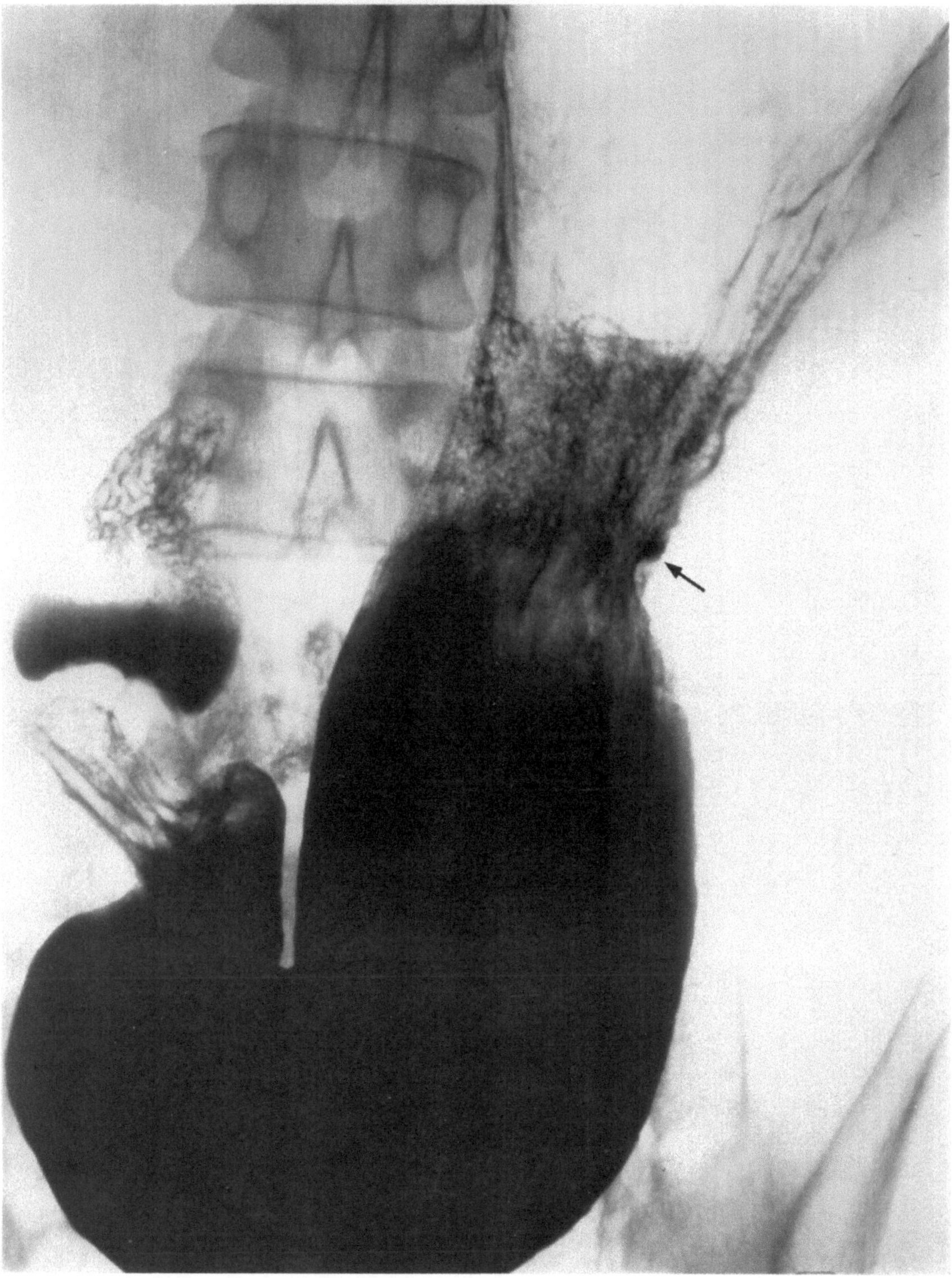

Fig. 105a Barium filled stomach. A small pea-sized niche is seen on the greater curvature of the depressed upper gastric body.

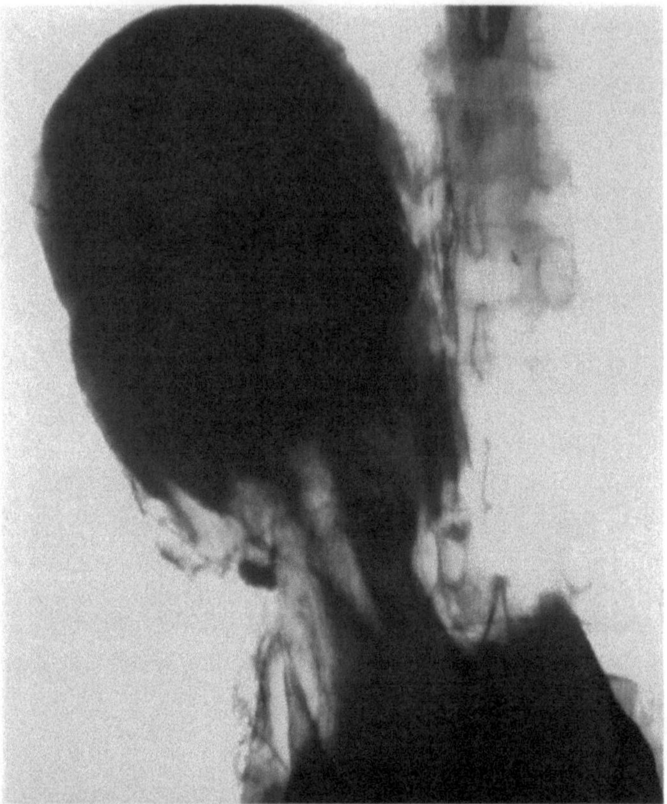

105b

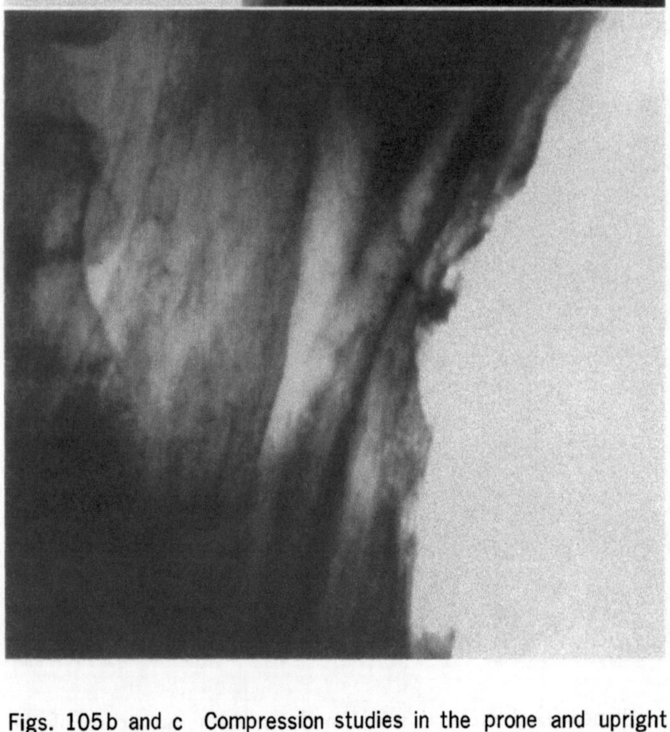

105c

Figs. 105b and c Compression studies in the prone and upright positions. A benign-appearing niche surrounded by rugged, rigid mucosal folds is seen. In the profile view, it is revealed as a niche on the depressed wall (niche en castre).

105 d

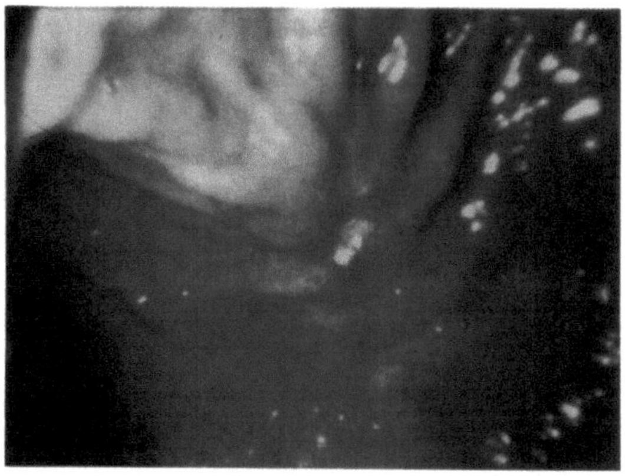

Fig. 105 d Endoscopic picture. Note the abruptness of the mucosal folds. After the biopsy study the lesion was erroneously diagnosed as benign.

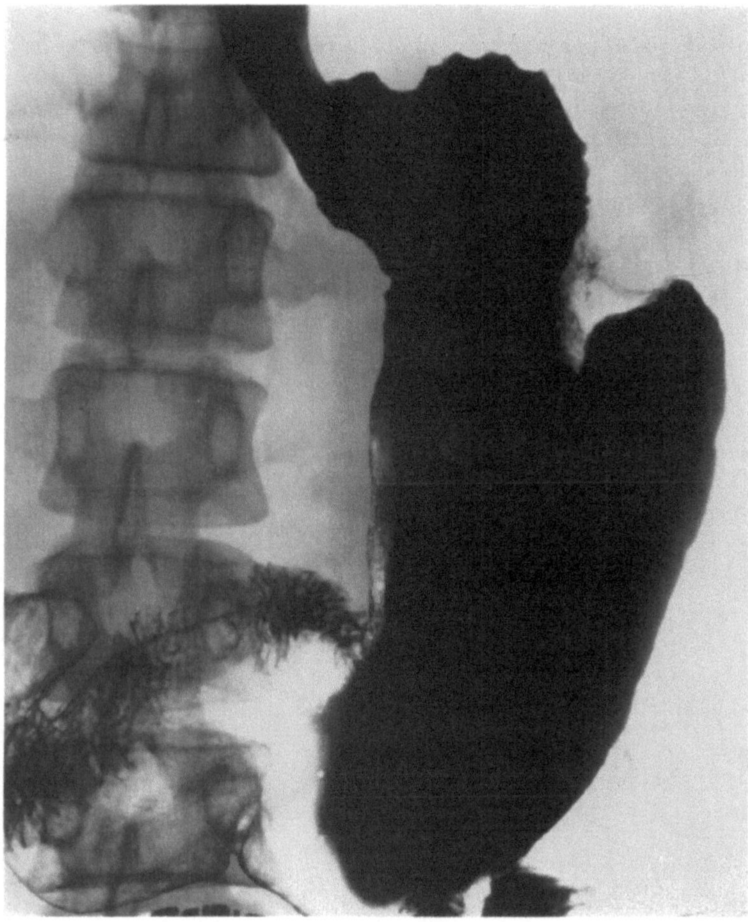

105 e

105 f

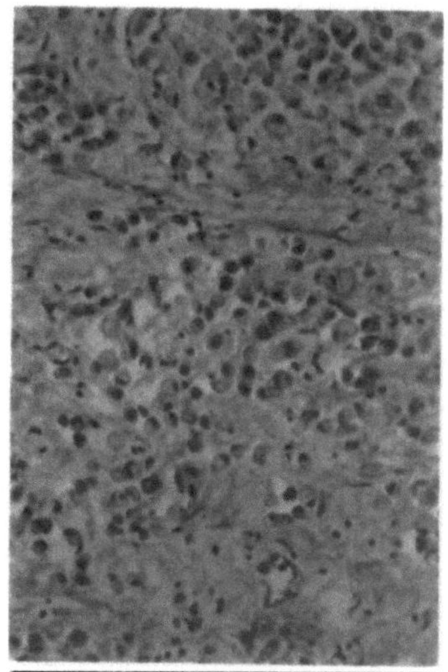

Fig. 105 e X-ray picture four months later. Typical features of a scirrhous carcinoma are demonstrated.
Fig. 105 f Histopathological findings four months later.

4. Widespread type IIa early gastric cancer (in which it is difficult to show the presence of an excavation)

It is important to examine whether or not there is an excavation in the center of polypus lesions, particularly in a type IIa early cancer. In the case of carcinomas exhibiting ulceration in the center of plain protuberant lesions, carcinomatous infiltrations may often reach the lower layer. However, most type IIa early cancers without ulceration on the protuberant surfaces are mucosal carcinomas. These facts have already been described in the section on protruding lesions. In practice, however, there are cases which are difficult to distinguish from one another.

Case 39

c.c.: Fullness in the epigastrium and general lassitude.

66 year-old male.

The barium filled stomach (Fig. 106 a) revealed a large filling defect from the lesser curvature of the lower gastric body to the antrum and a markedly serrated margin. The filling defect was more clearly demonstrated in the barium filled stomach with the patient prone (Fig. 106 b). This showed the lesion to be chiefly located on the anterior wall and it appeared to be a large polypoid lesion.

The double-contrast picture (Fig. 106 c) and compression study (Fig. 106 d) revealed a widespread, IIa type early cancer in the same area mentioned above. This lesion consisted of many lobulated, partially elevated polypoid lesions from the angle to the antrum. On the compression study a round collection of barium was demonstrated in the center of this lesion. It was difficult to conclude whether this fleck was an ulceration on the top of the large protruding lesion or only a barium accumulation in the depression of a polypoid lesion. This lesion was diagnosed as a concave, ulcerative lesion of the IIa or IIa+IIc type of early carcinoma.

Endoscopic examination did not enable us to diagnose the lesion correctly. Gross specimen and histopathological findings revealed this lesion to be a large, IIa type early cancer (Fig. 106e). However, no ulceration was found on the surface of the lesion. A niche-like barium fleck in the compression study was made by the depressions of the lobulations of the polypoid lesion. Endoscopically, this lesion was misread as the roentgenologic interpretation was. The misleading factor was the exogeneous mucus observed in the center of the lesion. Histopathologic examination revealed the lesion to be an adenocarcinoma tubulare invading only the mucosal layer (Figs. 106 f and g).

106 a

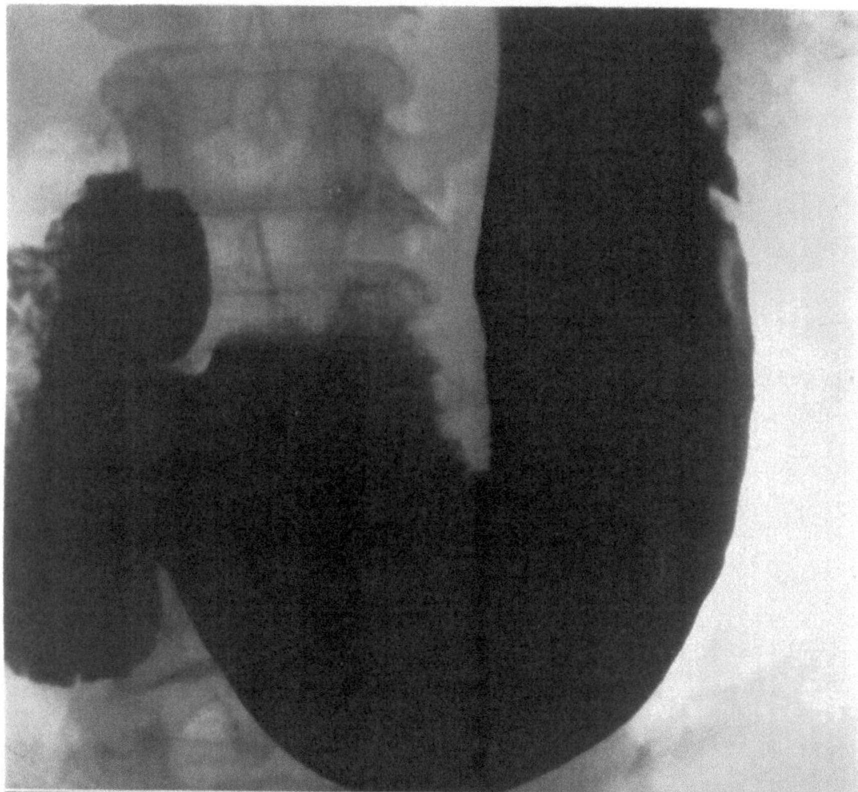

106 b

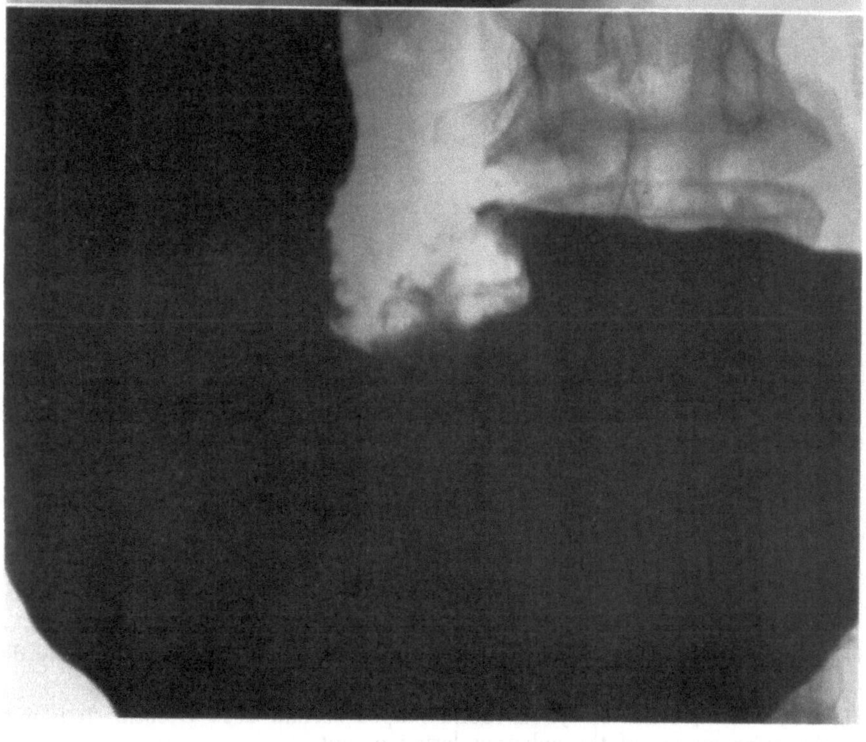

Fig. 106 a Barium filled stomach in the upright position.

Fig. 106 b Barium filled stomach in the prone position. The filling defects are effectively demonstrated.

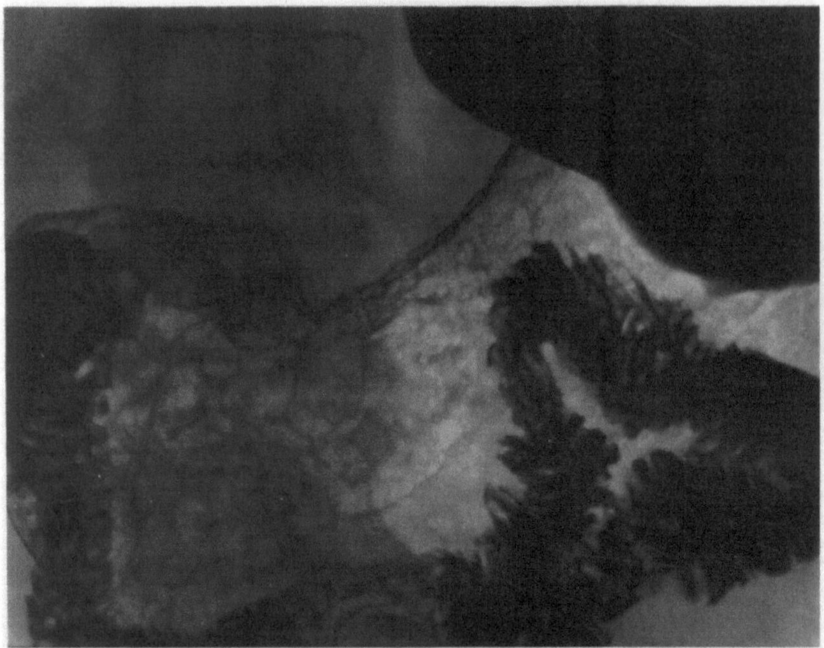

106c

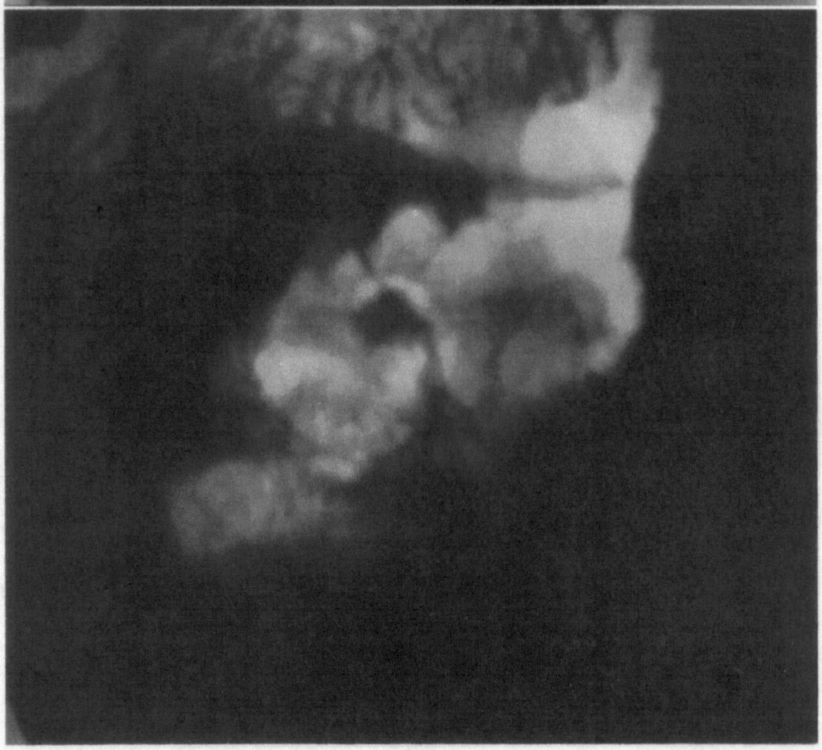

106d

Fig. 106c Double-contrast study. A widespread IIa type early cancer clearly demarcated from the normal mucosa is seen.

Fig. 106d Compression study. A round shaped barium fleck is seen. It is unclear whether there is ulceration on top of the polypous lesion or not.

106 e

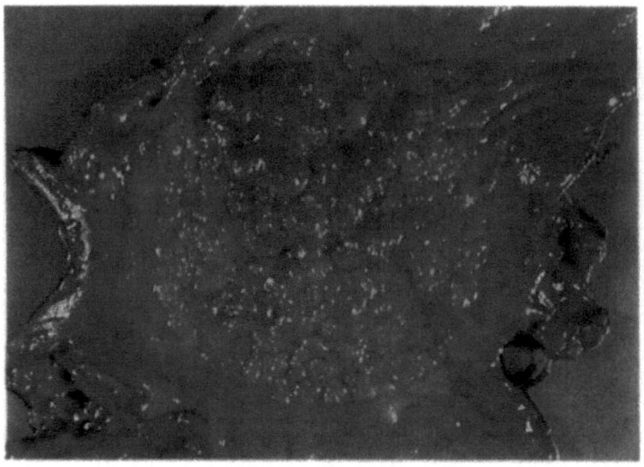

106 f

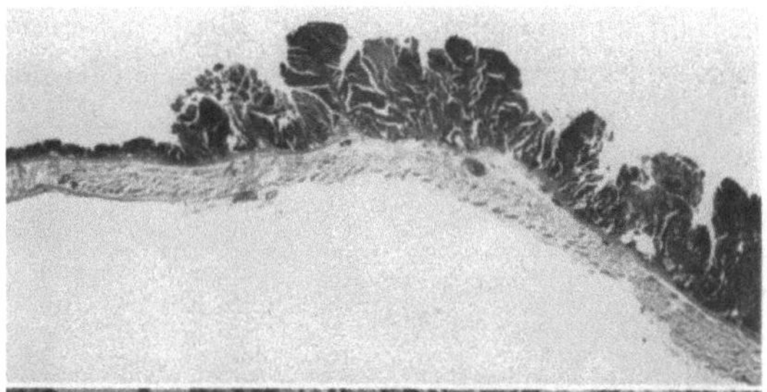

106 g

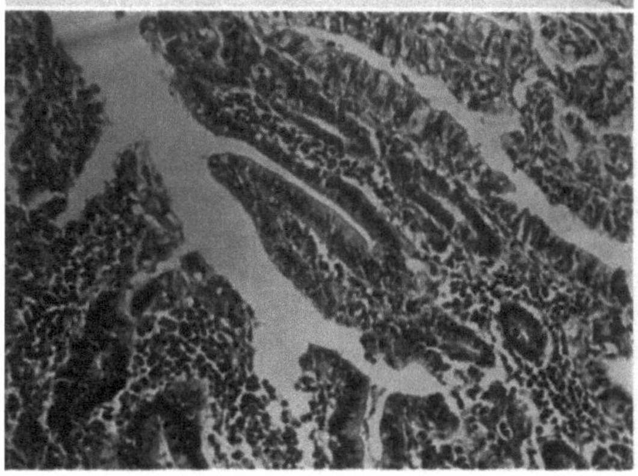

Fig. 106 e Resected stomach. Typical macroscopic finding of a type IIa is seen. There is no ulceration on the surface of this lesion.

Figs. 106 f and g Histopathological findings. Histologically, the lesion is revealed to be an adenocarcinoma tubulare limited to the mucosa.

C. Rare cases

1. Sarcoma of the stomach (Depressed type)

Generally speaking, there are two types of gastric sarcomas, one arising from lymphoid tissue and the other from smooth muscle. Macroscopic classifications have been variously described by many authors. Previously stated SKANDALAKIS's classification or PALMER's classification will suffice for practical use.

Such classifications are oversimplified. Mixed forms are frequently seen, but the classification is helpful diagnostically. X-ray and gastrofiberscopic findings such as localized giant mucosal folds, a thickening and rigidity of the gastric wall, and a rubbery mass with ulceration are suggestive; but differentiation from a diffuse carcinoma or a peptic ulcer with surrounding inflammation and syphilis of the stomach may be impossible. Cytological or biopsy procedures are necessary for preoperatative confirmation.

Case 40

c.c.: Epigastric pain and loss of appetite.

31 year-old male.

The barium filled stomach (Figs. 107 a, b) exhibited a remarkably deformed stomach with antral narrowing. Fair extension with a serrated, irregular wall on the lesser curvature of the body and retraction on the greater curvature were noted in the upright, filled study. From this picture, a widespread lesion was suspected, but it was very difficult to determine whether the lesion was a carcinoma or another malignant disease. However, it is important that a scirrhous carcinoma of the stomach is demonstrated by a more marked rigidity.

In the double-contrast study (Fig. 107 c), the characteristics of this lesion were clearly demonstrated. An irregularly shaped, shallow depression surrounded by hypertrophied mucosal folds was observed on the posterior wall of the gastric angle. Converging mucosal folds were markedly hypertrophied especially on the greater curvature, and various sized polypoid protrusions were demonstrated. Moreover, there were pea-sized granules on the floor of the depression. With compression fluorscopy, smooth, mucosal protrusions were clearly observed on the antrum. Endoscopically (Fig. 107 d), a superficial depression with a white coating was demonstrated on the gastric angle, but was not sharply demarcated. The surface of the lesion seemed to be smooth, rather than uneven, and somewhat rubbery.

Pathological examination of the gross specimen revealed a widespread, superficial depression, surrounded by hypertrophied folds and well-defined nodules scattered in the pyloric region (Fig. 107 e). The mucosal folds at the margins of the depression were thickened and rolled. The bottom of the depression was rugged and more granular, compared with the IIc type early cancer. Histologically (Fig. 107 f), the tumor was composed predominantly of immature lymphoid and reticulum cells, and was diagnosed as a reticulum cell sarcoma of the stomach.

107 a

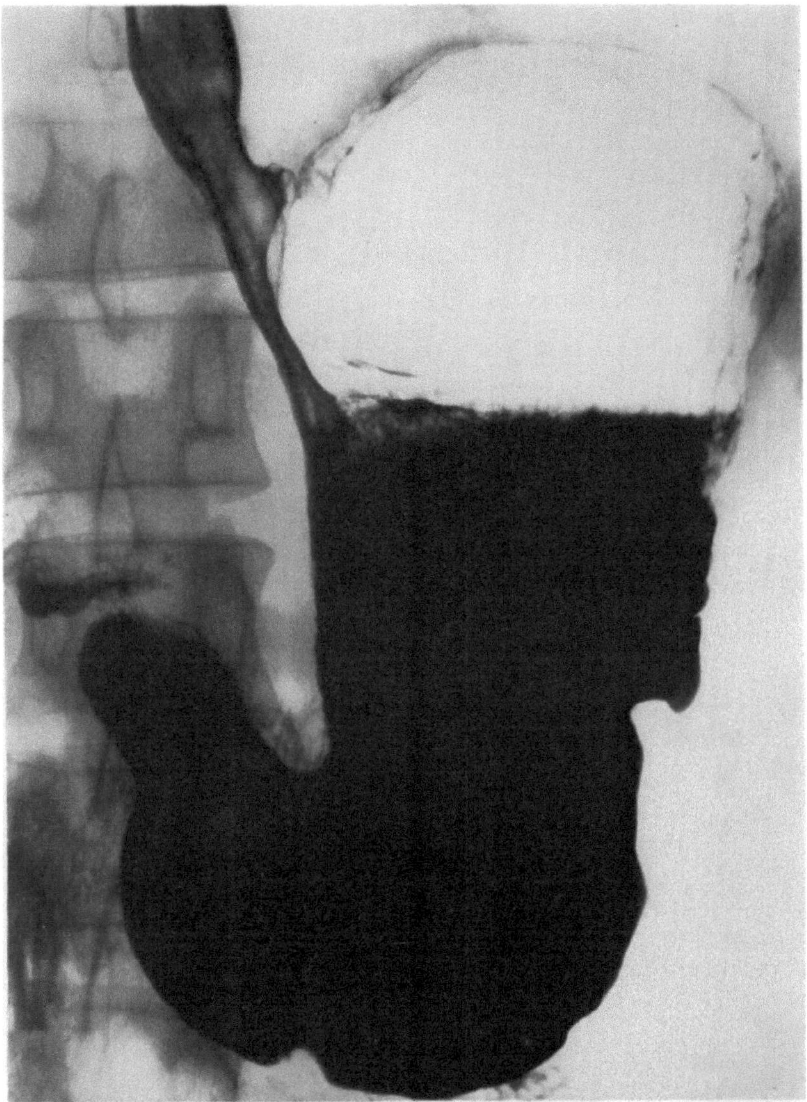

107 b

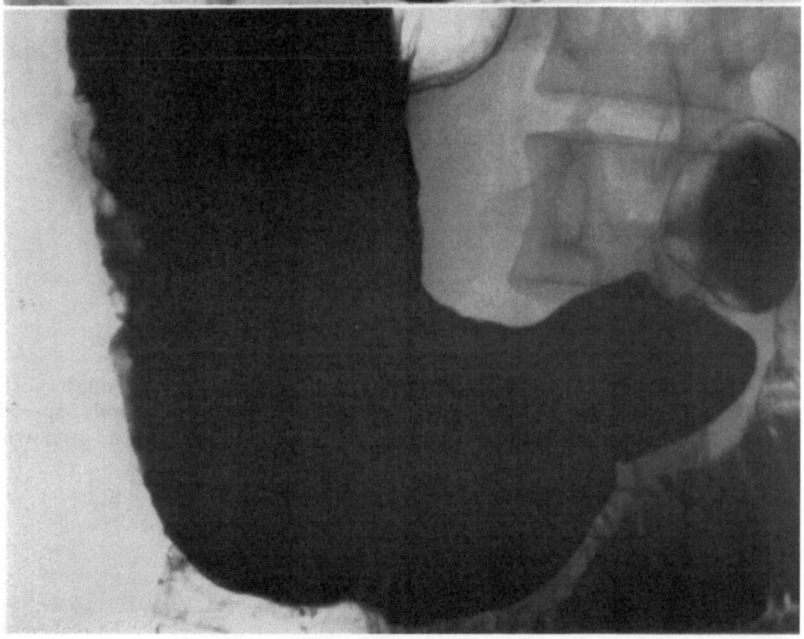

Figs. 107 a and b Barium filled stomach in the upright and prone position. These stomachs are markedly deformed, however, rigidity of the gastric wall is not very severe. These findings are suspicious of a noncancerous lesion.

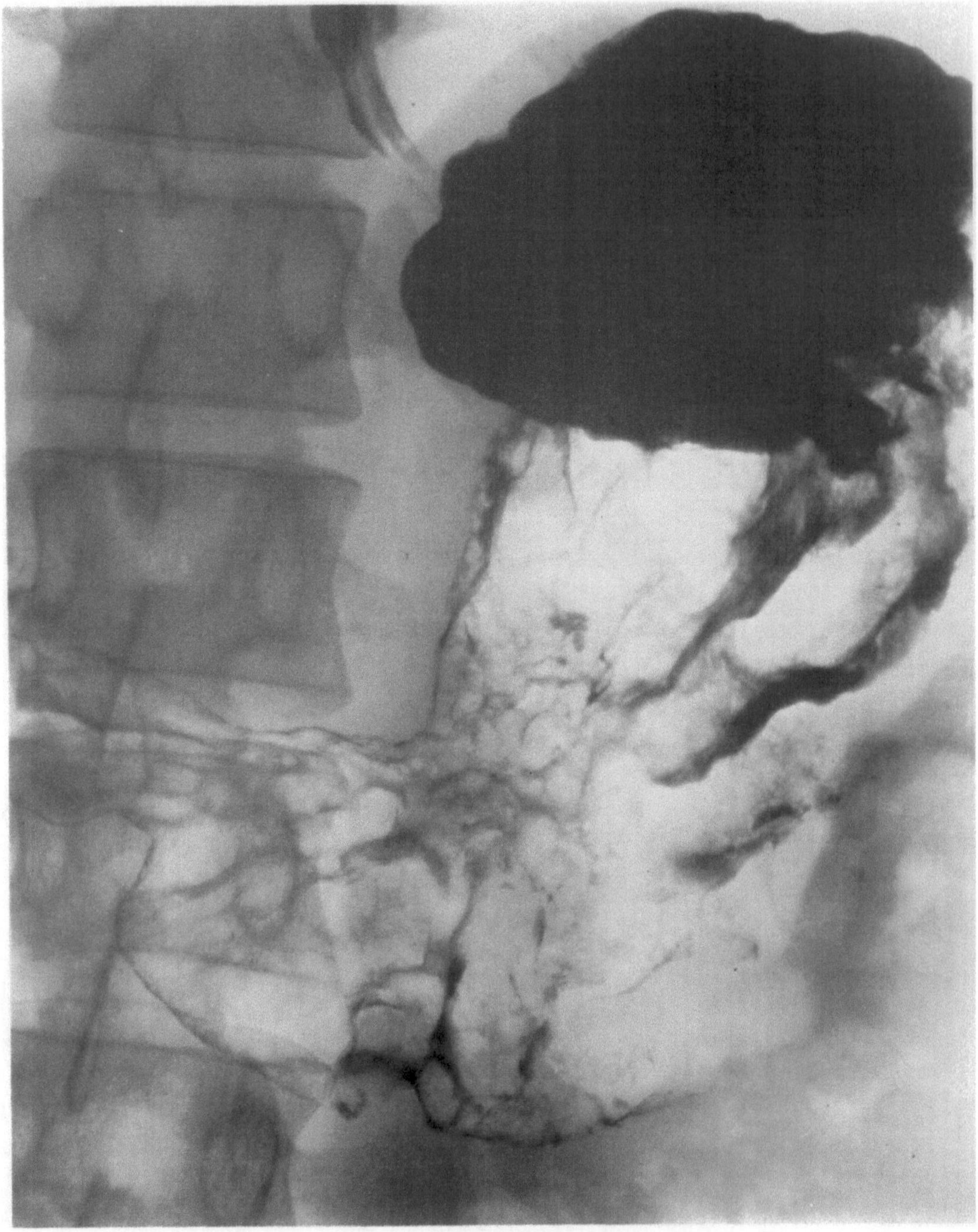

Fig. 107c Double contrast study in the supine position. A rough surfaced, nodular appearing depression is seen on the posterior wall of the lower gastric body, spreading to the antrum. The surrounding mucosal folds are markedly thickened and appear somewhat like a localized polypous protrusion.

107 d

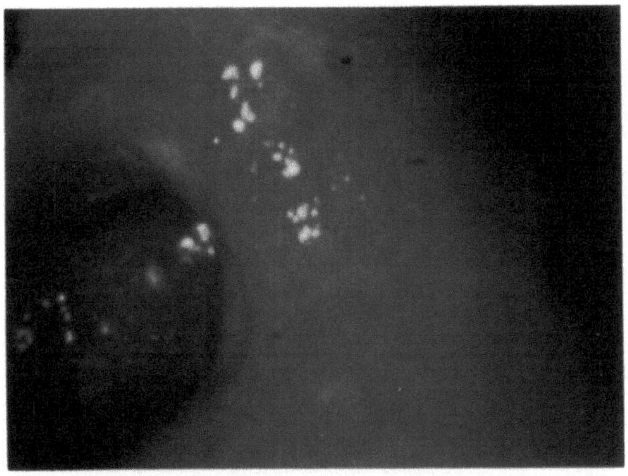

107 e

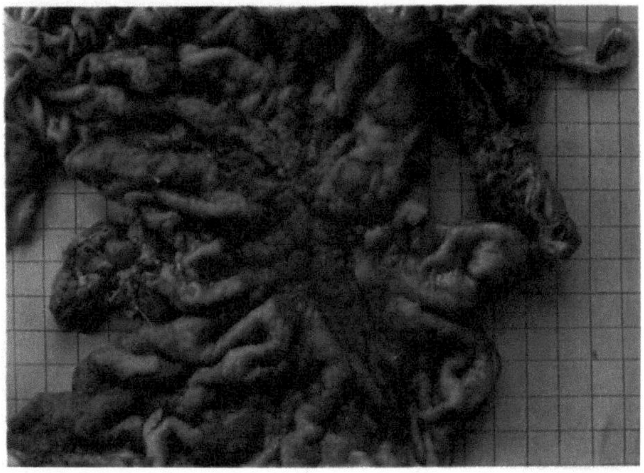

107 f

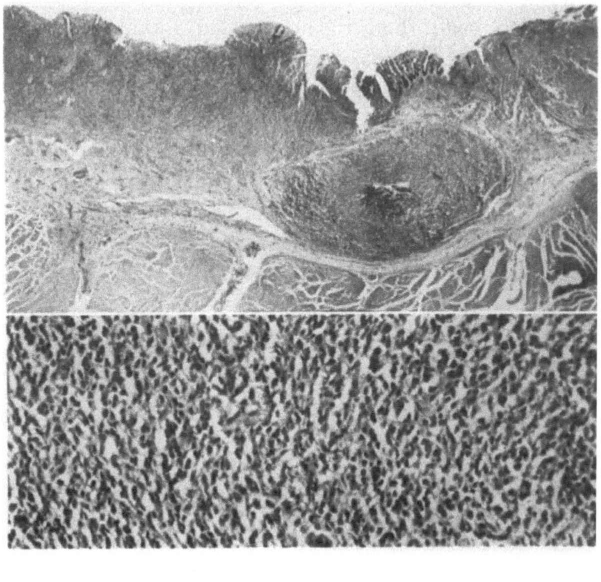

Fig. 107 d Endoscopic picture. A hazy, not clearly demarcated depression is seen on the thickened and broadened gastric angle. The surface mucosa of the lesion appears rather smooth and rubbery.

Fig. 107 e Resected stomach. Multiformed, partly depressed, and other protruding lesions are demonstrated in this picture. It seems difficult to differentiate this from a diffusely infiltrating carcinoma.

Fig. 107 f Histopathological findings. Histologically, the lesion was proved to be a reticulum cell sarcoma.

2. Reactive lymphoreticular hyperplasia

In 1958, SMITH and ELWIG suggested that this reaction of the stomach was being misinterpreted as a true lymphoma.

Several synonymous terms have been used for this disease: "chronische lymphatische Gastritis" (KONJETZNY), "lymphoid hyperplasia" (FARRIS), "reactive lymphoid hyperplasia" (SMITH), "Pseudolymphoma" (JACOB), "chronic lymphoid gastritis" (SCHINDLER), and others.

In our country in 1966, NAKAMURA *et al.* defined this reaction as a "reactive lymphoreticular hyperplasia", and classified into two types:

1) Localized, hypertrophic form originating from a gastric ulcer
2) Diffuse, flat form originating from a chronic gastritis

It is important that this reaction macroscopically resembles a IIc type early cancer or malignant lymphoma.

a. Localized hypertrophic form

Case 41

c.c.: Nausea and epigastric pain.

47 year-old male.

The compression study (Fig. 108 a) revealed a lineally shaped niche on the greater curvature of the antrum. The marginal zone of the area of the lesion seemed somewhat rigid and slightly indented. The mucosa around the niche was thickened and granular. Gastrofiberscopy (Fig. 108 b) revealed a lineally shaped, sharply demarcated, shallow ulceration with protrusion and interrupted mucosal folds on the greater curvature of the antrum.

Lavage cytology was negative for malignancy. Gastrectomy was performed because of the endoscopic diagnosis of a IIc type early gastric carcinoma. The macroscopic findings of the resected stomach (Fig. 108 c) revealed a shallow, lineally shaped depression surrounded by interrupted mucosal folds and a well-defined mucosal protuberance. This lesion was diagnosed macroscopically as a IIa+IIc type early cancer.

Histological findings demonstrated a tumor mass consisting of a well-differentiated, mature, lymphoid cellular infiltration (Fig. 108 d). Few diffuse, germinal centers were indentified. This case was finally diagnosed as a localized hypertrophic form of a reactive lymphoreticular hyperplasia, probably originating from a chronic gastric ulcer.

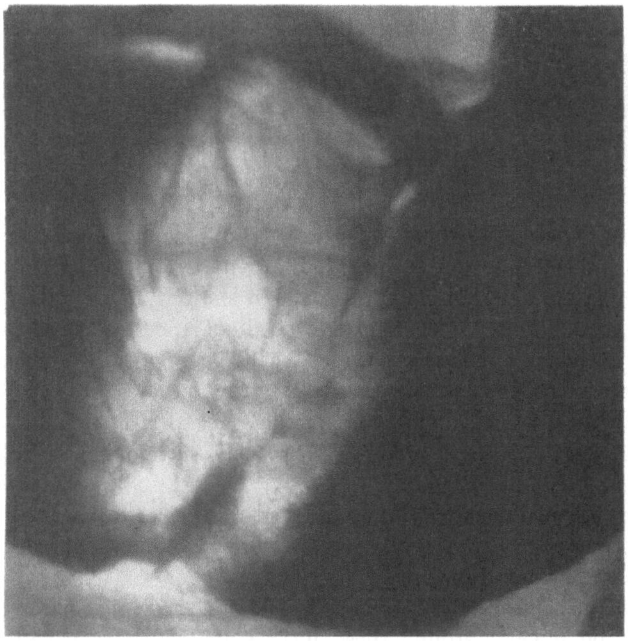

108 a

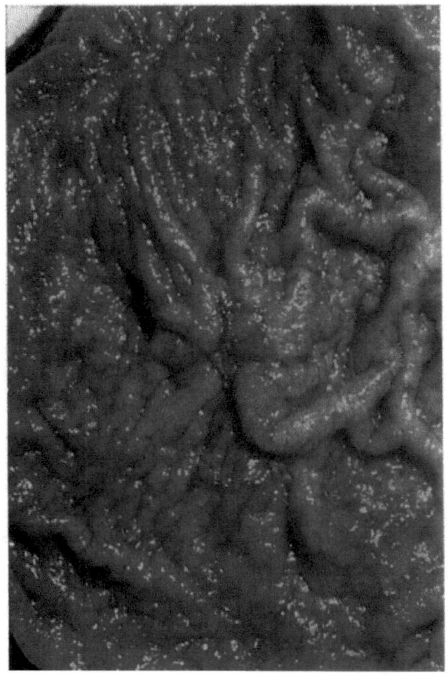

108 c

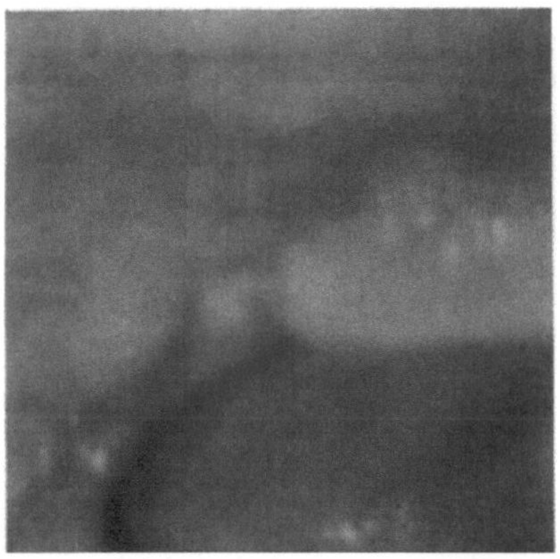

108 b

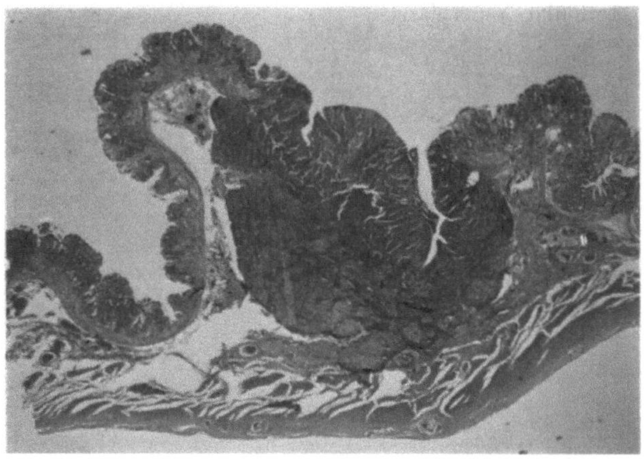

108 d

Fig. 108 a **Compression study.** A linear ulceration is clearly demonstrated on the greater curvature of the antrum. Note the mucosal granularity and thickening around the niche.

Fig. 108 b **Endoscopic picture.** A IIc appearing, shallow depression is revealed in this picture. It was positively diagnosed as a IIc type early cancer.

Fig. 108 c **Resected stomach.** This lesion was macroscopically misinterpreted as a IIa+IIc type early cancer. Even retrospectively, macroscopic differentiation is difficult.

Fig. 108 d **Histopathological findings.** Localized, massive lymphoid infiltration is seen.

b. Diffuse flat form

Case 42

c.c.: Heartburn and epigastric pain.
44 year-old male.

Physical examination revealed no abdominal masses or tenderness. The radiograph of the barium filled stomach in the upright position (Fig. 109 a) appeared essentially normal. The double-contrast study with a relatively small amount of barium (Fig. 109 b) showed an irregular, superficial depression with converging mucosal folds on the posterior wall of the lower body. Another double-contrast study showed (Fig. 109 c) a diffusely outlined, shallow depression in the same region. These x-ray findings suggested that this lesion was an infiltrative process, IIc type early cancer or a malignant lymphoma. However, the endoscopic picture (Fig. 109 d) revealed a benign-appearing, scarring ulcer on the lesser curvature of the gastric body surrounded by a hyperplastic, engorged mucosa.

Gastric lavage cytology was negative for malignancy, but isolated, large cells with scanty cytoplasm and prominent nuclei were observed. Gastrectomy was performed because of the possibility of malignancy, especially a IIc type early cancer.

Pathologically (Fig. 109 e), two gastric ulcer scars were found in a kissing arrangement on the lesser curvature of the lower body. The mucosa around these ulcer scars was uneven and somewhat reticular. A microscopic study (Fig. 109 f) revealed an ulcer scar (Ul-III) with extensive lymphocytic, inflammatory cell infiltration in the gastric mucosa and submucosa. The final diagnosis was made clinico pathologically as ulcer scars with a diffuse form of reactive lymphoreticular hyperplasia.

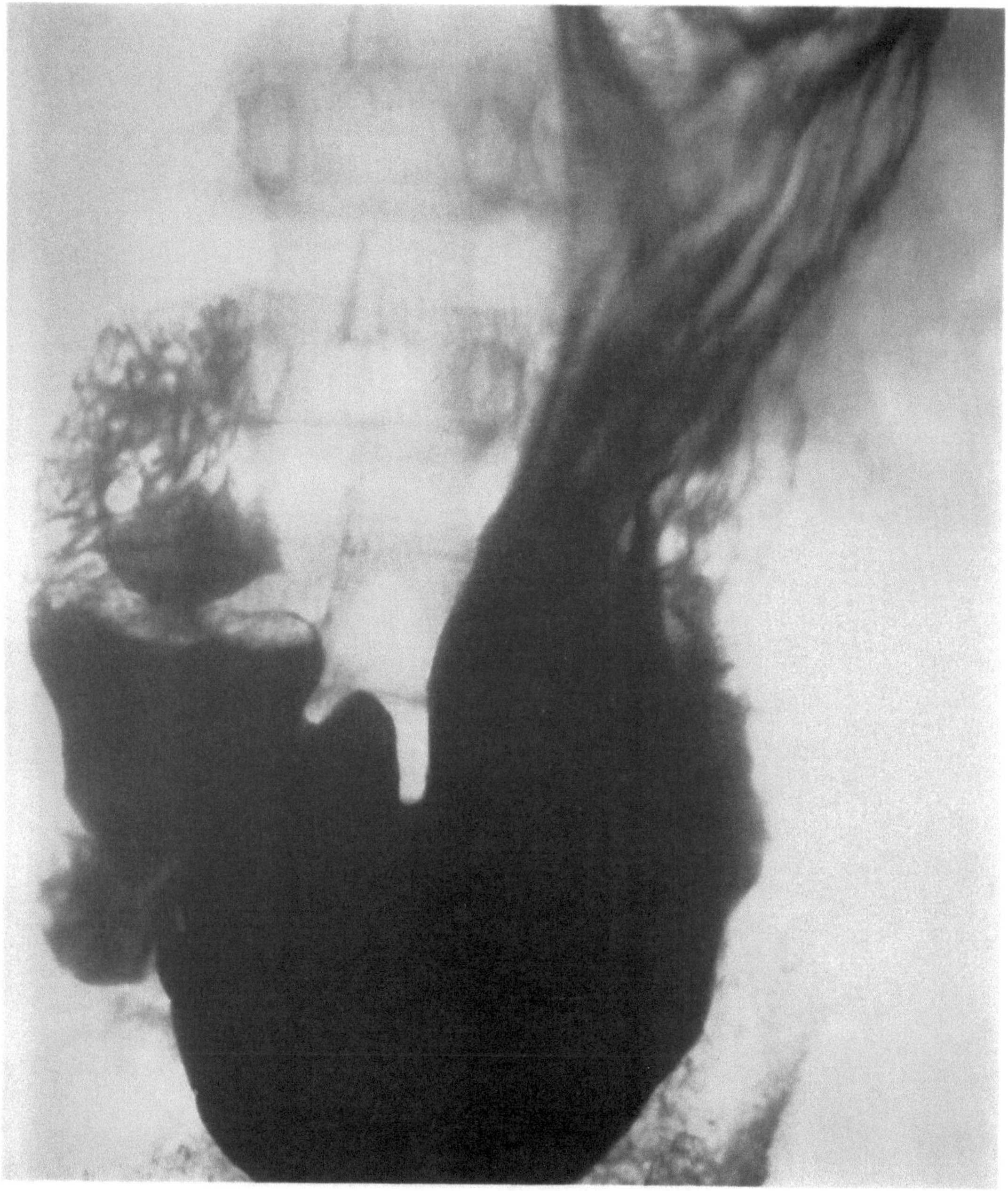

Fig. 109a Radiograph of the barium filled stomach in the upright position. A normal contour of the stomach is seen.

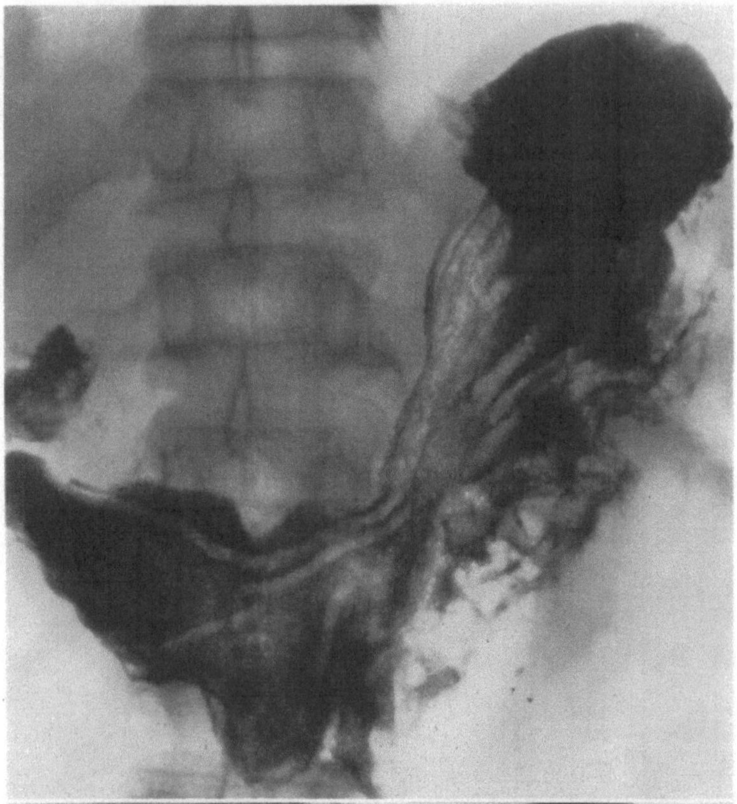

109 b

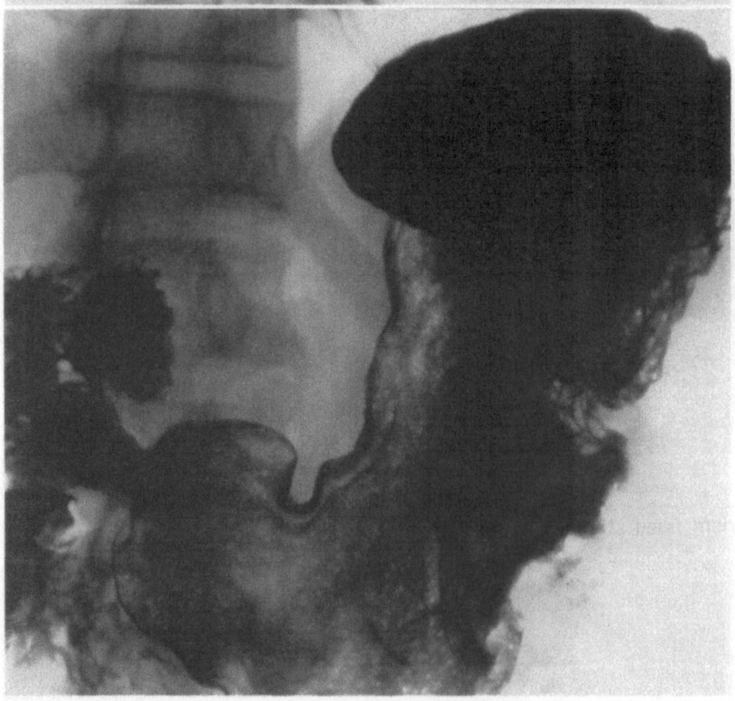

109 c

Figs. 109 b and c Double-contrast studies. Note the IIc appearing depression on the posterior wall of the lower gastric body.

109 d

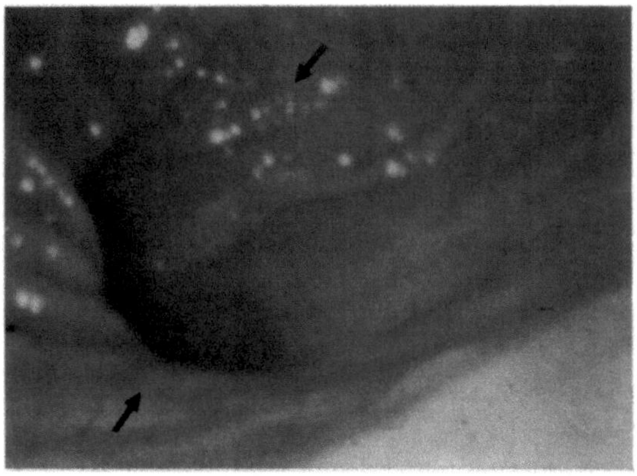

109 e

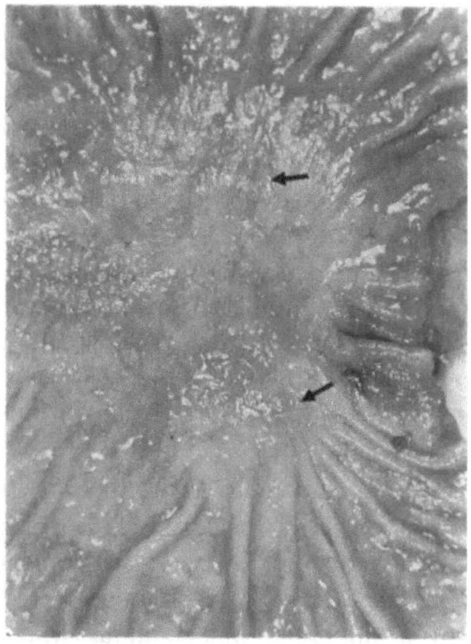

109 f

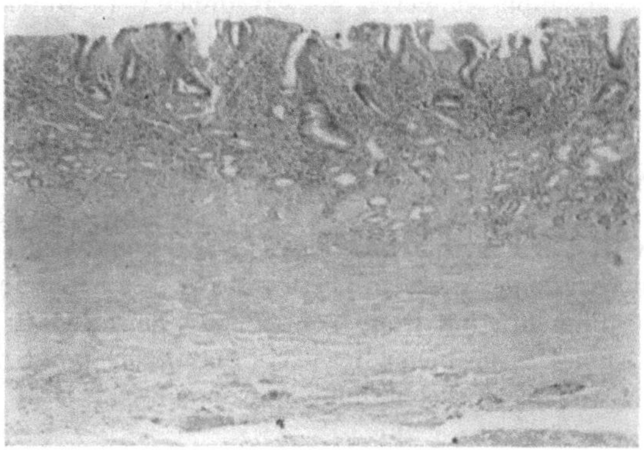

Fig. 109 d Endoscopic picture. An ulcer scar with engorgement on the lesser curvature and convergence of the mucosal folds on the posterior wall is seen (arrow). This finding suggests that this lesion may be benign.

Fig. 109 e Resected stomach. A kissing arrangement of ulcer scars surrounded by uneven, reticular mucosa with rugal convergance is seen (arrow).

Fig. 109 f Histopathological findings. Heavy, lymphocytic infiltration of the gastric wall is seen.

3. Acute phlegmonous gastritis

This is a purulent inflammation of the gastric wall, which originates from a gastric ulcer, a gastric carcinoma, or a metastatic hematogenous infection. For clinicopathological consideration, these are two types of phlegmonous gastritis. The localized form is recognized as an abscess, and the other as diffuse inflammations. In general, the clinical picture is that of a serious peritoneal disease, usually accompanied by chills, high fever, epigastralgia, and vomiting. Generally speaking, most patients with this disease die within a few days.

Case 43

c.c.: Nausea and general fatigue.

52 year-old male.

A leukocyte count of 10,000 was obtained, but a bacterial blood culture proved negative. On x-ray examination, a slight irregularity of the lesser curvature and a marked serration of the greater curvature were seen on the gastric body in the barium filled study in the upright position (Fig. 110 a). The double-contrast study with a relatively small amount of barium demonstrated a rugal radiation and a rigidity of the greater curvature of the body (Fig. 110 b).

In another double-contrast study (Fig. 110 c), an uneven, reticular appearance was demonstrated with granular shadows. Erosive lesions were suggested by this picture, but differentiation from a benign flat erosion, a purulent erosion, and a superficial carcinoma was difficult. The photograph taken by a GTF-A (Fig. 110 d) revealed two depressed lesions on the posterior wall of the lower gastric body. Endoscopically a triangular-shaped, reddish lesion, apparently an ulcer-scar, and a white coated, flat ulceration were seen. There seemed to be a diffuse thickening of the gastric wall.

We could not exclude a IIc type early cancer because of the endoscopic picture, in spite of obtaining a cytologically negative report for malignancy. Gastrectomy was performed under the diagnosis of a probable IIc type early cancer. Macroscopically (Fig. 110 e), a small ulcer, 0.5× 0.5 cm in size, and scar-like reddening were recognized on the posterior wall of the body surrounded by a thickened phlegmonous wall. Histopathologically (Fig. 110 f), it proved to be a localized type of phlegmonous gastritis. The most objective information was obtained by endoscopic examination, however, it was difficult to differentiate this disease from other erosive, ulcerative diseases.

4. Granulomatous diseases of the stomach

It is well-known that tuberclosis, syphilis, and other granulomatous diseases are infrequently found in the stomach wall. These diseases are often found to be of the ulcerative and erosive type, so differentiation from gastric carcinoma, especially from a IIc type early carcinoma, is difficult. For this problem, Bleruath and Frick point out that the lessened rigidity of the ulcer margin is valuable for confirming the diagnosis.

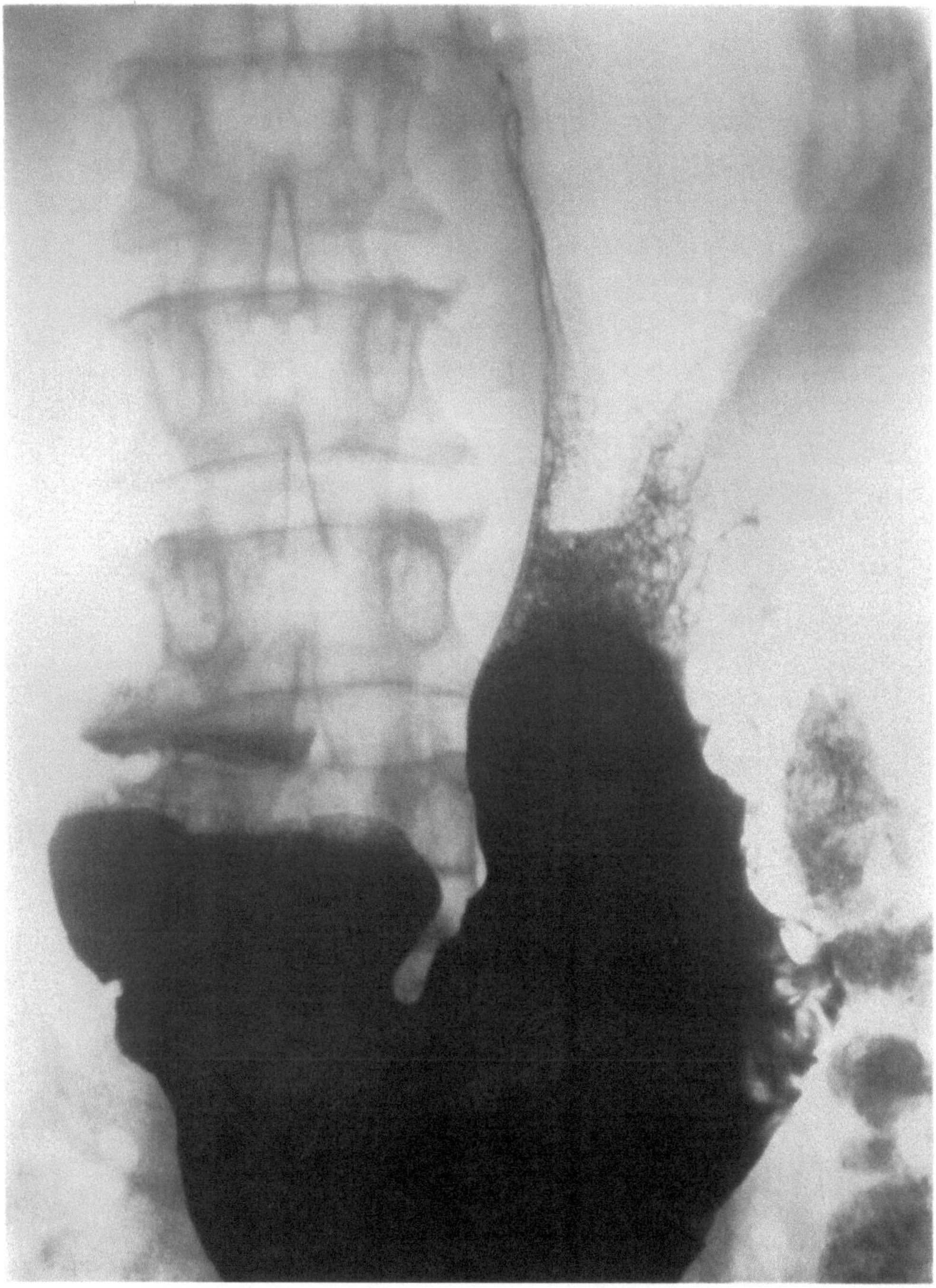

Fig. 110a Barium filled stomach in the upright position. A smooth, irregular wall on the lesser curvature of the lower body can be seen, however. rigidity of the gastric wall is absent. Serration of the greater curvature is impressive.

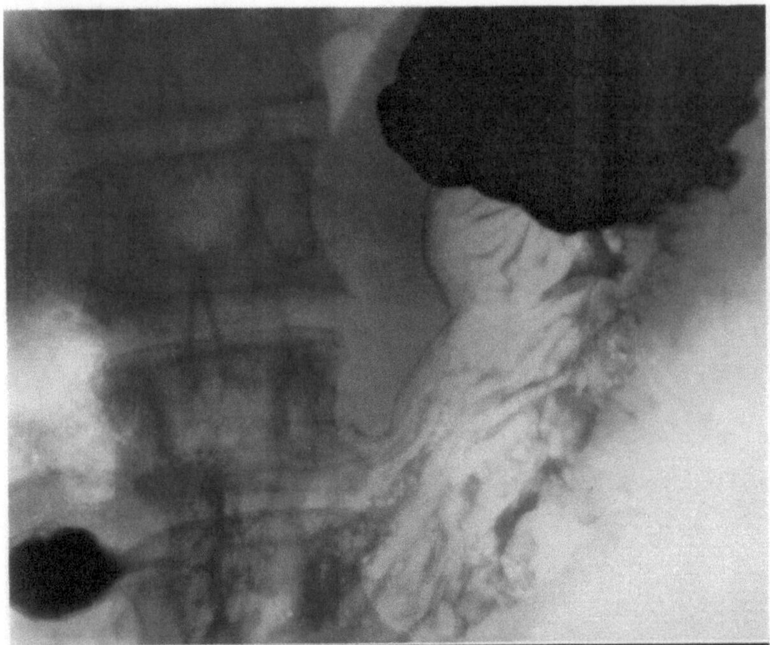

110b

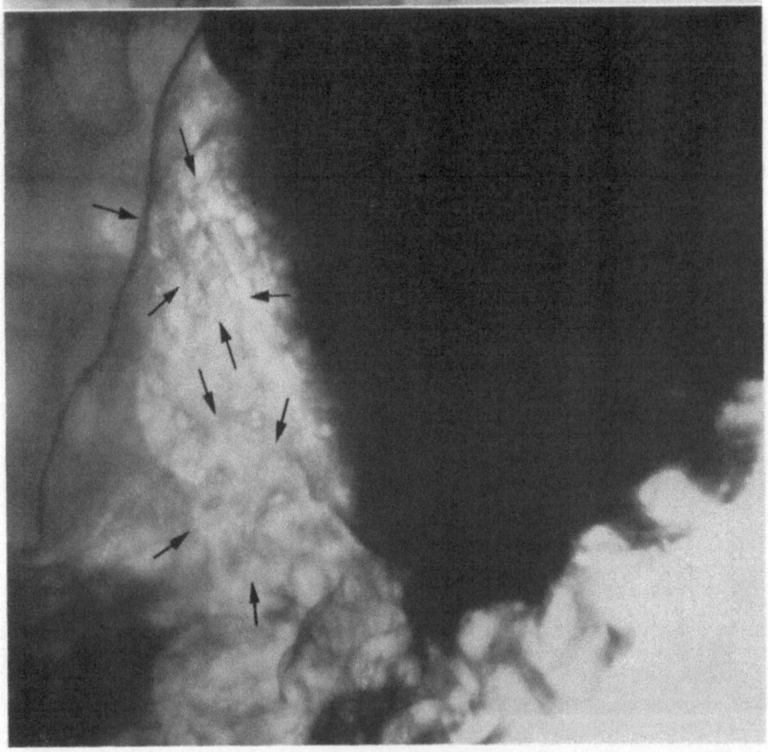

110c

Fig. 110b Double-contrast study (small amount of air). On the lesser curvature of the gastric body, converging mucosal folds and abnormal, oblique running rugae are present. In general, radiologically it may be considered an ulcer scar or a scarring ulcer.

Fig. 110c Double-contrast study. A faint barium fleck and a granular appearance are seen (arrows).

110d

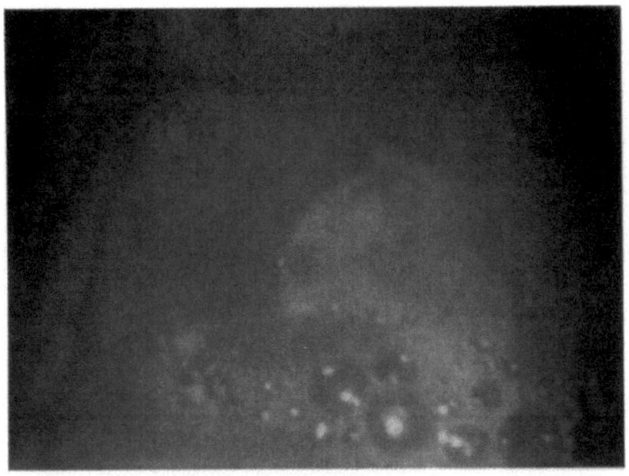

110e

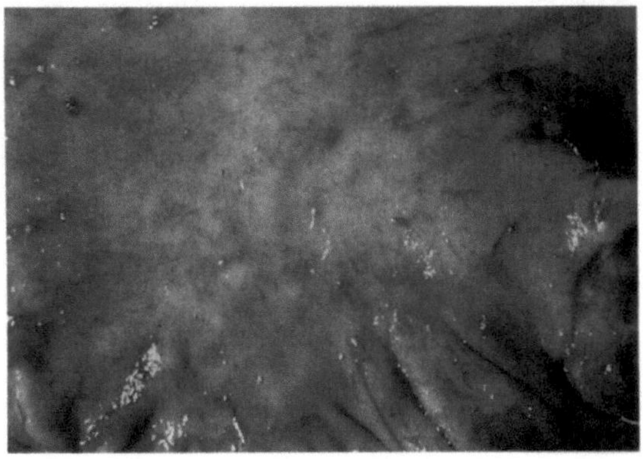

110f

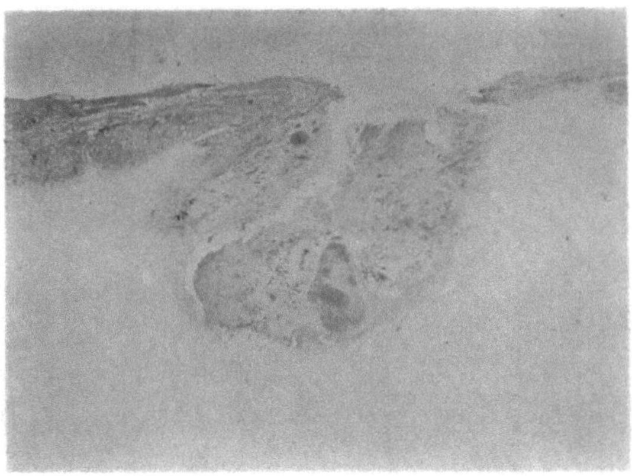

Fig. 110d Endoscopic picture. On the lesser curvature, we can see a scarring ulcer with converging mucosal folds. On the other wall, a thin, whitish-coated ulceration is visible. The surrounding mucosa seems normal or slightly elevated.

Fig. 110e Resected stomach. A small, flat ulcer, 0.5×0.5 cm in size, with mucosal convergence is revealed on the posterior wall, surrounded by a yellowish, discolored, thickened mucosa.

Fig. 110f Histopathological findings The lesion is diagnosed as a localized abscess. Its surface is slightly ulcerated.

References

ALLEN, A. W., et al.: Primary malignant lymphoma of the gastrointestinal tract. Amer. Surg., 140: 428-438, 1954.

AOYAMA, T.: Reactive lymphoreticular hyperplasia (in Japanese). Stomach and Intestine, 2: 1283-1291, 1967.

ASAKURA, M. et al.: Clinical and histological studies of gastric polyp (in Japanese). Jap. J. Clin. Surg., 22: 31, 1960.

ASHIZAWA, S.: Some diagnostic problems about gastrocamera (in Japanese). Stomach and Intestine, 1: 341-346, 1966.

ASHIZAWA, S. et al.: Atlas of gastroscopy (in Japanese). Bunkodo, Tokyo, 1968.

BALFOR, D. C., HENDERSON, E. F.: Benign tumors of the stomach. Ann. Surg., 85, 354-362, 1927.

BALFOUR, D. C., McCANN, J. C.: Sarcoma of the stomach. Surg, Gynec. and Obst., 50: 948-953, 1930.

BARTON, K. M. and KIRSNER, J. B.: Gastric ulcer. Med. Clin. North America, 48: 103, 1964.

BENEDICT, E. B. and Allen, A. W.: Adenomatous polyp of the stomach with special reference to malignant degeneration. Surg. Gynec. & Obst., 58: 79-84, 1934.

BENTIVEGNA, S. and PANAGOPOULAS, P. G.: Adenomatous gastric polyps. Amer. J. Gastroenterol., 44: 138-148, 1965.

BENZER, H.: Gutartige Neubildungen des Magens. Wien Med. Wscher., 109: 159-163, 1959.

BERG, J. W.: Histological aspects of the relation between gastric adenomatous polyp and gastric cancer. Cancer, 11: 1149-1155, 1958.

BOCKUS, H. L.: Gastroenterology. Vol. 1, 817-833, Saunders Co., Philadelphia & London, 1963.

BONFIELD, R. E. and MARTEL, W.: The problem of differentiating benign antral ulcers from intramural tumors. Radiology, 106: 25-27, 1973.

BORRMANN, R.: Geschwülste des Magens und Duodenums. Handbuch der Spez. Pathol. Anatomie u. Histologie, 4 (1): 838-855, Springer, Berlin, 1926.

BOWDEN, L.: Adenocarcinoma in a small gastric polyp. Cancer, 15: 468-471, 1962.

BRUNN, H. and PEARL, F.: Diffuse gastric polyposis-adenopapillomatosis gastrica. Surg. Gynec. & Obst., 43: 559-598, 1926.

BUCKER, J.: Die Frühdiagnose des Magenkrebses im Röntgenbild Fortschr. Röntgenstr., 63: 1-28, 1941.

CALENOFF, L. and SPARBERG, M.: Gastric pseudolesions; Roentgenographic-gastrophotographic correlation. Amer. J. Roentgenol. Radium Thera. Nucl. Med., 113: 139-146, 1971.

CAREY, J. B., and HAY, L. J.: Gastric polyps. Gastroenterology, 14: 280-286, 1950.

CARLSON, E. and WARD, J. G.: Surgical consideration in gastric polyps, gastric polyposis and giant hypertrophic gastritis in 74 cases. Surg. Gynec. & Obst., 107: 727-738, 1958.

CASTLEMANN, B.: Current approach to the polyp-cancer controversy. Gastroenterology, 51: 108-112, 1966.

CHIBA, H. and ISHIKAWA, K.: A case of "comfrey" bezoar treated with the aid of a fiberscope for biopsy (in Japanese). Stomach and Intestine, 5: 1145-1149, 1970.

D'AUNOY, R. and ZOELLER, A.: Sarcoma of the stomach. Amer. J. Surg. 9: 444-464, 1930.

DAWSON, P. J., COOPER R. A. and RAMBO, O. N.: Diagnosis of malignant lymphoma. A clinicopathological analysis of 158 cases. Cancer, 17: 1405-1413, 1964.

DOUGLOUS, J.: Benign tumors of the stomach. Ann. Surg., 77: 580-589, 1923.

EDWARDS, R. V. and BROWN, C.: Benign gastric polyps and their relation to carcinoma of the stomach. Gastroenterology, 16: 531-538, 1950.

EKLÖF. O.: Benign tumors of the stomach and duodenum. Acta Chirurgica Scand. Suppl., 291: 6-27, 1962.

ELIASON, E. L., PENDERGRASS, E. P. and WRIGHT, V. W. M.: The roentgenray diagnosis of pedunculated growth and gastric mucosa prolapsing through pylorus. Amer. J. Roentgenol. & Rad. Therapy. 15: 295-322, 1926.

ELIASON, E. L. and WRIGHT, V. W.: Benign tumors of the stomach. Surg. Gynec. & Obst., 41: 461-472, 1925.

EUSTERMAN, G. B. and SENTY, E. G.: Benign tumors of the stomach. Surg. Gynec. & Obst., 34: 5-15, 1922.

FARIS, T. D. and SALTSTEIN, S. L.: Gastric lymphoid hyperplasia. Cancer. 17: 207-212, 1964.

FERRUCCI, J. T.: Gastric polyps followed 20 years. J. A. M. A., 199: 207-209, 1967.

FLOOD, C. A. et al.: Recurrence in gastric ulcer under medical management. Gastroenteology, 16: 57-72, 1950.

FRANK, A.: Zur Röntgensymptologie des Retothelsarcoms des Magens. Fortschr. Röntgenstr., 83: 200-204, 1955.

FRANZER, J. W.: Malignant lymphomas of gastrointestinal tract. Surg. Gynec. & Obst., 108: 182-190, 1959.

FRIK, W. und ZEIDNER, A.: Röntgenuntersuchungen des Magenfeinreliefs. 1. Mitt. Forschr. Röntgenstr., 79: 681-692, 1953.

FRIK, W.: Lehrbuch der Röntgendiagnostik. 5: pp. 184-186, Thieme, Stuttgart, 1965.

FRIK, W.: Röntgenuntersuchungen des Magenfeinreliefs. 2, Mitt. Forschr. Röntgenster., 88: 546-557, 1958.

FRIK, W.: Zur Differentialdiagnostik Zwischen Magengeschwür und Kleinem Magenkarzinom. Fortschr. Roentgenstr., 105: 322-330, 1966.

FRIK, W. and HESSE, R.: Die Röntgenologische Darstellung von Magenerosionen. Dtsch. Med. Wschr., 81: 1119-1121, 1956.

FURUSAWA, M. and HIYAMA, T.: The relationship between endoscopic findings and histopathology of gastric polyps (in Japanese). Stomach and Intestine, 1: 783-792, 1966.

GIESELER, H.: Zur Klinik und Pathologie der Magenopolypen. Langenbecks Arch. Klin. Chir., 299: 637-653, 1962.

GOLDEN, R.: Non-malignant tumors of the duodenum. Amer. J. Roentgenol., 20: 405-413, 1928.

GOLDEN, R. and STOUT, A. P.: Smooth muscle tumors of the gastrointestinal tract and retroperitoneal tissues. Surg. Gynec. & Obst., 73: 784-810, 1941.

GOLDEN, R. and STOUT, A. P.: Superficial spreading carcinoma of the stomach. Amer. J. Roentgenol. 59: 157-167, 1948.

GONOI, T. et al.: Radiologic findings of gastric ulcer-scar (in Japanese). Jap. J. Clin. Radiol., 10: 589-594, 1965.

GÜTGEMANN, A. und SCHREIBER, H. W.: Die Chirurgie des Magensarkoms. Thieme, Stuttgart, 1960.

GUTMANN, R. A.: Le diagnostic du cancer d'estomac á la période utile. G. Doin, Paris, 1956.

GUTZEIT, K. und TEITIGE, H.: Die Gastroskopie. Urban & Schwarzenberg, München, 1954.

HAROLD, C. K. and GELLER, J. S.: Gastric polyp to carcinoma. Gastroenterology, 17: 442-444, 1951.

HAY, L. J.: Polyps and adenomas of the stomach. Surgery, 33: 446-467, 1953.

HAY, L. J.: Surgical management of gastric polyps and adenomas. Surgery, 39: 114-119, 1956.

HEINZ, H.: Über Polyposis Ventriculi. Brun's Beitr. Klin. Chir., 93: 228-250, 1914.

HAUSER, G.: Die Peptischen Schädigungen des Magens, des Duodenums und der Speiseröhre und des peptische postoperative Jejunalgschwür. In Henke-Lubarsch der speziellen pathologischen Anatomie und Histologie. Bd. IV, 1. Teil, Julius Springer, Berlin, 1926.

HAYASHIDA, T. et al.: Gastrocamera and its application (in Japanese). Bunkodo, Tokyo, 1966.

HEINKEL, K.: Diagnostik der malignen Magentumoren. Chirurg., 43: 537-542, 1972.

HENNING, N.: Die Polyposis Ventriculi. Lehrbuch der verdkrh., 341-349, Thieme, Stuttgart, 1949.

HIGURASHI, K.: X-ray diagnosis of early gastric cancer. Jap. J. Gastroenterol., 64: 71-88, 1967; 64: 197-213, 1967.

HORINOUCHI, K. et al.: On evolution of depressed type early gastric cancer considered from the standpoint of internal medicine (in Japanese). Stomach and Intestine, 5: 7-14, 1970.

HOLMES, E. J.: Morphogenesis of gastric adenomatous polyps transformation to invasive carcinoma of intestinal type. Cancer, 19: 794-802, 1966.

HUPPLER, E. G., PRIESTLEY, J. T., MORIOCK, C. G. and GAGE, R. P.: Diagnosis and results of treatment in gastric polyps. Surg. Gynec. & Obst., 110: 309-313, 1960.

ICHIKAWA, H. et al.: Radiologic diagnosis of gastric multiple-ulcers (in Japanese). Jap. J. Clini. Radiol., 8: 392-397, 1963.

ICHIKAWA, H. et al.: Practical roentgenology of the stomach (in Japanese). Bunkodo, Tokyo, 1964.

IDA, K. et al.: Roentgenography of the gastric tumor prolapsing into the duodenal bulb (in Japanese). Jap. J. Clin. Radiol., 15: 609-615, 1970.

ISHIHARA, K., TANAKA, H. and FUKUTOMI, S.: Biopsy diagnosis of protractable gastric ulcer (in Japanese). Stomach and Intestine, 2: 1029-1034, 1967.

ISHIOKA, K. et al.: Biopsy under direct vision and cytological diagnosis (in Japanese). Stomach and Intestine, 5: 829-836, 1970.

IUY, A. G., GROSSMAN, M. I. and BACHRACH, W. H.: Peptic ulcer. The Blakiston Co., Philadelphia and Tronto, 1950.

JOSEPH, J. I. and LATTES, R.: Gastric lymphosarcoma, clinicopathologic analysis of 71 cases and its relation to disseminated lymphosarcoma. Amer. J. Clin. Path., 45: 653-669, 1966.

KAGITANI, T. et al.: Primary gastric sarcoma (in Japanese). Jap. J. Cancer Clinics, 6: 141-151, 1960.

KALK, H. und BRÜHL, W.: Leitfaden der Laparoskopie und Gastroskopie. Thieme, Stuttgart, 1951.

KASUGAI, T. et al.: Sarcoma of the stomach, with special reference to its endoscopic diagnosis (in Japanese). Stomach and Intesitne, 5: 287-299, 1970.

KATSCH, G. und PICKERT, H.: Polypöse Geschwülste des Magens. Handbuch der inn. Medicine, 4(3): 758-761, Springer, Berlin-Göttingen-Heidelberg, 1953.

KAWAI, K.: Diagnosis of early gastric cancer. Endoscopy, 3: 23-27, 1971.

KAWAI, K.: Validity rate of concerted diagnosis using various methods. Gann Monograph on Cancer Research 11, Early Gastric Cancer, University of Tokyo Press, 1971.

KAWAI, K.: The significance of endoscopy for the gastric disease. Endoscopy 4, 39-43, 1972.

KAWAI, K., Y. AKASAWA, F. MISAKI, K. MURAKAMI and M. MASUDA: Gastrofiberscopic biopsy on early gastric cancer. Endoscopy 2: 82-87, 1970.

KAWAI, K., MURAKAMI, K. and MISAKI, F.: Endoscopical observation of the gastric ulcer. Endoscopy, 1: 97-101, 1969.

KAWAI, K., TAKADA, H. and SHIRAKABE, H.: Double contrast radiograph on routine examination of the stomach, Amer. J. Gastroenterol. 53: 147-153, 1970.

KAWAI, K. et al.: X-ray diagnosis of the gastric ulcer (in Japanese). Stomach and Intestine, 2: 485-495, 1967.

KAWAI, K. et al.: The process of gastric polypoid lesions (in Japanese). Gastroenterological Endoscopy, 10: 281-223, 1968.

KAWAI, K. et al.: Radiological diagnosis of gastric submucous tumors (in Japanese). Jap. J. Clin. Radiol., 13: 18-27, 1968.

KAWASHIMA, S.: Applied gastroenterology (in Japanese). Kanehara-Shoten, Tokyo, 1966.

KIDOKORO. T. et al.: Surgery and gastric biopsy (in Japanese). Stomach and Intestine, 5: 803-815, 1970.

KIRKLIN, B.R.: Roentgenologic diagnosis of neoplastic disease of the stomach. Amer. J. Cancer, 16: 1134-1143, 1932.

KOGA, M.: On gastric bezoar in Japan (in Japanese). Stomach and Intestine, 4: 575-587, 1969.

KONJETZNY, G.E.: Die Entzündung des Magens: Henke-Lubarsch. Handbuch der spez. pathol. Anatomie u. Histologie, 4(2): 780, 1928.

KONJETZNY, G.E.: Der oberflächliche Schleimhautkrebs des Magens. Chirurg., 12: 192-202, 1940.

KOZEN, G., TANAGUCHI, H., IWANAGA, T., OKUDA, S., MITSUEDA, T., MORII T. and H. KOYAMA: Lymphnode metastasis of the protruding types of gastric carcinoma. J. Jap. Society for Cancer Therapy, 4: 222, 1969.

KUMAKURA, K.: Atlas of radiological diagnostics of gastric diseases (in Japanese). Kanehara-Shuppan, Tokyo, 1968.

KUMAKURA, K. et al.: X-ray diagnosis of anterior wall lesions of the stomach (in Japanese). Jap. J. Clin. Radiol., 10: 789-796, 1965.

KÜMMERLE, F. und SCHMITT-KÖPPLER, A.: Magen polypen, Morphologie und Therapie. Deutsch. med. Wschr., 96: 1485-1489, 1971.

KUROKAWA, T.: Collection of gastrointestinal disease by roentgenography (in Japanese). Nakayama-Shoten, Tokyo, 1956.

LAWRENCE, J.C.: Gastrointestinal polyps. Amer. J. Surg., 31: 499-505, 1936.

LINDHEIMER, W.: Syphilitische Erkrankung des Magens. Münch. med. Wschr., 109: 638-643, 1967.

LOOKWOOD, B.C.: Benign tumors of the stomach with report of cases. J.A.M.A., 98: 969-973, 1932.

MAJIMA, S., YOSHIDA, K., TESHIMA, T. and KARUBE, K.: Histopathological study on gastric polyps and their malignant degeneration. Tohoku J. Exper. Med., 80: 355-369, 1963.

MARSHAK, R.H.: The pedunculated adenomatous polyp. Amer. J. Digestive Disease, 10: 958-967, 1965.

MARSHAK, R.H. and FELDMAN, F.: Gastric polyps. Amer. J. Digestive Disease, 10: 909-930, 1965.

MARSHALL, S.F. and MEISSNER, W.A.: Sarcoma of the stomach. Ann. Surg., 131: 824-837, 1950.

MARUYAMA, M. et al.: Gastric lesions associated with secondary syphilis: a case suspected of gastric sarcoma by x-ray and endoscope (in Japanese). Stomach and Intestine, 3: 195-202, 1968.

MASON, J.I. and DWYER, M.F.: Benign tumor of the stomach. Ann. Surg., 88: 866-869, 1928.

MASSA, J.: Le petit cancer l'estmac. Masson, Paris, 1961.

MASUDA, M., KAWAI, K., UEMATSU, T., IDA, K., WAKABAYASHI, T., AKASAKA, Y., KOBAYASHI, Y., MORI, Y., SHIMAMOTO, K., KOHLI, Y., MISAKI, F. and MURAKAMI, K.: Clinical considerations of early gastric cancer. J. Kyoto Pref. Univ. Med., 79: 363-374, 1970.

MASUDA, M. et al.: Radiological diagnosis of gastric polypoid lesions, especially as to protruded type of early gastric cancer (in Japanese). Naika, 26: 22-37, 1970.

MATSUMOTO, S. and OOTA, K.: Gastric neoplasms other than carcinomas: A histological and statistical study on 1489 resected stomachs. Gann, 47: 143-152, 1956.

MCNEER, G. and BERG. J.W.: The clinical behavior and management of primary malignant lymphoma of the stomach. Surgery, 46: 829-840, 1959.

MEUWISSEN, F.J.: X-ray atlas and manual of esophagus, stomach and duodenum. Amsterdam, Elsevier, 1955.

MEYER, A.: Gutartige Geschwülste des Magen Darm-Traktes. Klinik und Therapie, Münch. med. Wschr., 20: 1101-1108, 1966.

MILLER, T. G., ELIASON, E. L. and WRIGHT, V. W.: Carcinomatous degeneratien of polyp of the stomach. Arch. Int. Med., 46: 841–878, 1930.

MING, S. C. and GOLDMAN, H.: Gastric polyps: A histogenetic classification and its relation to carcinoma. Cancer, 18: 721–726, 1965.

MITCHELL, R. M. and BRALOW, S. P.: Acute erosive gastritis due to early syphilis. Ann. Intern. Med., 61: 933–938, 1964.

MOCHIZUKI, T. et al.: Considerations on the malignant change of gastric polyps (in Japanese). Stomach and Intestine, 3: 720–724, 1968.

MONACO, A. P., ROTH, S. I., GASTLEMEN, B. and WELCH, C. E.: Adenomatous polyps of the stomach; A clinical and pathological study of 153 cases. Cancer, 15: 456–467, 1962.

MONAT, T. B.: Two cases of polypus of stomach. Brit. J. Surg, 13: 165–168, 1925.

MOORE, A. B.: A roentgenologic study of benign tumors of the stomach. Amer. J. Roentgenol., 11: 61–66, 1924.

MORSON, B. C.: Gastric polyps composed of intestinal epithelium. Brit. J. Cancer, 9: 550–557, 1955.

MURAKAMI, T.: Pathologic studies on early gastric cancer (in Japanese). Jap. J. Cancer Clinics, 3: 233–242, 1957.

MURAKAMI, T.: Gastric polyp (in Japanese). Surgical Pathology, Vol. 2. Igaku Shoin, Tokyo, 1963.

MURAKAMI, T. and SUZUKI, T.: Histopathological studies on gastroduodenal ulcer and healing (in Japanese). Jap. J. Gastroenterol., 58: 1181–1186, 1957.

MURAKAMI, T. et al.: Linear ulcers of the stomach and the duodenum (in Japanese). J. Clinical Digestive Diseases, 1: 83–95, 1959.

MURAKAMI, T. et al.: Malignant changes in gastric polyps (in Japanese). Naika, 17: 1027–1034, 1966.

MURAKAMI, T. et al.: Gastric polypoid lesions (in Japanese). Surgery, 29: 1360–1368, 1967.

MURAKAMI, T. et al. (ed.): Diagnostic methodology of early gastric cancer (in Japanese). Bunkodo, Tokyo, 1967.

MURAKAMI, T. et al.: About the development of human gastric cancer involving very small early gastric cancer (in Japanese). Stomach and Intestine, 3: 779–785, 1968.

MUTO, T.: Study on polypogenesis and malignant degeneration of adenomatous polyps of the stomach (in Japanese). Jap. J. Cancer Clinics, 95–111, 1970.

NAKAYAMA, K. et al.: Gastric polyps in our clinic for the past twelve years (in Japanese). Operation, 12: 760–768, 1958.

NAKAMURA, K., SUGANO, H., TAKAGI, K. and FUCHIGAMI, A.: Histological study of an early carcinoma of the stomach. Criteria for diagnosis of atypical epithelium. Gann, 57: 613–620, 1966.

NAKAMURA, K. et al.: Reactive lymphoreticular hyperplasia (in Japanese). Jap. J. Cancer Clinics, 12: 691–696, 1966.

NAKAMURA, T.: Gastric polyp (in Japanese). Jap. J. Clin. Med., 22: 1979–1987, 1964.

NEBESAR, R. A. and POLLARD, J. J.: Polypoid lesion of the stomach. J. A. M. A., 188: 678–679, 1964.

NELSON, R. S. and LANZA, F. L.: Eodoscopy in the diagnosis of gastric lymphoma and sarcoma. Amer. J. Gastroenterol, 50: 37–46, 1968.

NIEMETZ, D. and WHARTON, G. K.: Benign gastric polyps. Ann. Int. Med., 42: 339–344, 1955.

NISHIZAWA, M.: Endoscopic studies on early gastric cancer (in Japanese). Gastroenterological Endoscopy, 8: 203–221, 1966.

NISHIZAWA, M. et al.: The x-ray demonstrability of microcarcinoma (in Japanese). Stomach and Intestine, 5: 951–959, 1970.

OCHSNER, S. F. and JANETOS, G. P.: Benign tumors of the stomach. J. A. M. A., 191, 881–887, 1965.

OGATA, T. et al.: General pathology (Vol. 2) (in Japanese). Nanzando, Tokyo, 1936.

OHTA, K.: Diseases of the stomach (in Japanese). Clinical Pathology. Kyorin-Shoin, Tokyo, 1956.

OI, M.: Gastric ulcer (in Japanese). Nankodo, Tokyo, 1957.

OI, M. et al.: Non-cancerous gastric tumor—Statistical studies of cases from 93 medical institutes in Japan (in Japanese). Surgery, 29: 112–131, 1967.

OKABE, H. et al.: Clinical and histopathological studies on the course of peptic ulcerations coexisting with gastric carcinoma (in Japanese). Stomach and Intestine, 3: 1673–1682, 1968.

OKUDA, S. et al.: Depth of involvement and mode of development of early gastric cancer studied by the endoscopic method (in Japanese). Stomach and Intestine, 4: 313–236, 1969.

PALMER, E. D.: The sarcomas of the stomach. A review with reference to gross pathology and gastroscopic manifestations. Amer., J. Digestive Disease, 17: 186–195, 1950.

PALMER, E. D.: Course and prognosis of sarcoma of the stomach: 21 Cases. Gastroenterology, 33: 389–394, 1950.

PALMER, E. D.: Benign intramural tumors of the stomach: A review with special reference to gross pathology. Medicine, 30: 81–181, 1951.

PALMER, E. D.: Clinical gastroenterology. Harper & Brothers, New York, 1963.

PALMER, W. and SCHINDLER, R.: Syphilis of the stomach. Ann. Int. Med., 18: 393–396, 1943.

PALMER, W. L. and HUMPHREYS, E. M.: Gastric carcinoma: Observation on peptic ulceration and healing gastroenterology, 3: 257-274, 1970.

PATTERSON, G. and MILFORD, O.: Description of gastroscopic appearance of luetic gastric lesions in late aquired syphilis. Gastroenterology, 10: 474-485, 1948.

PAUL, W. D. and LOGAN, W. P.: Polyps of the stomach with reference to gastroscopic findings. Gastroenterology, 8: 592-606, 1947.

PEARL, F. L. and BRUNN, H. B.: Multiple gastric polyposis: supplementary report of 41 cases, including 3 new personal cases. Surg. Gynec. & Obst, 76: 257-269, 1943.

PERRY, T. and SHEKARACHI, K.: Polypoid adenomas of the stomach. Amer. J. Surg., 101: 440-446, 1961.

PLACHTA, A. and SPEER, F. D.: Gastric polyps and their relationship to carcinoma of the stomach: Review of the literature and report of 65 cases. Amer. J. Gastroenterol., 28:160-175, 1957.

PRÉVOT, R. und LASSRICH, M. A.: Röntgendiagnostik des Magen-Darmkanals. Thieme, Stuttgart, 1959.

REIFFERSCHIED, M.: Die gutartigen Tumoren des Magens und Dünndarms. Med. Klin., 54: 41-46, 1959.

RIGLER, L. G.: Roentgenologic observations on benign tumors of the stomach. Amer. J. Surg., 8: 144-150, 1930.

RIGLER, L. G., BLANK, L. and HEBEL, R.: Granuloma with eosinophils. Benign inflammatory fibroid polyps of the stomach. Radiol., 66: 169-176, 1956.

RIGLER, L. G. and ERICKSON, L. G.: Benign tumors of stomach: Observation on their incidence and malignant degeneration. Radiol., 26: 6-15, 1936.

RIGLER. L. G., KAPLAN, H. S. and Fink, C. D.: Pernicious anemia and the early diagnosis of tumors of the stomach. J. A. M. A., 128: 426-432, 1945.

ROBERTS, J. M., NOHLGREN, J. E. and LOOMIS, J. W.: Gastric adenomas. A clinicopathologic study. Amer. J. Surg., 98: 223-228, 1959.

ROSATO, F. E. and NOTO, J. A.: Gastric polyps. Amer. J. Surg., 3: 647-650, 1966.

SANGI, E. et al.: Clinico-pathological investigation of gastric polyp. Clinical Gastro-Enterology, 8: 169-178, 1960.

SANO, R.: Histopathology of multiple gastric ulcers (in Japanese). Stomach and Intestine, 2: 1175-1180, 1967.

SANO, R.: Classification of gastric adenomatous polyp and its malignant change (in Japanese). Stomach and Intestine, 3: 725-728, 1968.

SANO, R. et al.: Pathology of gastric sarcoma (in Japanese). Stomach and Intestine, 5: 311-322, 1970.

SCHINDLER, R.: Gastroscopy. 2nd edition, The University of Chicago Press, Chicago, New York, 1950.

SCHINZ, H. R.: Roentgen diagnosis. Vol. 4, Grune & Stratton, New York, 1954.

SHIDA, S. et al.: Diagnosis of gastric submucosal tumor (in Japanese). Jap. J. Clin. Med., 22: 1967-1978, 1964.

SHINDO, T.: Histochemical study on gastric polyps (in Japanese). Med. J. Osaka Univ., 16: 233-240, 1964.

SHIRAKABE, H. et al.: X-ray and macroscopic findings of erosive gastritis. Nipp. Act. Radiol., 15: 1182-1183, 1956.

SHIRAKABE, H. and KUMAKURA, K.: X-ray diagnosis of gastroduodenal ulcer. Jap. J. Gastroenterol., 58: 1187-1191, 1961.

SHIRAKABE, H., ICHIKAWA, H., KUMAKURA, K., NISHIZAWA, M., HIGURASHI, K., HAYAKAWA, H. and MURAKAMI, T.: Atlas of x-ray diagnosis of early gastric cancer. Igaku Shoin, Tokyo, 1966.

SHORT, W. F. and YOUNG, B. R.: Roentgen demonstration of prolapse of benign polypoid gastric tumors into the duodenum, including a dumbbell-shaped leiomyoma. Amer. J. Roentgenol. & Rad. Therapy, 103: 317-320, 1968.

SI-CHUN, M. and GOLDMAN, H.: Gastric polyps. A histologic classification and its relation to carcinoma. Cancer, 18: 721-726, 1965.

SKANDALAKIS, J. E., GRAY, S. W. and SHEPERD, D. S.: Smooth muscle tumors of the stomach. Internat. Abstr. Surg., 110: 209-226, 1960.

SMITH, J. L., JR. and HELWIG, E. B.: Malignant lymphoma of the stomach. Amer. J. Path., 34: 553, 1958.

STEWART, M. J.: Observations on the relation of malignant disease to benign tumors of the intestinal tract. Brit. Med. J., 2: 567-569, 1929.

STOUT, A. P.: Superficial spreading type of carcinoma of the stomach. Arch. Surg., 44: 651-657, 1942.

STOUT, A. P.: Atlas of tumor pathology. Sect. 6, Fasc. 21, Armed Force Institute of Pathology, Washington, 1953.

SUGANO, H. et al.: Morphogenesis and frequency of cancer and atypical epithelium found in the polypoid lesions of the gastric mucosa (in Japanese). Stomach and Intestine, 3: 729-736, 1968.

SYDNEY, J. H. and HARPER, R. A. K.: Shortening of lesser curvature in gastric ulcers. Brit. J. Radiol., 25: 451-461, 1952.

TACHDJIAN, V.: Benign tumors of the stomach. Bockus' Gastroenterology, Vol. 1, Saunders Co., Philadelphia, 1963.

TAKAGI, K.: Gastric biopsy (in Japanese). Stomach and Intestine, 2: 93-101, 1967.

TAKAGI, K.: Gastric biopsy (in Japanese). Stomach and Intestine, 2: 261-268, 1967.

TAKAGI, K.: IIa and atypical epithelium (in Japanese). Stomach and Intestine, 3: 15-25, 1968.

TAKAGI, K., KUMAKURA, K., SUGANO, H. and NAKAMURA, K.: Clinico-pathological study on polypoid lesions of the stomach with special reference to atypical epithelial lesions. Jap. J. Cancer Clinics, 13: 809-817, 1967.

TANAKA, H.: Endoscopic diagnosis of early gastric cancer (in Japanese). Gastroenterological Endoscopy. 8: 5-7, 1966.

TANAKA, H.: Diagnosis on the wide-spreading IIa type early gastric cancer (in Japanese). Stomach and Intestine, 5: 1697-1700, 1970.

TANAKA, H.: Problems involving early gastric cancer of the depressed type (in Japanese). Stomach and Intestine, 6: 175-183, 1971.

TANAKA, H.: Endoscopic diagnosis of a gastric ulcer-scar (in Japanese). Series of medicine, No. 2—Gastroduodenal ulcer. pp. 226-238, Nanzando, Tokyo, 1971.

TANAKA, H.: Practice of clinical diagnosis for early gastric cancer (in Japanese). Stomach and Intestine, 7: 139-321, 1972.

TANAKA, H.: Endoscopic diagnosis of an early protruded type of gastric cancer (in Japanese). Series of medicine, No. 8—Early gastric cancer (in Japanese). 200-211, Nanzando, Tokyo, 1972.

TANAKA, H., OKITA, E., SAKAMOTO, K., KURIHARA, T. and MIURA, K.: Endoscopic diagnosis of gastric lesions on the anterior wall (in Japanese). Stomach and Intestine, 6: 1419-1424, 1971.

TANAKA, H., FUKUMOTO, SH., OKITA, E., SAKUMOTO, K. and ISHIHARA, K.: Bioptische Diagnostik des Magenfrühkarzinom. Leber Magen Darm, 3: 69-72, 1973.

TANAKA, H. et al.: X-ray studies on the double-contrast technique of the anterior wall of the stomach (in Japanese). Jap. J. Clin. Radiol., 11: 952-961, 1966.

TANAKA, M.: The endoscopic diagnosis of a gastric ulcer scar (in Japanese). J. Yonago Med. Ass, 19: 1-19, 1968.

TESCHENDORF, W.: Lehrbuch der röntgenologischen Differentialdiagnostik. p. 2 (4), Thieme, Stuttgart, 1954.

THOMPSON, H. L. and OYSTER, J. M.: Neoplasms of the stomach. Gastroenterology, 15: 185-243, 1950.

TSUNEOKA, K. et al.: Tuberculosis of the stomach (in Japanese). Stomach and Intestine, 4: 601-617, 1969.

URELES, A. L., ALSCHIBAGA, T., LODICO, D. and STABIUS, S. J.: Idiopathic eosinophilic infiltration of the gastrointestinal tract; diffuse & circumscribed. Amer. J. Med., 30: 899-909, 1961.

WALK, L.: Erosive Gastritis. Gastroenterolgia, 84: 87-98, 1955.

YAMADA, T. et al.: Gastric polypoid lesions (in Japanese). Stomach and Intestine, 1: 145-150, 1966.

YAMAGATA, S.: Current internal medicine (in Japanese). Vol. II b, Gastrointestinal diseases. Nakayama-Shoten, Tokyo, 1962.

YAMAGATA, S.: Atlas of endoscopic diagnosis (in Japanese). Nakayama-Shoten, Tokyo, 1969.

YARNIS, H., MARSHAK, R. H. and FRIEDMAN, A. I.: Gastric polyps. J. A. M. A., 148: 1088-1094, 1952.

YOSHIKAWA, Y.: Radiological studies on gastric polypoid lesions (in Japanese). J. Chiba Medical Society, 43: 358-387, 1967.

WATSON, R. J. and O'BRIEN, M. T.: Gastric pseudolymphoma (lymphofollicular gastritis). Ann. Surg., 17: 98-106, 1970.

WILLIS, R. A.: Pathology of tumors. Butterworth, London, 1960.

Index

MIX
Papier aus verantwortungsvollen Quellen
Paper from responsible sources
FSC® C105338

If you have any concerns about our products,
you can contact us on
ProductSafety@springernature.com

In case Publisher is established outside the EU,
the EU authorized representative is:
Springer Nature Customer Service Center GmbH
Europaplatz 3, 69115 Heidelberg, Germany

Printed by Libri Plureos GmbH
in Hamburg, Germany